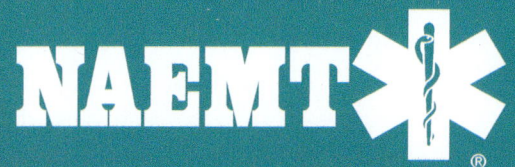

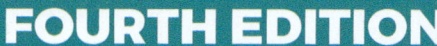

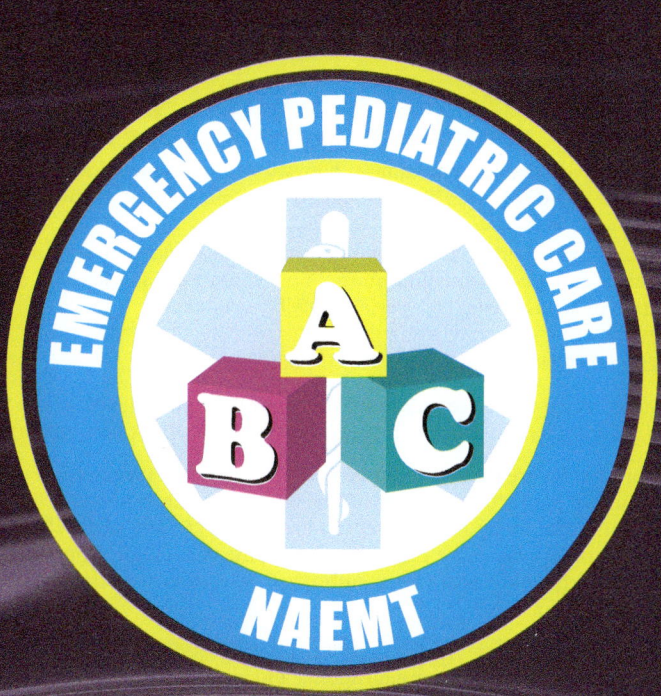

# Emergency Pediatric Care

## Course Manual

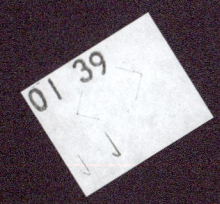

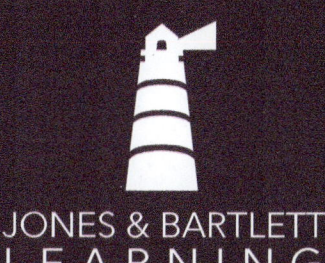

JONES & BARTLETT
LEARNING

*World Headquarters*
Jones & Bartlett Learning
25 Mall Road
Burlington, MA 01803
978-443-5000
info@jblearning.com
www.jblearning.com
www.psglearning.com

Jones & Bartlett Learning books and products are available through most bookstores and online booksellers. To contact Jones & Bartlett Learning Public Safety Group directly, call 800-832-0034, fax 978-443-8000, or visit our website, www.psglearning.com.

Substantial discounts on bulk quantities of Jones & Bartlett Learning publications are available to corporations, professional associations, and other qualified organizations. For details and specific discount information, contact the special sales department at Jones & Bartlett Learning via the above contact information or send an email to specialsales@jblearning.com.

**Production Credits**

VP, Product Management: Marisa R. Urbano
VP, Content Strategy and Product Implementation: Christine Emerton
Director, Content Management: Donna Gridley
Content Strategist: Alexander Belloli
VP, International Sales, Public Safety Group: Matthew Maniscalco
Manager, Product Management: Kristen Rogers
Project Manager: Madelene Nieman
Digital Project Specialist: Angela Dooley

Director of Marketing: Brian Rooney
VP, Manufacturing and Inventory Control: Therese Connell
Composition and Project Management: S4Carlisle Publishing Services
Cover and Text Design: Scott Moden
Media Development Editor: Troy Liston
Rights Specialist: Benjamin Roy
Cover Image (Title Page): © Ralf Hiemisch/fStop/Getty Images
Printing and Binding: LSC Communications

**Library of Congress Cataloging-in-Publication Data**
Library of Congress Cataloging-in-Publication Data unavailable at time of printing.

ISBN: 978-1-284-22837-3

6048

Printed in the United States of America
26 25          10 9 8 7 6 5 4 3

# Brief Contents

**Acknowledgments**    **ix**

CHAPTER 1    **Pediatric Development and Assessment**    **1**

CHAPTER 2    **Respiratory Emergencies**    **23**

CHAPTER 3    **Trauma**    **57**

CHAPTER 4    **Pediatric Shock**    **89**

CHAPTER 5    **Pediatric Medical Emergencies**    **107**

CHAPTER 6    **Pediatric Cardiac Events**    **137**

CHAPTER 7    **Toxicologic Emergencies**    **165**

CHAPTER 8    **Pediatric Maltreatment**    **181**

CHAPTER 9    **Obstetric/Newborn Care and Congenital Birth Defects**    **201**

CHAPTER 10    **Children With Special Healthcare Needs**    **237**

CHAPTER 11    **Pediatric Behavioral Health**    **255**

**Index**    **269**

# Contents

**Acknowledgments**    **ix**

**CHAPTER 1**    **Pediatric Development and Assessment**    **1**

Introduction    1
Developmental Milestones    1
Pediatric Vital Signs    1
Scene Size-Up    4
General Patient Impression    4
   The Pediatric Assessment Triangle    5
   The Pediatric Glasgow Coma Scale (PGCS)    11
The Pediatric Management Diagram    12
   The "Quick" Patient    13
   The "Not Quick" Patient    13
   "Quick" Versus "Not Quick"    14
The Primary Survey    14
   Exsanguination    15
   Airway    15
   Breathing    15
   Circulation    16
   Disability    16
   Exposure and Environment    16
Secondary Assessment    17
Treatment Plan    18
Pediatric Transport    19
Family-Centered Care    20

**CHAPTER 2**    **Respiratory Emergencies**    **23**

Introduction    23
The Pediatric Respiratory System    23
   Physiology    23
   Anatomy    24
Assessing Severity of Respiratory Emergencies    25
   Respiratory Distress    25
   Respiratory Failure    26
   Respiratory Arrest    27

Classification of Respiratory Emergencies by Etiology     27
   Upper Respiratory Emergencies     27
   Lower Respiratory Emergencies     33

**CHAPTER 3     Trauma     57**

Introduction     57
Kinematics of Pediatric Trauma     57
   Seat Belts and Motor Vehicle Crashes     58
   Falls     58
   Bicycle Collision Injuries     59
The Trauma Triad of Death     59
   Hypothermia     59
   Acidosis     59
   Coagulopathy     60
   Managing the Triad     60
Types of Injuries     61
   Hemorrhage     61
   Airway Injuries     62
   Chest Injuries     63
   Head Injuries     66
   Fractures     68
   Burns     68

**CHAPTER 4     Pediatric Shock     89**

Shock     89
   Causes of Shock     89
   Compensated Shock     91
   Decompensated Shock     92
   Types of Shock     92
   Hypovolemic Shock     94
   Distributive Shock     94
   Cardiogenic Shock     96

**CHAPTER 5     Pediatric Medical Emergencies     107**

Introduction     107
Altered Mental Status     107
   Assessing Mental Status     107
   AEIOU-TIPS     108
Hypoglycemia     111
   Signs of Hypoglycemia     111
   Pathophysiology of Hypoglycemia     112
   Hypoglycemia Severity     112

Mild to Moderate Hypoglycemia Management | 112
Severe Hypoglycemia Management | 113
**Hyperglycemia** | **114**
Diabetes Mellitus | 114
Hyperglycemic Emergencies | 114
Hyperglycemia Management | 116
**Fever** | **117**
Fever Myths | 117
Fever Emergencies | 117
Fever Management | 117
**Seizures** | **118**
Commonly Encountered Seizure Emergencies | 119
Seizure Management | 120

CHAPTER 6 | **Pediatric Cardiac Events** | **137**
**Introduction** | **137**
**The Normal Pediatric ECG** | **137**
Normal QRS and Expected Axis | 137
T Waves | 138
Q Waves | 138
**Pediatric Cardiac Rhythms** | **138**
Tachycardia | 139
Bradycardia | 149

CHAPTER 7 | **Toxicologic Emergencies** | **165**
**Introduction** | **165**
Routes of Exposure | 165
**Assessment of Toxic Exposures** | **166**
**Common Substances** | **167**
**Button Battery Ingestion** | **168**
**Illicit Substance Abuse** | **168**
**Scene Safety** | **169**
**Poison Control** | **170**

CHAPTER 8 | **Pediatric Maltreatment** | **181**
**Introduction** | **181**
**Types of Child Maltreatment** | **181**
**Epidemiology, Demographics, and Risk Factors** | **182**
**Red Flags for Abuse** | **182**
Scene Size-Up | 183
Caregiver Behavior | 183
Child Behavior | 184

Bruising in Children                                      184

Pattern Marks                                            187

Abusive Head Trauma                                      187

Burns                                                    189

    Abusive Burns                    190

Pediatric Human Trafficking                              191

Conditions Mistaken for Maltreatment                     192

    Congenital Dermal Melanocytosis   192

    Coining (Cao Gio/Gua Sha/Kerikan) 192

    Cupping                           193

History Taking                                           193

    Mandated Reporting                194

**CHAPTER 9    Obstetric/Newborn Care and Congenital Birth Defects    201**

Introduction                                             201

    Circulatory Changes               201

    Respiratory Changes               201

    Renal Changes                     201

    Gastrointestinal Changes          201

    Endocrine Changes                 202

Fundal Height and Viability                              202

    Age of Viability                  202

Documentation of Pregnancy History                       204

High-Risk Deliveries                                     204

    Multiple Previous Births          204

    Prematurity                       204

    Multiple Gestation Pregnancies    204

    Meconium                          205

    Placental Abnormalities           205

    Preeclampsia                      207

    Eclampsia                         208

    Abnormal Fetal Presentations      208

Congenital Heart Defects                                 226

Cyanotic Heart Defects                                   226

    Tetralogy of Fallot               228

    Transposition of the Great Arteries 229

    Truncus Arteriosus                229

    Tricuspid Atresia                 229

Acyanotic Heart Defects                                  229

    Septal Defects                    229

Obstructive Heart Defects ..... 230
    Coarctation of the Aorta ..... 230
Sign and Symptoms of Congenital Heart Defects ..... 230

**CHAPTER 10  Children With Special Healthcare Needs ..... 237**

Introduction ..... 237
Cognitive Versus Physical Disabilities ..... 237
Assessment ..... 238
Tracheostomy Tubes ..... 238
Cerebrospinal Fluid Shunts ..... 239
Central Venous Catheters ..... 239
Feeding Tubes ..... 240
Vagal Nerve Stimulator ..... 241
Additional Forms of Assistive Technology ..... 241

**CHAPTER 11  Pediatric Behavioral Health ..... 255**

Introduction ..... 255
Attention Deficit/Hyperactivity Disorder (ADD/ADHD) ..... 255
Anxiety ..... 256
Depression ..... 257
Bipolar Disorder ..... 257
Schizophrenia ..... 258
Posttraumatic Stress Disorder (PTSD) ..... 258
Suicide Attempts and Suicidal Ideation ..... 258
Autism Spectrum Disorder ..... 259

**Index ..... 269**

# Emergency Pediatric Care, Fourth Edition

## NAEMT Emergency Pediatric Care Committee

**Katherine Remick, MD, FAAP, FACEP, FAEMS**
NAEMT EPC Committee Medical Director
Associate Professor, Departments of Pediatrics
and Surgery
Associate Chair for Quality, Innovation, and Outreach
Co-Director, National EMS for Children Innovation
and Improvement Center
Medical Director, San Marcos/Hays County EMS
System
Dell Medical School, The University of Texas at Austin

**Mark X. Cicero, MD, FAAP**
Associate Professor of Pediatrics
Director, Pediatric Disaster Preparedness
Co-Lead, Pediatric Pandemic Network Education
Committee
Section of Pediatric Emergency Medicine
Department of Pediatrics
Yale University School of Medicine

**Ann M. Dietrich, MD, FAAP, FACEP**
Division Chief Pediatric Emergency Medicine
PRISMA
Professor of Pediatrics and Emergency Medicine
University of South Carolina College of Medicine

**Emily Nichols, MD**
Associate Medical Director, New Orleans EMS
Physician, Ochsner Medical Center

**Sylvia Owusu-Ansah, MD, MPH**
Assistant Professor of Pediatrics and Emergency
Medicine
Associate Vice Chair of Diversity, Equity, and Inclusion
Prehospital-EMS Medical Director (Medical Command
Physician MD-22)
UPMC Children's Hospital of Pittsburgh
Assistant Professor of University of Pittsburgh
School of Health and Rehabilitation Services
Pediatric Liaison, Division of EMS, Department
of Emergency Medicine

**Sabine Sagner, MBA, RN, CCNRP**
St. Louis Children's Hospital

**Jeremy Sidlauskas, MPA, CFO, EFO, NREMT-P**
Deputy Fire Chief, Pasco County (FL) Fire Rescue
Adjunct Professor, Eastern Oregon University

**Shannon Watson, MHA**
NREMT-P, Critical Care, Community Paramedic
Assistant Chief, Christian Hospital EMS

**Jonathan Willoughby, DET, BSN, NRP, RN**
NAEMT State Education Coordinator—Iowa
Staff Nurse, Emergency Department
Mercy Hospital

## Editorial Consultant to NAEMT for Emergency Pediatric Care Course Manual, Fourth Edition

**Wm. Travis Engel, DO, MSc, Paramedic, FP-C, CCP-C**
Pediatric Critical Care Medicine Fellow
Children's Mercy Hospital

# National Association of Emergency Medical Technicians 2021 Board of Directors

# CHAPTER 1

# Pediatric Development and Assessment

## LESSON OBJECTIVES

- Explain the developmental and physiologic differences in pediatric patients based on their age.
- Understand the Pediatric Assessment Triangle (PAT).
- Explain the interplay of appearance, breathing, and circulation in the child.
- Demonstrate the pediatric assessment.
- Understand the use of family-centered care.

## Introduction

Emergency calls involving ill or injured children are a low-frequency event within emergency medical services (EMS) systems in the United States. It is estimated that 10% of EMS calls for service will involve a pediatric patient, and of those calls, significantly fewer will involve a patient with a critical level of illness or injury. The number of pediatric patients presenting to general emergency departments, whether by private vehicle or by ambulance, is similarly low. This results in patient encounters that are low frequency, but high risk.

The goal of the NAEMT Emergency Pediatric Care (EPC) course is to provide learners with the skills and confidence necessary to reduce the risk involved in these low-frequency events.

## Developmental Milestones

Understanding developmental milestones is important for prehospital practitioners, because it allows them to adapt their approach to patient assessment and treatment based on what is appropriate for the patient's age. Development in the motor and cognitive domains is rapid in the first 6 years of life. As children enter adolescence, development is most noticeable in the social and emotional domains, with motor development having been largely completed.

Knowledge of age-appropriate milestones can also aid the prehospital practitioner in assessing whether or not the patient is at their baseline for level of consciousness. If a child does not seem developmentally appropriate for their age, it may be helpful to ask the caregiver if they think the patient is acting normally, or if their illness or injury has affected their behavior (**Figure 1-1**). Study **Table 1-1** to become familiar with major milestones for various age groups.

### LATE BLOOMERS...

**Pediatric growth and development is a continuous process. Although milestones are traditionally broken into discrete age ranges, it is reasonable to expect that some children will meet certain milestones sooner than expected, whereas others may attain milestones later than other children in their age range.**

## Pediatric Vital Signs

The expected normal range for vital signs in pediatric patients varies greatly with age (**Table 1-2**). Infants and children have faster pulse and respiratory rates while at rest, and the average blood pressure is lower. Lower cardiac stroke volumes and respiratory tidal volumes

**Table 1-1** Developmental Milestones

| Age | Motor Skills | Speech Development | Social/Emotional Development | Comments/Red Flags |
|-----|-------------|-------------------|------------------------------|--------------------|
| 0–2 Months | ▪ Complete head lag when pulled from supine to upright position<br>▪ Able to lift head up momentarily while lying prone<br>▪ No visual tracking of objects | ▪ Crying is primary communication | ▪ Sleeps often<br>▪ Peak fussiness seen around age 6 weeks | ▪ Fewer than 6 wet diapers in 24 hours is concerning for dehydration.<br>▪ First signs of illness are often lethargy, decreased feeding, decreased wet diapers.<br>▪ Fever in this age range (100.4°F or higher measured rectally) is an emergency. |
| 2–4 Months | ▪ Visual tracking present | ▪ Cooing (vowel sounds) present | ▪ Social smile is present | ▪ Lack of visual tracking is concerning neurologic injury or deficit. |
| 4–6 Months | ▪ No head lag when pulled from supine to upright position<br>▪ Rolling begins<br>▪ Increased control of head and neck | | ▪ Increased social smile and laughing<br>▪ Will seek attention with actions other than crying<br>▪ May begin sleeping through the night | ▪ Injuries from rolling off of furniture prior to age 4 months should raise suspicion. |
| 6–8 Months | ▪ May begin to sit unassisted<br>▪ Scooting then crawling | ▪ Cooing evolves into babbling | ▪ Stranger anxiety | ▪ Performing as much of the exam as possible with the infant and parent together may be helpful. |
| 8–12 Months | ▪ Mobility increases<br>▪ May pull from sitting to standing<br>▪ Cruising along furniture | ▪ May say mama, dada, and other simple words | ▪ Temper tantrums begin<br>▪ Curiosity increases<br>▪ Will play peek-a-boo (object permanence)<br>▪ Waves bye-bye<br>▪ May show or share a toy with an adult when prompted | ▪ As mobility and curiosity increases, injuries from falls, pulling objects onto themselves from elevated surfaces, and ingestion of toxic substances increases dramatically. |
| 12–18 Months | ▪ Standing unassisted<br>▪ Walking progresses<br>▪ Able to scribble | ▪ Understands one-step commands<br>▪ 3- to 6-word vocabulary | ▪ Separation anxiety | |
| 18–24 Months | ▪ Running progresses | ▪ 25- to 50-word vocabulary | ▪ Parallel play develops | |

| Age | | | | |
|---|---|---|---|---|
| 2–4 years | ■ Draws a circle then a cross | ■ 50-to-100-word vocabulary<br>■ 50% of speech should be understandable<br>■ 3-word sentences | ■ Cooperative play develops<br>■ Toilet training typically near completion by 4 years old | ■ Magical thinking may lead to children blaming themselves for being sick or injured.<br>■ Reassurance that being sick or injured is not a punishment is important. |
| 4–6 years | ■ Can balance and hop on one foot unsupported<br>■ Able to skip (closer to 6 years)<br>■ Uses a fork and spoon<br>■ Dressing self<br>■ Progressively develops ability to draw a square then a triangle, then a diamond | ■ 4+-word sentences<br>■ 100% of speech should be understandable | ■ Ability to tell fantasy from reality develops<br>■ Can play games with rules closer to 6 years<br>■ Association of actions and consequences | |
| 6–12 years | ■ Ties shoelaces | | ■ Enjoy independence from parents<br>■ Regression when stressed is common | ■ Signs of puberty may be present as early as 10 years old.<br>■ Practitioners should fully describe procedures before performing them, especially painful procedures.<br>■ Allow them to help manage their own pain or discomfort by breathing deeply, holding still, or squeezing someone's hand. |
| 12–17 years | | | ■ Generally more concerned about the possibility of disfigurement or permanent injury<br>■ Will want more privacy during history and exam, increased sense of modesty<br>■ Risk-taking behavior increases<br>■ Social and peer pressure plays a larger role in behavior and decision making | ■ Vital signs will begin to approach standard adult ranges.<br>■ Allow these patients to participate in decision making when possible.<br>■ Examination of patients at this age may need to be private, and a single practitioner should not be alone with them. |

in the pediatric population mean that the pulse and respiratory rate must be increased at baseline to maintain adequate perfusion and ventilation.

It is important not only to recognize abnormal vital signs, but also to consider them in context with the entire patient presentation. Occasionally, vital signs outside of the normal range may be expected in certain patients. Hypotension and hypoxia in an asthmatic patient is extremely concerning, whereas decreased blood pressure and lower oxygen saturation in a child with an unrepaired congenital heart defect may be their baseline. It is essential to involve family members and caregivers when assessing every patient and allow them to assist you in forming an overall impression.

> Caregiver or family member concern about the child's condition should always be respected and prompt further evaluation and assessment.

| Table 1-2 Vital Signs for the Pediatric Patient | | | |
|---|---|---|---|
| Age | Pulse | Respiratory | Systolic BP |
| 0–6 months | 100–190 | 30–60 | >60 |
| 6–12 months | 100–160 | 30–60 | >60 |
| 1–3 years | 90–150 | 20–30 | 80–100 |
| 3–5 years | 80–140 | 20–25 | 80–100 |
| 6–12 years | 70–120 | 15–20 | 80–110 |
| 13–17 years | 60–100 | 12–20 | 90–110 |

© Jones & Bartlett Learning.

## CASE STUDY

**You are assessing a preschool-age patient (3 years old) who complains of left arm pain after falling on the playground.**

### Case Questions

- What are the differences between adult and pediatric assessment regarding the following?
  - Scene size-up
  - General patient impression
  - Primary survey and treatment
- Secondary survey and treatment

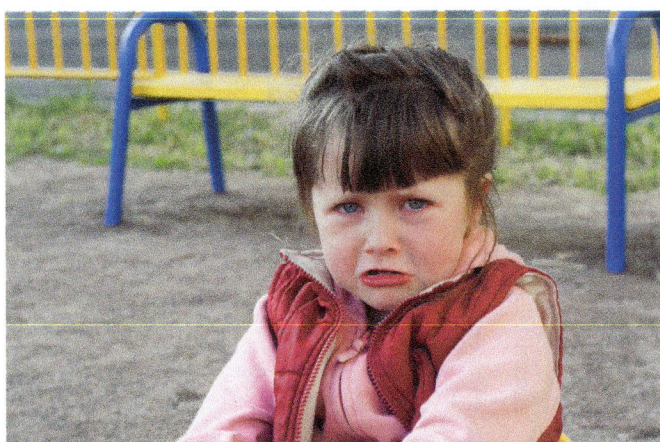

**Figure 1-1** A 3-year-old would be expected to express pain after a playground fall.
© Ruslan Merzliakov/Shutterstock.

# Scene Size-Up

The initial tasks of scene size-up and ensuring scene safety are largely the same regardless of the patient's age. The prehospital practitioner should always maintain an increased level of awareness for potential hazards and safety concerns when entering any scene. In addition to looking for potential safety hazards, identifying concerns specific for pediatric patients is important. Visibly dirty or soiled living environments, along with patients who do not appear to have been bathed for an extended period of time should raise concern for potential neglect. As you scan the environment, pay special attention for any cleaning agents, medications, drug paraphernalia, or other substances that could have potentially been ingested by the patient. If the call involves a patient who has been injured, evaluate the environment and assess whether the reported mechanism of injury matches the pattern and severity of injury that the patient has suffered. When there is any concern that the scene is not safe or that abuse or neglect may have occurred, law enforcement backup should be contacted per local protocols.

# General Patient Impression

The first step—before the prehospital practitioner even makes physical contact with the pediatric patient—is to form a general impression based on a rapid visual assessment that can be performed at a distance. As more experience is gained with pediatric patients, this "across the room" assessment becomes second nature and can be accomplished in seconds. The primary purpose of this assessment is to determine if immediate lifesaving interventions are necessary, or if there is time to perform further assessment and evaluation. This general impression can also aid in determining if rapid intervention and transport are required (quick) or if there is time to perform interventions on scene prior to initiating transport (not quick). A useful tool that describes the elements required to form a general impression is the Pediatric Assessment Triangle (PAT).

## The Pediatric Assessment Triangle

The Pediatric Assessment Triangle focuses on the observation of three distinct categories: General **appearance**, work of **breathing**, and **circulation** (**Figure 1-2**).

When using the Pediatric Assessment Triangle, each element is assessed individually, and then an overall general impression is formed by combining the assessment findings (**Table 1-3**).

When all sides of the Pediatric Assessment Triangle are reassuring and there are no concerning findings on the initial impression, the patient is likely compensating appropriately and the likelihood that a life-threatening illness or injury is present is very low. This gives the practitioner time to perform the primary assessment, take vital signs, obtain a history, and focus on family-centered care. Children with a normal appearance, but abnormal general impression findings in the respiratory

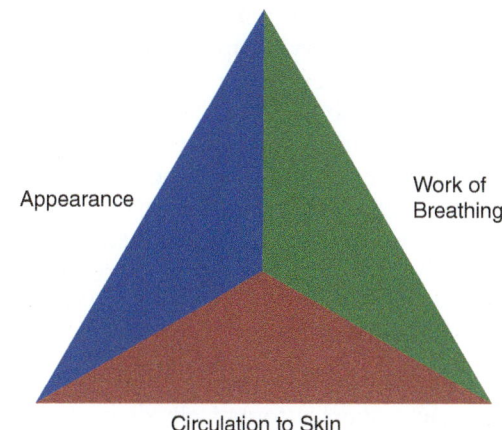

**Figure 1-2** The Pediatric Assessment Triangle is a useful tool to form a general impression of the pediatric patient.

Used with permission of the American Academy of Pediatrics, Pediatric Education for Prehospital Professionals, © American Academy of Pediatrics, 2000.

| Table 1-3 General Impression Based on Pediatric Assessment Triangle Findings | | | |
|---|---|---|---|
| **Appearance** | **Breathing** | **Circulation** | **Impression** |
| Reassuring | Reassuring | Reassuring | The patient is fully compensated and there is a low likelihood that life-threatening illness or injury is present. |
| Reassuring | Reassuring | Abnormal | The patient is likely compensating well. Further evaluation for possible circulatory emergency is necessary. |
| Reassuring | Abnormal | Reassuring | The patient is likely compensating well. Further evaluation for possible respiratory emergency is necessary. |
| Reassuring | Abnormal | Abnormal | The patient is compensated, but there is a *very* high risk of decompensation if life-threatening conditions are not rapidly treated. |
| Abnormal | Reassuring | Abnormal | The patient has clear circulatory compromise and is decompensating. |
| Abnormal | Abnormal | Reassuring | The patient has clear respiratory compromise and is decompensating. |
| Abnormal | Abnormal | Abnormal | The patient has full cardiopulmonary collapse and there is a high likelihood of impending arrest. |

Categories highlighted in green represent reassuring findings, where there is low level of concern. Areas highlighted in red represent abnormal findings, where the level of concern is high and immediate intervention is needed. Areas highlighted in yellow, where the appearance is normal, but there is respiratory or circulatory concern, will require case-by-case evaluation to determine if rapid transport versus initiation of stabilization and treatment at the scene is warranted.

or circulatory categories are likely compensating appropriately but require further evaluation and treatment of their illness or injury to prevent decompensation.

Patients with a reassuring appearance, but signs of circulatory and respiratory compromise represent children who are on the verge of decompensating. Immediate intervention to prevent life-threatening cardiopulmonary collapse is required in these patients.

Patients with an abnormal appearance and signs of circulatory and respiratory compromise are the most severely ill or injured. They are already experiencing cardiopulmonary collapse and they have exhausted their ability to compensate. If immediate interventions are not taken, the patient will likely experience cardiopulmonary arrest. Although a rare event, when pediatric cardiopulmonary arrest occurs, the likelihood of survival without neurologic impairment decreases rapidly.

## General Appearance

Assessment of the general appearance is likely the first thing most practitioners automatically do when they encounter a pediatric patient (**Figure 1-3**). The general appearance is used to determine how the child is tolerating their illness or injury overall, and whether they appear to be compensating appropriately. The TICLS (think "tickles") mnemonic is useful for assessing the general appearance of the pediatric patient and is endorsed by the American Academy of Pediatrics (AAP; **Table 1-4**).

When there is any abnormality or nonreassuring findings on the general appearance of the pediatric patient, it is an indication that they are not compensating. Rapid evaluation for circulatory or respiratory compromise is essential.

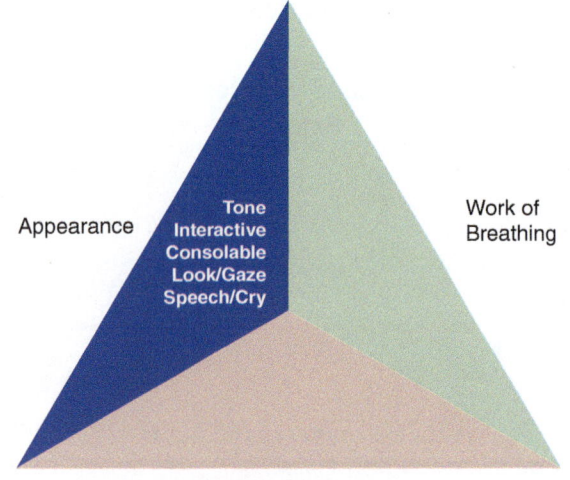

**Figure 1-3** General appearance is the first side of the Pediatric Assessment Triangle to assess.

Used with permission of the American Academy of Pediatrics, Pediatric Education for Prehospital Professionals, © American Academy of Pediatrics, 2000.

| Table 1-4 The TICLS Mnemonic for Assessment of General Appearance | |
| --- | --- |
| **T**one | Is the child actively moving? |
| | Does the child resist when you examine them? |
| | Is the child listless and limp? |
| **I**nteractiveness | Does the child interact with you or caregivers appropriately? |
| | Does the child respond to sounds, movements, or when touched during the exam? |
| | Will the child reach for a favorite toy or cling to caregivers? |
| **C**onsolability | Is the child's level of distress appropriate for the situation? |
| | Can the parent or caregiver calm or soothe the child? |
| | Is the level of stranger and separation anxiety developmentally appropriate for the child's age? |
| **L**ook | Is the child's gaze intentional, or is the child unable to focus? |
| | Does the child appear to be interested or engaged in seeing what is happening? |
| | Will the child look at or follow a lighted object? |
| **S**peech | Is the child able to speak or make sounds that are developmentally appropriate for age? |
| | In children who are verbal, does the content of the child's speech make sense, or does it seem confused and agitated? |

© Jones & Bartlett Learning.

## Work of Breathing

Accurate assessment of the work of breathing is especially critical in pediatric patients (**Figure 1-4**). The majority of pediatric cardiac arrest cases are precipitated by respiratory compromise and arrest. One of the first compensatory mechanisms that pediatric patients will exhibit when experiencing respiratory distress is the

The child appears to have good tone and interacts with you by establishing eye contact as you approach her. She appears scared but is not crying. She is cradling her left arm.

### Case Questions

- Is the general appearance of this patient reassuring or compromised?
  - This patient has good tone and is appropriately interactive. She is scared, which is appropriate given the situation. She appears to be aware that she is injured, and she is responding to the pain appropriately.

The general appearance of this patient is reassuring.

use of accessory muscles and positioning themselves in such a way to maximize inhaled tidal volumes.

A useful mnemonic to aid in recalling the elements to look for when assessing the work of breathing is FRAP (**Table 1-5**).

### Flaring

The nares represent the area of highest resistance in the pediatric upper airway. It is for this reason that prehospital practitioners will often note significant nasal flaring in pediatric patients as they attempt to decrease upper airway resistance and maximize inhaled tidal volumes while reducing inspiratory effort. Nasal flaring in infants and neonates with respiratory distress is an ominous sign. The appearance of nasal flaring can be

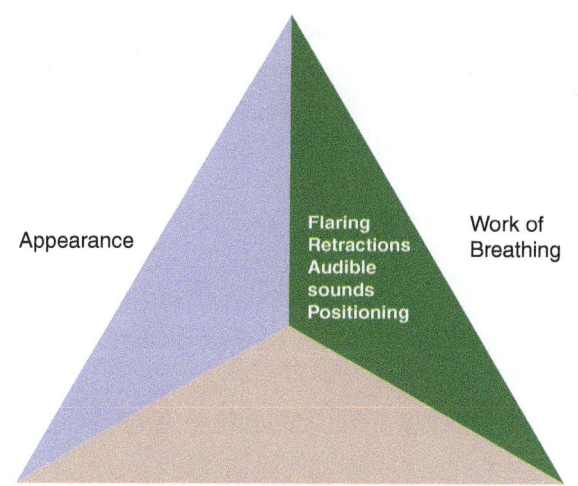

**Figure 1-4** A pediatric patient's work of breathing can be an indicator of respiratory compromise or distress.

Used with permission of the American Academy of Pediatrics, Pediatric Education for Prehospital Professionals, © American Academy of Pediatrics, 2000.

| **Table 1-5** FRAP Assessment of Work of Breathing | |
|---|---|
| **F**laring | Pediatric patients will flare their nostrils in an attempt reduce upper airway resistance and maximize inspiratory air flow. The presence of nasal flaring is an ominous sign, particularly in neonates and infants. |
| **R**etractions | Accessory muscle use progresses from superior to inferior as severity of respiratory distress increases. The presence of subcostal retractions and abdominal breathing indicates severe respiratory compromise. |
| **A**udible breath sounds | Any breath sounds that can be heard without the use of a stethoscope indicate that respiratory distress is present. |
| **P**ositioning | Pediatric patients will often assume a tripod position to reduce inspiratory effort when they have maximized accessory muscle use. It is a sign that they are getting tired and at risk for respiratory failure and arrest. |

© Jones & Bartlett Learning.

very subtle, especially in neonates, and requires careful and intentional observation to notice on examination.

### Retractions

Inhalation is an active process that primarily involves the use of the diaphragm. As respiratory distress progresses and respiratory effort increases, pediatric patients will recruit additional muscles to aid in respiration. To observe the use of accessory muscles, start at the neck and work down. First observe the suprasternal notch and note any tracheal tugging that may be present. Then look laterally to the clavicles and observe for supraclavicular retractions (**Figure 1-5**). Next, have the caregiver raise the patient's shirt and directly observe the chest and abdomen. Any visible retractions between the ribs indicate that the patient is using the intercostal muscles to aid in increasing inhaled tidal volumes. Finally, observe the subcostal area and abdomen. Subcostal retractions and paradoxical abdominal movement with inspiration and exhalation (seesaw breathing) indicate a significant level of respiratory distress and accessory muscle use.

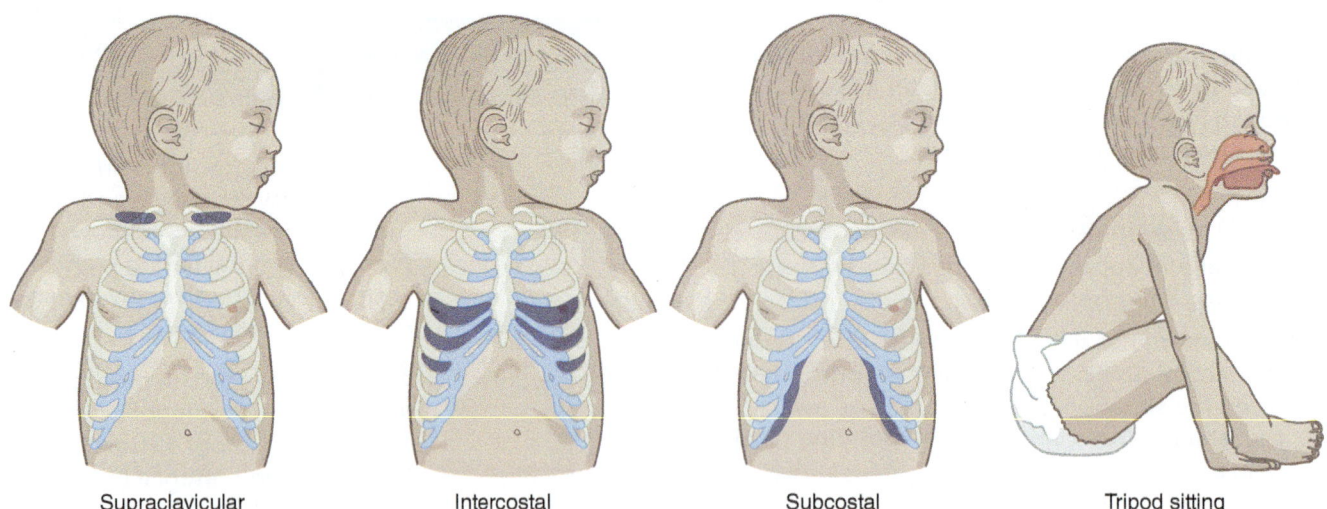

| Supraclavicular | Intercostal | Subcostal | Tripod sitting |

**Figure 1-5** As accessory muscle use moves inferiorly, the severity of respiratory distress is likely increasing.

© Jones & Bartlett Learning.

## Audible Breath Sounds

Audible breath sounds are those that can be heard without the aid of a stethoscope; they are usually heard while approaching the patient. These sounds can be categorized as inspiratory, expiratory, or biphasic (both inspiratory and expiratory; **Table 1-6**).

The most common inspiratory breath sound heard in pediatric patients is stridor. Stridor is a high-pitched, brassy sound that is caused by narrowing of the upper airway. When stridor is present, a high index of suspicion for upper airway obstruction should be present. Stridor can also be heard on exhalation in some cases, especially when the patient generates a significant exhalation force such as coughing, crying, or sneezing. Biphasic stridor indicates significant narrowing of the upper airway and is often seen in severe upper airway obstructive disease processes.

Expiratory breath sounds often include wheezing, crackles, and rhonchi. Wheezing is heard when there is narrowing of the lower airways that results in turbulent airflow, often at the end of exhalation. As the narrowing of the lower airways becomes more severe, the wheezing may progress to cover the entire exhalation phase, and it can be present on inhalation and exhalation (biphasic) in severe lower airway obstruction. Crackles most often are associated with fluid or congestion in the lower airways and may be indicative of pneumonia or congestive heart failure. Rhonchi are similar to crackles in that they are caused by congestion and fluid; however, they are more often associated with the larger airways, as opposed to crackles, which tend to be heard with small airway disease. Rhonchi can be heard in more severe pneumonia, cystic fibrosis, and anaphylaxis where significant edema and congestion are present in the large airways.

Grunting is a specific expiratory breath sound often heard in neonates and infants. It can be heard at the end of exhalation and indicates that the patient is trying to generate positive end expiratory pressure (PEEP) to splint open their lower airways. Grunting may be heard in newborns with transient tachypnea of the newborn (TTN), infants with bronchiolitis or reactive airway disease, and any other pathology in which the lower airways are prone to collapse at the end of exhalation.

**The child is sitting in a normal position and appears comfortable. There is no nasal flaring present. You have the mother raise the patient's shirt so you can observe the patient's chest. There is no evidence of accessory muscle use. You cannot hear any concerning audible breath sounds.**

### Case Questions

- Does this patient have any signs of increased work of breathing?

  - Using the FRAP mnemonic, the following observations can be made:

    - There is no nasal flaring present.

    - No retractions were observed when the patient's shirt was lifted.

    - No audible breath sounds were heard

    - The patient appears to be sitting in a comfortable position and not tripoding.

This patient does not have a compromised work of breathing, and there appears to be no concern for respiratory distress.

**Table 1-6** Audible Breath Sounds

| Sound | Description | Location of Pathology | Common Association |
|---|---|---|---|
| Stridor | High pitched, brassy, "seal bark" | Upper airway | ■ Indicates upper airway pathology<br>■ Common causes include:<br>  ▪ Croup<br>  ▪ Epiglottitis<br>  ▪ Foreign body obstruction<br>  ▪ Anaphylaxis |
| Stertor | Snoring or snorting | Upper airway | ■ Indicates obstruction by tissues in the upper airway<br>■ Repositioning of the airway is often beneficial |
| Grunting | Humming noise at the end of exhalation | Lower airway | ■ Indicates that the patient is trying to generate positive end expiratory pressure to splint open lower airways<br>■ Common causes include:<br>  ▪ Transient tachypnea of the newborn<br>  ▪ Reactive airway disease<br>  ▪ Bronchiolitis |
| Wheezing | Fine, high pitched, musical in some cases | Lower airway | ■ Indicates lower airway obstruction due to bronchoconstriction<br>■ Common causes include:<br>  ▪ Asthma<br>  ▪ Anaphylaxis |
| Rhonchi | Rattling, gurgling, low pitched | Large airways of the lower respiratory tract | ■ Indicates congestion and edema of the large airways in the lower respiratory tract<br>■ Common causes include:<br>  ▪ Severe pneumonia<br>  ▪ Bronchiolitis<br>  ▪ Chronic bronchitis<br>  ▪ Pulmonary dysplasia<br>  ▪ Cystic fibrosis<br>  ▪ Chronic obstructive pulmonary disease |

© Jones & Bartlett Learning.

Grunting is highly suggestive of severe respiratory distress and compromise and indicates patients who are likely nearing the end of their ability to compensate.

It is important to note that hearing any single type of airway sound in isolation is rare, and patients with severe respiratory disease often have a combination of audible breath sounds. Combining the history of present illness with a thorough physical exam will aid in determining the primary respiratory pathology.

## Positioning

When accessory muscle use has been maximized, patients will often begin to assume a tripod position, leaning forward and propping themselves up on their extended arms. This elevates the thoracic cavity and reduces the amount of negative pressure that must be generated during inhalation, indicating that the patient is in distress and using all available compensatory mechanisms.

Patients will often extend their neck and position their upper airway to maximize inspiratory airflow.

## Circulation

Rapid assessment of circulatory status in the pediatric patient is critical (**Figure 1-6**). Positive outcomes are more likely when intervention for hemodynamic compromise is initiated with minimal delay. The primary method for assessing circulatory status in pediatric patients is a "quick look" at the patient's skin to assess the color. Quickly scan for cyanosis, pallor, and mottling.

Pallor is observed as pale-appearing skin. It is an indication that peripheral tissues are beginning to constrict to promote blood flow to the vital organs. Pallor may also be seen in patients who are anemic (low hemoglobin concentration). Assessing for pallor can be difficult in some cases. Some patients may be very fair skinned at baseline. It is important to ask caregivers if they feel that the patient appears pale. Pallor can be assessed in all patients by looking at the overall appearance of the skin. Examination of the conjunctiva, mucous membranes, and nailbeds may be particularly helpful when assessing for pallor in patients with darker complexions.

As the body continues to constrict the peripheral vasculature in an effort to perfuse vital organs, pallor will progress to mottling. Mottling is seen as a blotchy, net-like (reticular) pattern on the skin (**Figure 1-7**). It may begin in the distal extremities and progress toward the core. Mottling is a concerning finding and indicates severe compromise of the peripheral circulation. When

this level of peripheral circulatory compromise is present, the likelihood of poor perfusion to the vital organs is high. Mottling may also be seen in older children when they are cold and attempting to conserve body heat. When mottling is seen in an infant or neonate, there should always be an elevated suspicion for circulatory compromise and shock.

When circulatory function is depressed to the point that cardiac output is no longer sufficient to deliver oxygenated blood to the peripheral tissues, the prehospital practitioner may notice a dusky grey or blue appearance of tissues that normally have a rich blood supply. Tissues where cyanosis is most commonly seen include the lips, nail beds, hands, and feet (**Figure 1-8**). As cyanosis becomes more severe, it will progressively move toward the core. Cyanosis can be seen in respiratory or circulatory compromise. When cyanosis is present in the absence of signs of respiratory compromise, there is a high likelihood that the patient is experiencing circulatory compromise and can no longer adequately perfuse the peripheral tissues.

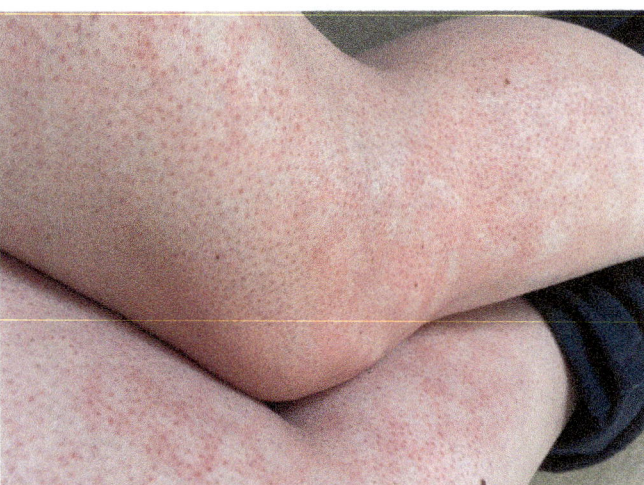

**Figure 1-7** Mottling appears as a blotchy, net-like pattern on the skin and indicates severe compromise of the patient's peripheral circulation.
© Lorna Roberts/Shutterstock

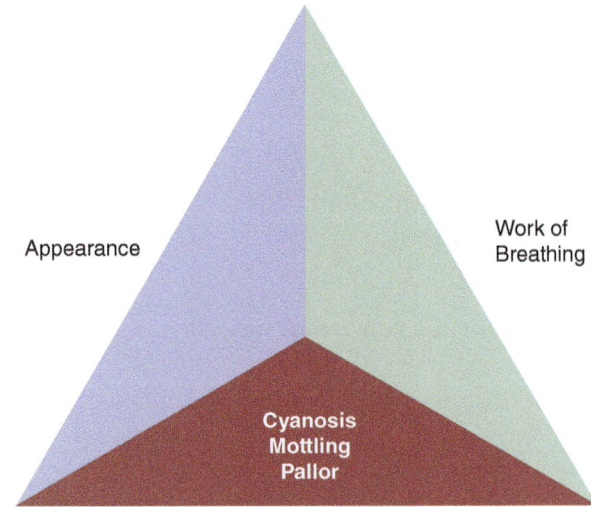

**Figure 1-6** A pediatric patient's circulation status can be assessed by quickly looking at the child's skin color and condition (e.g., mottling, pallor, cyanosis).

Used with permission of the American Academy of Pediatrics, Pediatric Education for Prehospital Professionals, © American Academy of Pediatrics, 2000.

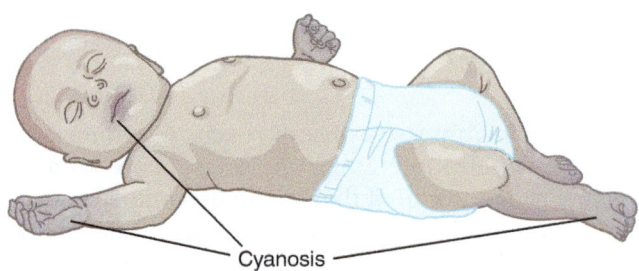

**Figure 1-8** Cyanosis is most commonly seen in the lips, nail beds, hands, and feet. It is an indication of respiratory or circulatory compromise.
© Jones & Bartlett Learning.

As you observe the child, you note that the skin color appears normal. There is no sign of pallor, mottling, or cyanosis.

### Case Questions

- Does this patient have any signs of compromised circulation?
  - There is no pallor, mottling, or cyanosis noted. The patient does not have any signs of compromised circulation based on this assessment.

The patient's general appearance, observed earlier, is also not concerning, further indicating that the circulatory status is intact.

## The Pediatric Glasgow Coma Scale (PGCS)

Another tool to use in forming the general impression is a Pediatric Glasgow Coma Scale (PGCS) score (**Table 1-7**). The Pediatric Glasgow Coma Scale assesses the same three domains as the standard Glasgow Coma Scale (eye opening, motor response, verbal response); however, it contains age-appropriate modifications in each domain. The highest possible PGCS score is 15, which is considered very reassuring. The lowest possible score is 3, which indicates a patient is completely unresponsive in all three domains and likely has a severe level of illness or injury. A PGCS score of less than 8 in any patient should be viewed as very concerning and will usually require rapid stabilization and transport.

**Table 1-7** Pediatric Glasgow Coma Scale

| | >1 Year | <1 Year | Score |
|---|---|---|---|
| **EYE OPENING** | Spontaneously | Spontaneously | 4 |
| | To verbal command | To shout | 3 |
| | To pain | To pain | 2 |
| | No response | No response | 1 |
| **MOTOR RESPONSE** | Obeys | Spontaneous | 6 |
| | Localizes pain | Localizes pain | 5 |
| | Flexion—withdrawal | Flexion—withdrawal | 4 |
| | Flexion—abnormal (decorticate rigidity) | Flexion—abnormal (decorticate rigidity) | 3 |
| | Extension (decerebrate rigidity) | Extension (decerebrate rigidity) | 2 |
| | No response | No response | 1 |

| | >5 Years | 2–5 years | 0–23 months | |
|---|---|---|---|---|
| **VERBAL RESPONSE** | Oriented | Appropriate words/phrases | Smiles/coos appropriately | 5 |
| | Disoriented/confused | Inappropriate words | Cries and is inconsolable | 4 |
| | Inappropriate words | Persistent cries and screams | Persistent inappropriate crying and/or screaming | 3 |
| | Incomprehensible sounds | Grunts | Grunts, agitated, and restless | 2 |
| | No response | No response | No response | 1 |

**TOTAL PEDIATRIC GLASGOW COMA SCORE (3–15):**

Your patient is opening her eyes spontaneously and looking around curiously at the emergency personnel. When the patient's mother asks her to say hello to the emergency personnel, she waves her right hand and says, "Hi!" loudly, she then says, "I fell and hurt my arm!"

## Case Questions

- What Pediatric Glasgow Coma Score would you assign to this patient?

  - This patient is greater than 1 year old and opening her eyes spontaneously. She should be assigned a score of 4 for eye opening.

  - This patient is greater than 1 year old and waved hello when asked to do so (obeying commands). She should be assigned a score of 6 for motor response.

  - This patient is between 2 and 5 years old and using appropriate words and phrases. She should be assigned a score of 5 for verbal response.

This patient should be assigned an overall score of 15 on the PGCS, which is very reassuring.

# The Pediatric Management Diagram

The Pediatric Management Diagram (PMD) is designed to give a general overview of the care and management of the pediatric patient (**Figure 1-9**). The general impression formed by using the Pediatric Assessment Triangle is the launching point for the PMD and will determine the appropriate pathway for the prehospital practitioner to follow.

A key element to be aware of is that pediatric patients who are ill have the ability to compensate for long periods of time and do not demonstrate steady decompensation like adults do. Pediatric patients are more likely to have a sudden deterioration after exhausting their ability to compensate for respiratory

Always analyze the risk of delaying transport to perform stabilizing care with the benefit that care may or may not provide to the patient. Consider what interventions can be accomplished safely during transport.

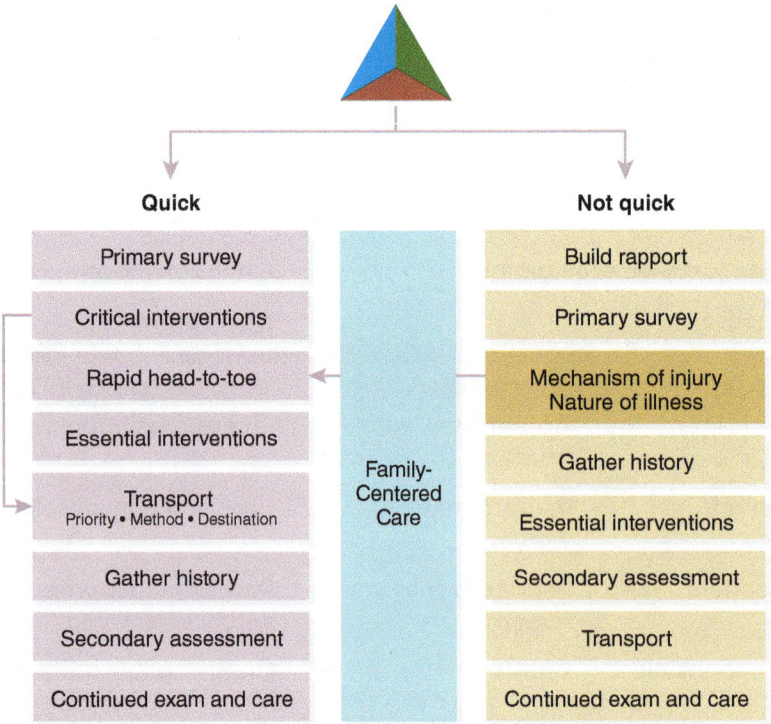

**Figure 1-9** The Pediatric Management Diagram helps prehospital practitioners with decision making about care and management of pediatric patients.

or circulatory compromise. Early recognition of life threats and the ability to determine which patients are at risk for decompensation are the key predictors of positive outcomes in ill and injured children.

## The "Quick" Patient

When the general impression is not reassuring and there is concern for cardiac or respiratory compromise, the prehospital practitioner should proceed down the "quick" pathway (**Figure 1-10**). This pathway implies that the patient requires immediate action. This may include goal-oriented care such as IV access and fluid administration or immediate transport.

Once it has been determined that a patient is "quick," begin the primary survey by assessing level of consciousness with the Alert, Voice, Pain, Unresponsive (AVPU) scale when appropriate and assessing the XABCs. Any life-threatening conditions encountered during the primary survey should be treated immediately and simultaneously with the exam when possible. Critical interventions to control external hemorrhage, support ventilatory status, and manage circulatory status should be performed without delay. Transport should be initiated as soon as possible, with the remainder of the assessment, including the head-to-toe (or toe-to-head) exam taking place en route to the hospital. When time permits, the prehospital practitioner should gather additional history and perform a secondary assessment. This may not always be possible depending on the severity of illness or injury, or when the transport destination

is a short distance away. Patients being treated on the "quick" pathway are considered critically ill or injured and require constant examination, reassessment, and care.

## The "Not Quick" Patient

When patients have a reassuring general impression based on the Pediatric Assessment Triangle, or in those who appear to be compensating well with no signs of imminent decompensation, the "not quick" pathway is appropriate for initial management (**Figure 1-11**). This pathway assumes that there is time to build rapport with the pediatric patient. Once adequate rapport has been built, a primary survey can be completed in similar fashion to the "quick" pathway. If the nature of illness is severe, or there is severe injury or significant mechanism of injury encountered during the primary survey, the prehospital practitioner can transition to the "quick" pathway, moving through a rapid head-to-toe exam and initiating critical interventions along with rapid transport when appropriate.

If no severe illness or injury is noted on the primary survey, then the prehospital practitioner should proceed down the "not quick" pathway by gathering more history and initiating any essential interventions as appropriate. A secondary assessment is then performed, and a transport decision made. While en route to the transport destination, continued examinations—including reassessment of vital signs—and care are required to prevent any further progression of illness or injury.

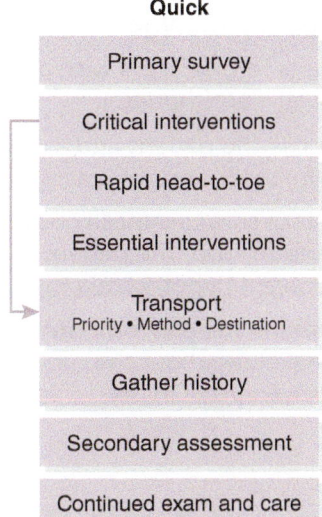

**Figure 1-10** Patients who are critically ill or injured should be treated along the "quick" pathway.
© Jones & Bartlett Learning.

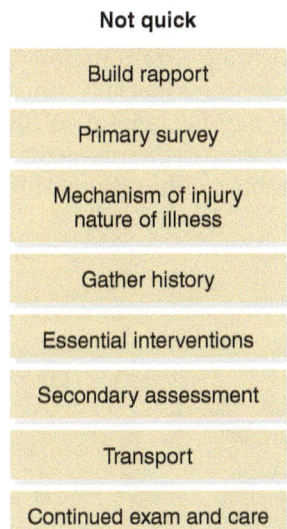

**Figure 1-11** Care for a pediatric patient with no severe illness or injury may be managed along the "not quick" pathway.
© Jones & Bartlett Learning.

No matter how critically ill or injured a child is, it is essential to communicate effectively with the caregivers about what is happening. When possible, assign a member of the crew to provide support and communication to the caregivers.

## "Quick" Versus "Not Quick"

The decision to declare a patient as "quick" versus "not quick" can be difficult, especially when prehospital practitioners have limited exposure and experience with pediatric patients (**Figure 1-12**). When there is *any* concern that immediate critical interventions are necessary or delaying transport may negatively impact the patient outcome, the patient should be considered "quick." Only when you are completely confident that the patient's status is reassuring and they do not require any critical interventions should you consider them "not quick."

## The Primary Survey

After forming a general impression with the Pediatric Assessment Triangle, the prehospital practitioner should proceed with the primary survey (**Table 1-8**). Whereas the PAT is focused on identifying patients in need of rapid treatment and transport, the primary survey is a systematic method for identifying what specific life-threatening conditions exist; the elements of the primary survey are known as the XABCDEs. Immediate care should be provided for life-threatening conditions encountered during the primary survey.

When performing examination and assessment of pediatric patients, especially those age 3 years and younger, it may be helpful to do the exam in a toe-to-head fashion. In general, pediatric patients will be less comfortable with examination of the head,

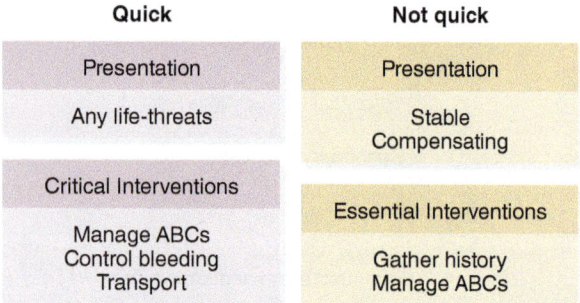

**Figure 1-12** The "quick" versus "not quick" decision is an important aspect of prehospital care for pediatric patients.
© Jones & Bartlett Learning.

| Table 1-8 | Elements of the Primary Survey |
|---|---|
| **X** | **E**xsanguination<br>• Check thoroughly for any life-threatening bleeding or hemorrhage.<br>• Identify suspicion for internal bleeding based on mechanism of injury or nature of illness. |
| **A** | **A**irway<br>• Ensure that the airway is open and patent.<br>• Examine the nose and mouth for any possible obstruction if clinically indicated. |
| **B** | **B**reathing<br>• Assess respiratory rate, $SpO_2$, and auscultate lung sounds.<br>• Optimize oxygenation and ventilation as soon as possible with supplemental oxygen or ventilatory assistance. |
| **C** | **C**irculation<br>• Palpate pulses.<br>• Assess capillary refill time.<br>• Feel skin temperature.<br>• Obtain blood pressure, if appropriate. |
| **D** | **D**isability<br>• Assess for any altered level of consciousness caused by the illness or injury. |
| **E** | **E**xposure/environment<br>• Assess temperature with a thermometer (rectal if appropriate).<br>• Expose the patient and assess all areas for injury or signs of illness.<br>  • Make sure to expose one area at a time and to cover the patient back up to prevent hypothermia.<br>• Examine the environment for any additional clues about the nature of illness or mechanism of injury. |

© Jones & Bartlett Learning.

neck, and chest until trust has been established. Starting at the feet and working toward the head allows the child to realize that the exam will not be painful, and the child will be less distressed when auscultating the

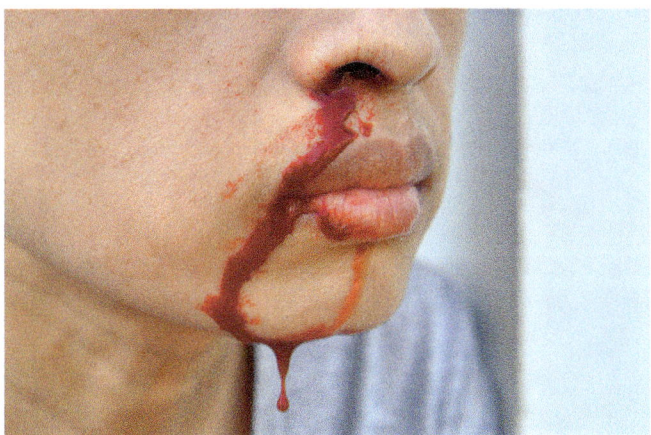

**Figure 1-13** Even a patient with epistaxis should be evaluated for large volume blood loss.
© BeautifulPicture/Shutterstock.

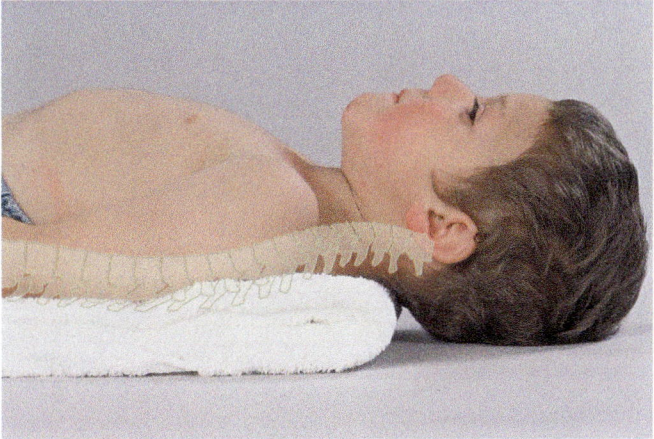

**Figure 1-14** Provide adequate padding under the child's torso, or use a spine board with a cutout for the child's occiput.
© National Association of Emergency Medical Technicians (NAEMT).

chest and examining the head. It is also helpful to start with noninjured body parts and examine any areas that may be injured at the end of the exam when possible.

## Exsanguination

Pediatric patients are particularly susceptible to hypotension and shock secondary to even small amounts of blood loss. The area around the patient should be quickly scanned for pooling blood. Any active bleeding that is encountered should be controlled immediately before continuing with the assessment.

Do not forget to maintain a high index of suspicion for internal bleeding and other occult sources of blood loss when the nature of illness or mechanism of injury warrants. Abdominal and pelvic injuries can lead to large volume loss. Patients with epistaxis can lose large amounts of blood that may not be visible because the patients swallow the blood in an effort to maintain a clear airway (**Figure 1-13**). It is important to carefully inspect the mouth and throat if you suspect upper airway bleeding.

## Airway

Ensuring an open and patent airway is second only to hemorrhage control when it comes to critical interventions. Unconscious and lethargic pediatric patients may have positional upper airway obstruction due to flexion of the neck. Pediatric patients have a larger occiput, which positions the chin closer to the chest when lying supine, leading to narrowing of the upper airway. Alternatively, hyperextension of the neck can also cause narrowing of the airway due to softer tracheal rings that are more susceptible to collapse when pressure is applied by overextending the neck. A small roll placed under the shoulders of the supine patient should be enough to bring the airway axis into appropriate alignment and maintain an open and patent airway (**Figure 1-14**).

## Breathing

The general assessment of the patient's work of breathing was performed initially while completing the Pediatric Assessment Triangle. During the primary survey, a more in-depth assessment of breathing is performed. The respirations in pediatric patients should be counted for a full minute when practical. Do not rely on automated calculations of respiratory rate from telemetry monitors until you have established a baseline respiratory rate by direct examination and counting of the respirations. Also take note of the depth of respiration. Auscultation of the chest should be performed next (**Figure 1-15**). Pay close attention to whether sounds are present on inhalation, exhalation, or both. This can be an important clue regarding what type of sounds you are hearing and where the respiratory pathology is located (upper versus lower airway).

Pulse oximetry should be examined when practical and can give the prehospital practitioner important information regarding the effectiveness of oxygenation. Supplemental oxygen should be applied any time respiratory distress is present with a target oxygen saturation of 94% to 99%.

Some patients, especially those with underlying congenital heart defects or chronic lung disease may have lower than normal baseline oxygen saturation. It is always important to ask the caregiver what is normal for a specific patient and consider the patient's past medical history during your assessment.

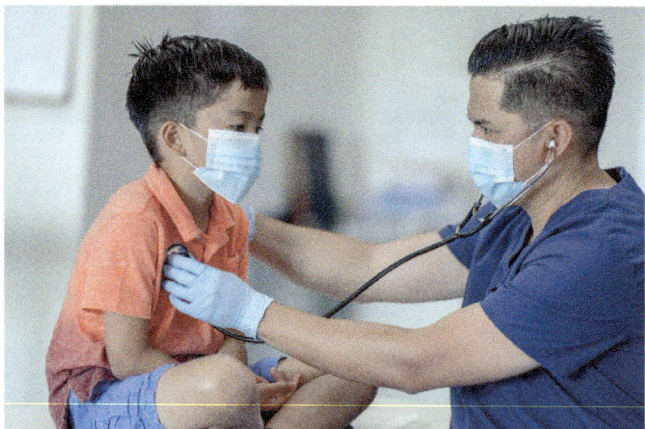

**Figure 1-15** Auscultation with a stethoscope can provide important information about the patient's work of breathing.
© FatCamera/E+/Getty Images.

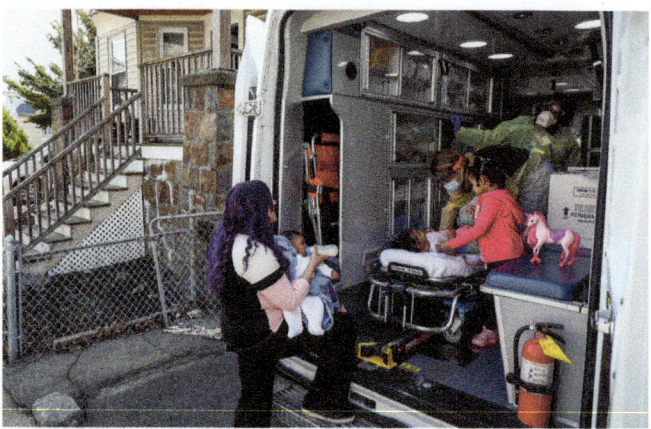

**Figure 1-16** If possible, move the child to a quiet area to continue your assessment.
© Erin Clark/The Boston Globe/Getty Images.

# Circulation

Assessment of circulation in the pediatric patient starts by placing a hand on the patient's skin and determining if the patient is maintaining an adequate body temperature. This can be done on one of the lower extremities, and the prehospital practitioner can immediately follow this by applying light pressure to blanch the skin to assess capillary refill time. Capillary refill time can also be assessed by applying pressure to the nailbeds. Capillary refill time greater than 2 seconds is considered delayed and should raise concern for circulatory compromise. Rapid capillary refill time that appears instantaneous ("flash" capillary refill) along with flushed skin and decreased blood pressure should raise concern for possible distributive shock.

After assessing skin temperature and capillary refill time, palpate distal pulses in the upper or lower extremities. In infants and neonates, it may be necessary to palpate the brachial or femoral pulses, as radial pulses might not be readily palpable in that age range. Assess the pulses for both rate and quality: Does the rate fall within the expected range? Does the quality of pulses feel appropriate? Weak or thready pulses may indicate the patient is compensating with peripheral vasoconstriction. Bounding pulses indicate the patient is hyperdynamic and the circulatory system is likely being stressed.

Obtaining a blood pressure reading may not be possible on every patient due to lack of patient cooperation or equipment limitations; however, it is important to obtain a blood pressure whenever possible and assess whether it falls within the expected range for the patient's age. When blood pressure readings are outside of normal limits, consider whether the reading is accurate based on how cooperative the patient is with the exam, and by assessing whether the other

circulation parameters, such as pulse rate, capillary refill, and skin temperature, also point to possible circulatory compromise. If the patient's blood pressure is abnormal and there are other signs of circulatory compromise present, they should be considered at risk for hemodynamic collapse and treated appropriately.

# Disability

When assessing for disability, a general understanding of pediatric milestones and the expected behavior for patients of various ages is helpful. If you suspect that a patient is not acting appropriately for their age, consider asking a caregiver or someone who knows the child well if their behavior is different than their baseline. When a child is not acting age appropriately, or they are acting differently than their baseline behavior, neurologic injury and decreased perfusion or oxygenation of the brain should be considered.

It can be difficult to assess for disability when a child is distressed by the commotion of an emergency situation. This may be compounded by the illness or injury. It may be helpful to safely move the child to a quiet area with the caregiver and continue the exam there, when appropriate (**Figure 1-16**).

# Exposure and Environment

The final portion of the primary survey is exposure of the patient and examination of the environment for additional clues. Expose the patient one region at a time and take care to cover them back up to prevent hypothermia. Examine them for any additional injuries that may have been missed or other clues that might help with treatment and stabilization. This is also a good opportunity to check the patient's temperature. Measurement of temperature rectally is preferred in infants and neonates. In older children, use of an oral thermometer is appropriate if they can follow commands. Measurement of axillary temperatures is not ideal, especially when fever is suspected, but may be necessary depending on the situation.

Take a moment to scan the environment around the patient in more detail. Observe for clues that may have been missed on your initial scene size-up. Take note of anything that could help clarify the mechanism of injury.

---

**As you perform your primary survey, you note the following:**

**X**—No obvious bleeding noted

**A**—Open and patent

**B**—Respiratory rate is 24 breaths/min, lung sounds are clear to auscultation bilaterally.

**C**—The skin is warm, capillary refill time is less than 2 seconds, the brachial pulse is strong.

**D**—GCS score is 15, the patient is acting appropriate for age and at her baseline behavior per mother.

**E**—Temperature is 98.7°F taken orally, there are no other obvious injuries noted, the patient is sitting on the ground next to the slide.

### Case Questions

- Are there any life-threatening injuries at this time?
  - Based on the information provided, it does not appear that the patient has any life-threatening injuries on the primary survey.
- What essential interventions should be provided before moving to the secondary assessment?
  - Treatment at this time should focus on managing the arm injury.
  - Splinting should be performed.
  - Distraction techniques to aid with pain management may be helpful.
  - Apply a cold pack to the area.

Provide pain medication if appropriate and within your scope of practice.

## Secondary Assessment

The secondary assessment involves taking a detailed history and combining that with the physical exam findings to build a more complete picture of the primary

---

cause of the patient's illness or injury. For example, although it may be obvious that the patient has lower airway obstruction, it is not until you have completed the secondary assessment that you learn they have a history of poorly controlled asthma and have recently run out of their maintenance medications.

One tool for assessing an acute process such as pain is the OPQRST mnemonic (**Table 1-9**).

When assessing a patient's pain, various age-appropriate pain scales are available. Visual pain scales can be used to overcome communication barriers or when patients are too young to fully articulate the pain they are experiencing (**Figure 1-17**).

Additional history can be elicited by using the SAMPLER mnemonic to prompt questions about the illness or injury (**Table 1-10**). Once the detailed history has been taken, the secondary assessment is completed by repeating both a focused exam of the area of interest,

| Table 1-9 OPQRST Memory Aid for History Taking | |
|---|---|
| **O**—Onset | ▪ When did the condition start? |
| | ▪ What was happening when the condition was first noticed? |
| **P**—Provocation/palliation | ▪ Does anything make the condition better or worse? |
| | ▪ Have you taken any medications or tried any treatment to help the condition? |
| **Q**—Quality | ▪ What does the condition feel like? |
| **R**—Radiation | ▪ Does the pain move to any other region or location? |
| **S**—Severity | ▪ Have the patient use an age-appropriate pain scale to rate the pain. |
| **T**—Timing | ▪ When did the condition start? |
| | ▪ Was it sudden, or has it been slowly worsening over time? |
| | ▪ What changed suddenly that caused you to seek emergency care now? |

## COMPARATIVE PAIN SCALE CHART
### Pain Assesment Tool

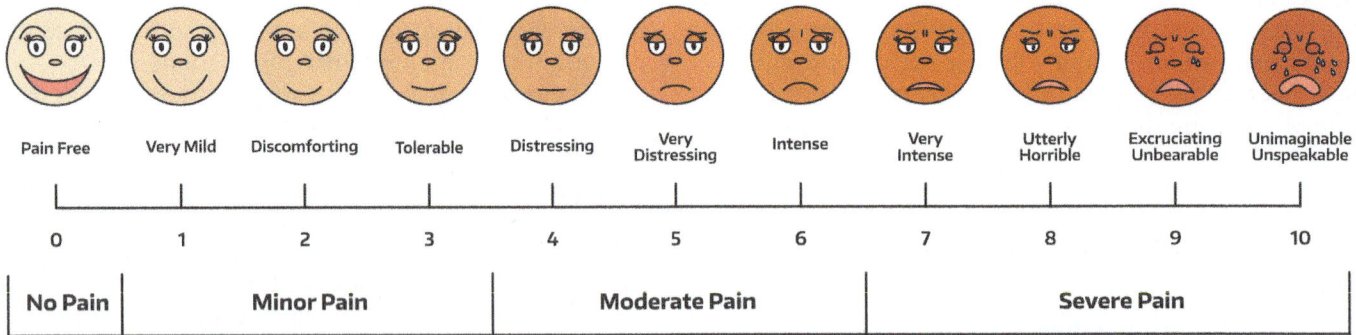

| | | | | | | | | | | |
|---|---|---|---|---|---|---|---|---|---|---|
| Pain Free | Very Mild | Discomforting | Tolerable | Distressing | Very Distressing | Intense | Very Intense | Utterly Horrible | Excruciating Unbearable | Unimaginable Unspeakable |
| 0 | 1 | 2 | 3 | 4 | 5 | 6 | 7 | 8 | 9 | 10 |

| No Pain | Minor Pain | Moderate Pain | Severe Pain |
|---|---|---|---|

**Figure 1-17** Visual pain scales are helpful when the patient is unable to verbally articulate their level of pain.
© Jones & Bartlett Learning.

**Table 1-10** SAMPLER Mnemonic for History Taking

| | |
|---|---|
| **S** | Signs and symptoms |
| **A** | Allergies |
| **M** | Medications |
| **P** | Past medical history |
| **L** | Last oral intake |
| **E** | Events leading up to the injury or illness |
| **R** | Risk factors |

© Jones & Bartlett Learning.

and a detailed head-to-toe (or toe-to-head) exam to identify additional injuries or medical concerns.

In the case of accident or injury, it is helpful to determine if there were any witnesses (teachers, caregivers) to the incident who can help complete the history of events provided by the patient. The patient should also be asked if they can remember the entire event. Be careful not to be distracted by the primary injury and miss other injuries. Ask the patient if they have any additional pain anywhere else.

## Treatment Plan

Once the secondary assessment is complete, a full treatment plan can be developed. In addition to the immediate interventions that were performed during the general impression and primary survey phases of care, ongoing treatment will be required in most cases. This treatment will be specific to whatever medical condition or injury is present. Further information on condition-specific treatment plans is included in later chapters.

**As you perform your secondary survey, OPQRST reveals the following:**

**O**—Acute onset after falling from a balance beam on the playground

**P**—Pain is provoked with movement of the arm and palliated when the arm is in a position of comfort.

**Q**—The patient describes the pain as throbbing.

**R**—The pain does not radiate anywhere.

**S**—The patient identifies the sad face corresponding with a rating of "7" on the FACES pain scale.

**T**—The pain has been present for about 15 minutes, since she fell off the slide.

**A SAMPLER history is obtained, and the following information is provided:**

**S**—Left arm pain with deformity

**A**—No known allergies to drugs, foods, or the environment

**M**—No medications

**P**—No significant past medical history

**L**—Patient ate breakfast at 0830 this morning—pancakes and cereal.

**E**—Fell approximately 4 feet from the slide while playing, remembers the whole event

**R**—None

## Case Questions

- At what point should you include the family or school in the assessment questions?
  - Obtaining additional history from bystanders who witnessed the accident or know more about the illness is always important.
  - Contacting the primary caregivers by phone if they are not available on scene can help fill in any pertinent past medical history such as medications, chronic medical conditions, and allergies.
- Can this patient still be treated if the parent or guardian is not present?
  - Consent for treatment of minors is generally implied when the parents or guardians are not available to provide direct consent.

Schools are generally allowed to provide consent when the child is in their care during the school day.

## Case Questions

- What additional treatment might be appropriate for this patient? How can these techniques be modified for older or younger children?
  - Physical comfort measures should be provided.
    - A sling or a splint should be applied.
    - Warm or cool packs can be used to reduce pain and swelling.
    - Neonates benefit from skin-to-skin contact.
    - Infants and toddlers may respond well to patting or rubbing (away from the injury site).
  - Distraction techniques can be used to reduce pain and anxiety.
    - The use of a phone or tablet to provide distracting music or videos may be helpful.
    - Bubbles, lighted toys, and books may be used in infants and toddlers.
    - Older children may benefit from video games, art, or other activities.
  - Coaching
    - Guided breathing activities and continuous dialogue may benefit some patients.
  - Analgesia
    - The previous activities and interventions may be useful on their own or can be combined with medications for pain.

Pain medication may be more effective, and lower doses may be required, when combined with interventions such as distraction, coaching, and physical comfort measures.

# Pediatric Transport

Multiple factors must be considered when initiating transport for the pediatric patient. The first consideration is when to begin transport. This is typically addressed in the general impression and primary survey phases of assessment when the patient is critically ill or injured. When the patient is stable, transport may be delayed while interventions such as IV access, pain control, bandaging, and splinting are performed on scene.

The mode of transport is also important to consider (**Figure 1-18**). In most urban and suburban environments, ground transport times may be fast enough to avoid the need for air medical transport. Traffic conditions in many urban and suburban locations may significantly increase ground transport times and should be taken into consideration. In rural areas, air transport will likely be the most rapid method to get the patient to the appropriate medical facility. Local protocols and case-specific circumstances will play a large role when choosing the most appropriate mode of transport.

When choosing a transport destination for the pediatric patient, the closest *appropriate* facility should be chosen whenever possible. Large tertiary pediatric care centers are generally the most skilled and specialized in dealing with acutely ill and injured children. In some circumstances, such as when a patient is unstable

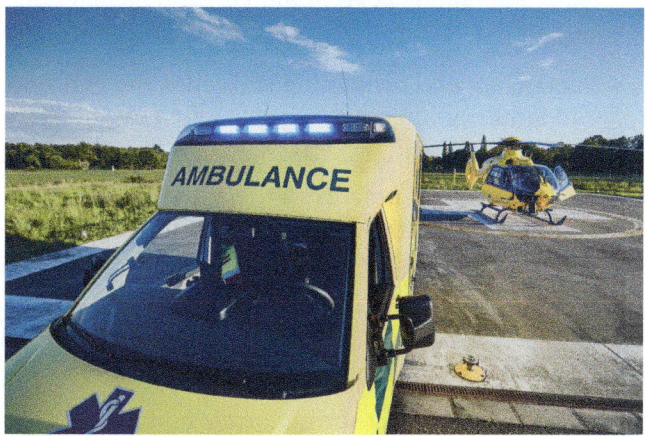

**Figure 1-18** Consider whether the patient requires air or ground transport.
© Jaromir Chalabala/Shutterstock.

and you are unable to establish an airway, it may be appropriate to transport to the closest available medical facility—even if that is a community hospital that does not specialize in pediatric patients. Local protocols and online medical direction can aid in making these decisions.

During the initial assessment and treatment of pediatric patients, it is appropriate for them to stay in the arms of their caregiver whenever possible. Once transport has been initiated, all ambulance occupants should be properly secured in their own seat. Parents should be informed that this is the safest means of transport, and pediatric patients should *never* be transported in the lap of a caregiver. An appropriately sized car seat or approved transport device should be utilized to properly secure the patient.

# Family-Centered Care

The principle of family-centered care is emphasized throughout the EPC course. Family-centered care is grounded in collaboration among patients, families and caregivers, physicians, nurses, and other healthcare professionals (**Figure 1-19**). The planning, delivery, and evaluation of the care provided to every pediatric patient relies on this collaboration. The collaborative relationship among these individuals is guided by the following principles:

- Respecting each child and their family

- Honoring racial, ethnic, cultural, and socioeconomic diversity encountered while caring for children and their families, and giving consideration to how these factors can influence the family's perception of the care they receive

- Recognizing and building on the strengths of each child and family, even in difficult and challenging situations

- Supporting and facilitating choice for the child and family about approaches to care and support

- Ensuring flexibility in organizational policies, procedures, and practices so services can be tailored to the needs, beliefs, and cultural values of each child and family

- Sharing honest and unbiased information with families on an ongoing basis and in ways they find useful and affirming

- Providing and/or ensuring formal and informal support (e.g., family-to-family support) for the child and parent(s) and/or guardian(s) during

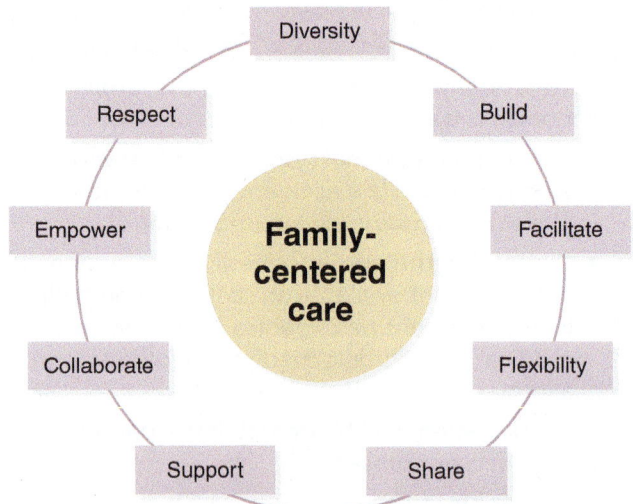

**Figure 1-19** Family-centered care is a critical component of all pediatric patient encounters.
© Jones & Bartlett Learning.

pregnancy, childbirth, infancy, childhood, adolescence, and young adulthood

- Collaborating with families at all levels of health care, in the care of the individual child and in professional education, policy making, and program development

- Empowering each child and family to discover their own strengths, build confidence, and make choices and decisions about their health

It is critical that all pediatric patients are considered within the context of their families. This is true whether the family members are blood relatives or other accustomed caregivers. Family members should be considered as part of the healthcare team.

The family can be included in multiple ways. Allowing a parent or caregiver to assist in providing care when appropriate is a highly effective approach to bringing them onto the healthcare team. Recognizing that caregivers are often knowledgeable about the condition of their child, and respecting their opinions, is another way to ensure that family members feel included. When possible, engage the family in shared decision making about the care being provided to the patient.

When family members are encouraged to work with the healthcare team, the effect is to prevent them from working *against* the healthcare team. Establishing trust and rapport with the family members of your pediatric patients is the first step toward initiating effective treatment and stabilization of the acutely ill or injured pediatric patient.

## LESSON WRAP-UP

There are many differences to be aware of when providing care to sick and injured children. Caring for critically ill and injured pediatric patients is a low-frequency, high-acuity event for prehospital practitioners. Familiarize yourself with the age-related differences in pediatric vital signs and assessment.

Practice forming a general impression using the Pediatric Assessment Triangle on every pediatric patient you see. The Pediatric Assessment Triangle is likely the single most important assessment tool that a prehospital practitioner can use to determine "quick" or "not quick." Being able to rapidly determine whether a pediatric patient is "quick" or "not quick" is a matter of life and death. Delaying transport for a critically ill or injured patient is likely to exacerbate the severity of their illness or injury. The key to rapid treatment and transport is rapid recognition.

Honesty and open communication are essential when treating pediatric patients and their families. Credibility and rapport must be established in order to communicate with all patients, regardless of age.

Building rapport with family members and encouraging them to participate in shared decision making when appropriate will improve healthcare delivery for all pediatric patients you encounter.

There are very few situations in which it is inappropriate to try and comfort a child by making them smile and laugh. A child's laughter is infectious and translates across all languages. You will often find that when a child laughs, it will bring a smile to everyone who hears it, including the parents and your teammates.

It is universal across all cultures to be compelled to instinctively help a child who is in distress. Caring for children who are critically ill or injured is about more than simply being an emergency prehospital practitioner, it is one of the core emotional responses that a human being possesses from birth. By participating in the EPC course, it is the hope of your instructors that you will be able to confidently and skillfully act on this most basic of human instincts—and save the life of a critically ill or injured child.

## REFERENCES

American Academy of Pediatrics, Committee on Pediatric Emergency Medicine; American College of Emergency Physicians, Pediatric Committee; Emergency Nurses Association, Pediatric Committee. Joint policy statement: guidelines for care of children in the emergency department. *J Emerg Nurs*. 2013;39(2):116-131.

Owusu-Ansah S, Moore B, Shah MI, et al.; Committee on Pediatric Emergency Medicine, Section On Emergency Medicine, EMS Subcommittee, Section on Surgery. Pediatric readiness in emergency medical services systems. *Pediatrics*. 2020;145(1):e20193308. doi:10.1542/peds.2019-3308

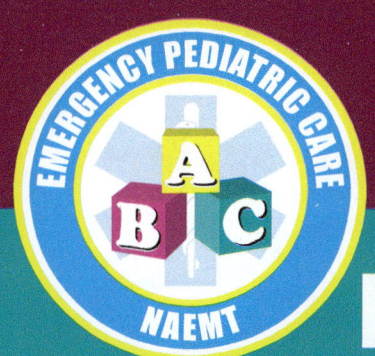

# CHAPTER 2

# Respiratory Emergencies

## LESSON OBJECTIVES

- Review the anatomy and physiology of the pediatric airway and ventilation.
- Differentiate between respiratory distress and failure in pediatrics.
- Discuss management of pediatric patients with respiratory emergencies using the Pediatric Assessment Triangle and XABCDE.
- Use the most appropriate pediatric airway management intervention based on the patient's assessment findings.

## Introduction

Respiratory emergencies are the most common medical emergency for children. When cardiac arrest is present, it is often preceded by respiratory distress and failure. Although respiratory emergencies are common throughout the entire year, they do demonstrate some seasonality. There is usually a respiratory season peak between the months of October and March in the Northern hemisphere.

## The Pediatric Respiratory System

An understanding of normal anatomy and physiology of the pediatric airway is necessary to assess and treat pediatric respiratory emergencies. Determining if the patient has pathology in the upper or lower airway can aid the prehospital practitioner in choosing what initial management may be effective. More important, it can aid in understanding what management may be ineffective, and valuable time can be saved for more effective treatments.

## Physiology

Several key physiologic differences exist between the adult and pediatric respiratory system. Children have significantly higher metabolic oxygen demand than adults. This increase in metabolic demand is most significant in newborns, and it decreases with age into adolescence, when it begins to mirror adult levels. Because of this increased metabolic oxygen demand, pediatric patients have reduced oxygen reserves, requiring them to recruit compensatory mechanisms sooner than adults.

To accommodate the increased metabolic oxygen requirement, pediatric patients must increase their minute ventilation. Minute ventilation is a function of inhaled tidal volume and respiratory rate. Because pediatric tidal volumes are comparatively lower than those seen in adults, respiratory rate is the primary mechanism used to increase minute ventilation. This means that when respiratory distress is present, many of the normal mechanisms used for compensation, such as increasing respiratory depth and rate, are already in use at baseline, and there is reduced capacity to compensate for extended periods. Respiratory distress in pediatric patients must be quickly identified and treated before compensatory mechanisms are exhausted.

Prior to age 6 months, infants are considered obligate nose breathers. This term is somewhat misleading, as neonates and infants are capable of breathing through their mouths when distressed; however, nasal breathing is the physiologic norm in this age group, and infants younger than 6 months who are seen breathing though their mouths are generally in respiratory distress.

**Minute Ventilation Equation**

$$V_E = V_T \times RR$$

$V_E$: **Minute ventilation**

$V_T$: **Tidal volume**

**RR: Respiration rate**

## Anatomy

The airway is divided into the upper and lower respiratory tracts, separated by the glottis (**Figure 2-1**). Both of these regions differ significantly from those of the adult airway.

The caliber of the upper airway in pediatric patients is smaller in comparison to adult airways, and even modest amounts of nasal congestion can cause significant respiratory distress due to increased airway resistance. In fact, reduction in airway size increases resistance to airflow by a factor of four. When nasal congestion is present, it can increase work of breathing significantly in pediatric patients.

The thoracic accessory breathing muscles are underdeveloped at birth. Newborns and infants rely heavily on the diaphragm for respiration and often appear to be belly breathing. Subcostal retractions in this patient population are highly concerning for this reason. This also affects their ability to adequately clear their airways. Mechanisms such as coughing and sneezing are generally ineffective when the thoracic and abdominal muscles cannot generate adequate force to produce thick secretions. As pediatric patients grow and develop, so do their thoracic accessory muscles. Around age 6 years, the musculature of the chest wall is developed to the point where accessory muscle use can be recruited for compensation when respiratory distress is present. These patients also have an increased ability to clear their own airways when secretions are present.

## Upper Airway

The upper airway includes all of the structures above the level of the glottis.

The nares of pediatric patients are smaller and more prone to obstruction due to congestion. Again, resistance is increased significantly as airway caliber is reduced due to constriction or congestion. The tongue is larger and the mandible is shorter in pediatric patients, making airway positioning and visualization during advanced airway maneuvers difficult. Thus, pediatric patients are much more susceptible to positional obstruction. The epiglottis is also larger and more "floppy" in pediatric patients, further complicating visualization

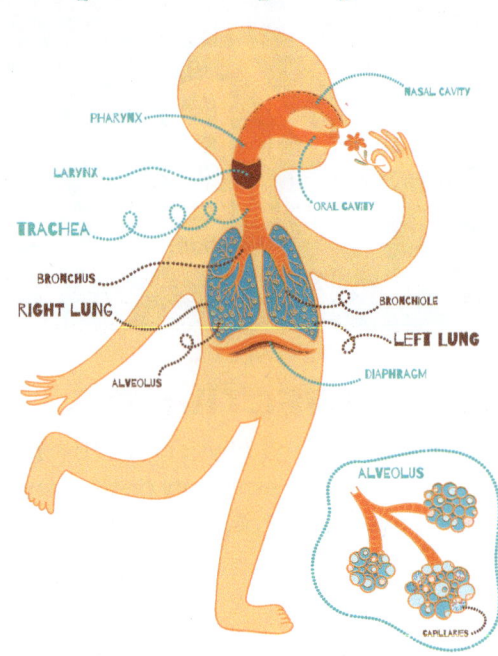

**Figure 2-1** The pediatric respiratory system.
© Shusha Guna/Shutterstock.

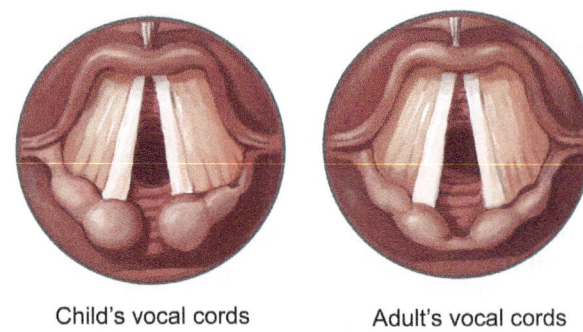

Child's vocal cords                    Adult's vocal cords

**Figure 2-2** Comparison of pediatric and adult vocal cords.
© Science History Images/Alamy Stock Photo.

of critical airway structures during advanced airway insertion (**Figure 2-2**).

The cartilage rings of the trachea are less rigid in children, resulting in narrowing when the airway is hyperextended, similar to how a straw or garden hose kinks when it is bent. This narrowing may be so profound that it can fully obstruct the upper airway. Careful attention to airway positioning is essential in pediatric patients. In addition, the cricoid ring is smaller and located more superiorly in pediatric patients. This increases the risk that an aspirated foreign body can cause critical airway narrowing and obstruction above the level of the carina, leading to loss of ventilation in both lungs.

**Table 2-1** Key Differences in Structures of the Pediatric Upper Respiratory Tract

| Nasal cavity | ■ Nares are smaller (increased resistance)<br>■ Obligate nose breathers younger than 6 months |
|---|---|
| Nasopharynx | ■ Prominent adenoids may cause obstruction |
| Tongue | ■ Proportionally larger and more likely to cause obstruction<br>■ More difficult to view structures critical for intubation |
| Mandible | ■ Proportionally shorter, making intubation more difficult |
| Oropharynx | ■ Prominent tonsils may cause obstruction<br>■ Tonsillar tissue more prone to infection and abscess |
| Epiglottis | ■ More "floppy" and difficult to control during intubation |
| Vocal cords | ■ Angle anterior-inferior to posterior-superior |

© Jones & Bartlett Learning.

**Table 2-1** describes critical anatomic considerations in the pediatric upper airway.

## Lower Airway

The lower airway includes all of the structures below the level of the glottis. The lower airways in pediatric patients are generally smaller, less rigid, and more prone to obstruction from secretions than the adult lower airway (**Figure 2-3**). Due to their underdeveloped accessory muscles, pediatric patients require deep suctioning when thick secretions are present.

The pediatric lower airway becomes more funnel shaped as it approaches the cricoid ring, which is located more superiorly than in adults. The cricoid ring causes the entry into the lower respiratory tract to be considerably narrower than that seen in adults. This creates an anatomic seal when endotracheal tubes are introduced and is one reason uncuffed tubes were used in the past for pediatric intubation. The most current guidelines recommend the use of cuffed endotracheal (ET) tubes when intubating infants and children. Local service and institution protocols should be followed.

### CUFFED VERSUS UNCUFFED ENDOTRACHEAL TUBES

Traditionally, uncuffed ET tubes were used in the pediatric population. The most current literature suggests that using cuffed ET tubes in infants and pediatric patients reduces the need for ET tube exchange and reintubation.

It is reasonable to choose cuffed over uncuffed ET tubes when intubating pediatric patients. Careful consideration should be given to size when using cuffed ET tubes.

# Assessing Severity of Respiratory Emergencies

Respiratory emergencies follow a progression of severity from distress to failure, ultimately leading to respiratory arrest. Identifying where the patient is on this continuum at any given point in time is critical so that proper interventions can be performed and further deterioration avoided. Proper use of the Pediatric Assessment Triangle (PAT), particularly the FRAP (flaring, retractions, audible sounds, positioning) mnemonic, to form an accurate general impression can be lifesaving (**Figure 2-4**). Deterioration from distress to failure and then arrest can happen rapidly and may be unexpected if the patient is not properly assessed throughout the encounter. The stages of progression from distress to failure often build upon each other. Identifying any progression is essential, and patients should be reassessed continuously.

## Respiratory Distress

Respiratory distress is a compensated respiratory emergency. The patient's overall appearance will often be normal, and their mental status will be intact because their brain is still receiving adequate oxygen.

Immediately on approaching the pediatric patient, use the FRAP mnemonic to assess the work of breathing by looking for nasal flaring and retractions, listening for audible breath sounds, and determining positioning. It is important to also complete the PAT and quickly assess for the presence of circulatory compromise. Circulatory compromise may be the primary cause of respiratory distress in some patients. Alternatively, some patients with significant respiratory

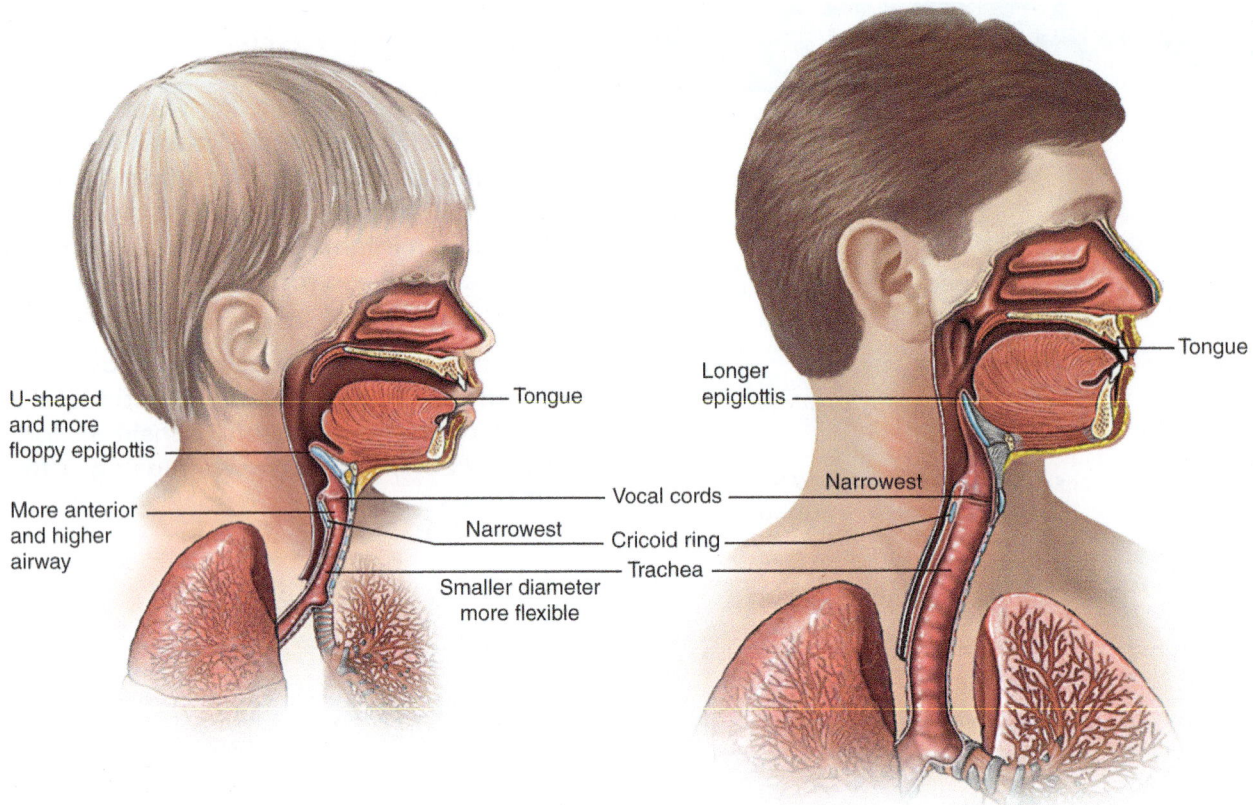

**Figure 2-3** Comparison of pediatric to adult respiratory tract.

© Jones & Barlett Learning.

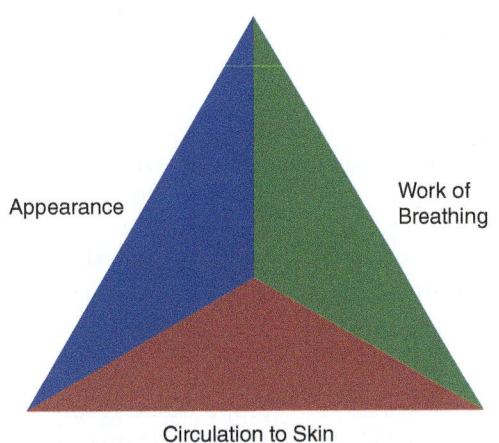

**Figure 2-4** Pediatric Assessment Triangle.

Used with permission of the American Academy of Pediatrics, Pediatric Education for Prehospital Professionals, © American Academy of Pediatrics, 2000.

compromise may overwhelm their circulatory compensatory mechanisms, and respiratory emergencies can then lead to circulatory collapse.

In patients with significant lower airway obstruction, such as asthma, hyperinflation can occur. The patient will be able to generate enough negative pressure to draw air into the lower airways; however, the swelling and congestion present in these airways prevents complete exhalation prior to the initiation of the next breath. This hyperinflation can lead to compression of the heart and great vessels in the mediastinum and reduce right-sided preload to the heart. This causes significant cardiac strain and can progress to circulatory collapse if not managed carefully.

The primary survey of a patient with respiratory distress will typically reveal tachypnea, abnormal airway sounds, and tachycardia. Obtain a full set of vital signs as soon as practical, including pulse oximetry, blood pressure, and temperature.

## Respiratory Failure

Patients who have exhausted their ability to compensate will progress to respiratory failure. Initially, these patients may be acutely agitated and unreasonable as they are air hungry and becoming progressively more hypoxic. They may not tolerate supplemental oxygen devices on or near their face. This agitation will deteriorate to a decreased level of consciousness if the hypoxia is not corrected, and their general appearance will be concerning when the Pediatric Assessment Triangle is evaluated. The patients will often be obtunded in late respiratory failure.

**Table 2-2** Respiratory Distress, Failure, and Arrest

| | Respiratory Distress | Respiratory Failure | Respiratory Arrest |
|---|---|---|---|
| **Respiratory rate** | Tachypnea | Tachypnea or bradypnea | Apnea |
| **Work of breathing** | Inadequate respiratory effort; nasal flaring, accessory muscle use | Increased or decreased respiratory effort | No respiratory effort |
| **Adventitial breath sounds** | Abnormal airway sounds; grunting, stridor | Abnormal airway sounds; grunting, stridor, wheezing, crackles, diminished air movement | No air movement |
| **Cardiovascular changes** | Tachycardia | Heart rate reduces as they become increasingly hypoxic; cyanosis, mottling | Bradycardia; cardiopulmonary arrest |
| **Mental status** | Normal | Decreased level of consciousness | Comatose |

© Jones & Bartlett Learning.

The overall work of breathing in patients with respiratory failure may be significantly increased in early failure and will quickly deteriorate if left untreated. These patients may become bradypneic with decreased respiratory effort as they progress toward respiratory arrest. Abnormal breath sounds will only be present if there is sufficient respiratory effort to generate these sounds. In cases of severe asthma or lower airway congestion, the lower airways may be so constricted or clogged with secretions that the chest will become silent even though the patient is trying to generate air movement. The silent chest, combined with significantly increased work of breathing, is an ominous sign and portends impending respiratory arrest.

As the patient becomes progressively more hypoxic, tachycardia will transition to bradycardia. The distal extremities may be cyanotic. This cyanosis will progress toward the core as respiratory failure becomes more severe. Peripheral vasoconstriction will proceed in an effort to perfuse vital organs, and mottling may be observed.

## Respiratory Arrest

Respiratory arrest will occur if respiratory failure is allowed to persist without intervention. Respiratory arrest is signified by inadequate or absent respiratory effort. The patient may be apneic or have agonal respirations. There will be completely insufficient work of breathing and breath sounds will be absent. The patient's level of consciousness will progress from obtunded to comatose as their brain is deprived of oxygen. Bradycardia will progress to dysrhythmias such as ventricular tachycardia or fibrillation, and ultimately to asystole. Circulatory collapse and cardiac arrest will ensue. The signs of respiratory distress, respiratory failure, and respiratory arrest are shown in **Table 2-2**.

# Classification of Respiratory Emergencies by Etiology

Classification of the respiratory emergency based on the most likely etiology can aid in knowing what initial interventions are most likely to be effective. When airway obstruction is present, the prehospital practitioner must determine if it is in the upper or lower airway. A thorough history will help determine if the patient has contracted an illness directly affecting the lung tissues. In some cases, a patient experiencing a respiratory emergency may have healthy lung tissues and airways; however, they are not breathing normally due to a disorder affecting the neurologic control of breathing. **Table 2-3** lists the major classifications of respiratory emergencies and the common causes of each.

## Upper Respiratory Emergencies

Upper respiratory emergencies are caused by direct blockage or dysfunction of the airway structures above the level of the glottis. Common causes of upper respiratory emergencies are listed in Table 2-3. Differentiating between infectious and obstructive causes is critical because they have different treatments.

**Table 2-3** Common Pediatric Respiratory Emergencies

| | | |
|---|---|---|
| Upper airway emergencies | Upper airway obstruction | ▪ Foreign body airway obstruction<br>▪ Anaphylaxis (angioedema) |
| | Upper airway infection | ▪ Croup<br>▪ Epiglottitis<br>▪ Retropharyngeal abscess<br>▪ Bacterial tracheitis |
| Lower airway emergencies | Lower airway obstruction | ▪ Asthma<br>▪ Reactive airway disease<br>▪ Anaphylaxis (bronchoconstriction) |
| | Lower airway infection or disease | ▪ Pneumonia<br>▪ Bronchiolitis<br>▪ Pertussis |
| Disordered control of breathing<br>(no airway disease present) | | ▪ Seizure<br>▪ Head injury<br>▪ Metabolic disorder (diabetic ketoacidosis)<br>▪ Toxicologic insult (ingestion, overdose)<br>▪ Excessive sedation (iatrogenic) |

© Jones & Bartlett Learning.

In many cases the history will be the biggest guide for management decisions.

## Upper Airway Obstruction

The major causes of upper airway obstruction are foreign body ingestion and airway narrowing due to anaphylaxis or infection. It is important to know what age groups are susceptible to choking and the major signs and symptoms of anaphylaxis to help differentiate the cause. In either case, patients with upper airway obstruction can quickly deteriorate into a "can't ventilate, can't oxygenate" scenario, and rapid recognition and treatment is essential.

### Foreign Body Airway Obstruction (FBAO)

Airway obstruction due to foreign body inhalation remains a leading cause of death in pediatric patients, particularly those between the ages of 1 and 3 years. This is primarily due to the developmental vulnerabilities present in that age range. As these patients begin to gain independence and explore the world, they tend to examine objects with their mouth. Patients who are teething may chew on objects for soothing purposes. Oral motor development and learning to safely eat a wider variety of solid foods also pose choking hazards to patients in this age range. As patients grow beyond 3 years old, their risk of choking decreases, but is not eliminated completely. Unintentional choking while eating or when objects are placed into the mouth continues to pose a hazard into adolescence.

Foods such as grapes, hot dog pieces, nuts, and hard candies are the ideal size to seat into the airway of pediatric patients and cause upper airway obstruction. Toys also pose a major hazard and balloons may be unintentionally inhaled into the airway, often with fatal consequences.

In some cases, the parent or caregiver will directly observe the onset of the child's choking episode while eating or playing and summon help immediately. It is more common, however, for parents to have their back turned or be otherwise preoccupied and note a sudden coughing, gagging, or choking sound coming from the patient. Inspiratory stridor may also be present along with respiratory distress, failure, or arrest.

When the patient is in a high-risk age range (1–3 years old), the onset of respiratory distress is sudden, and there is no fever or other sign of infection, it is reasonable to have a high index of suspicion for FBAO. Immediate treatment is necessary. If the patient can breathe, cry or speak, they have an incomplete obstruction. Assist them to a position of comfort and avoid agitation if possible. Agitation can lead to them unseating the object or inhaling it further into the airway. No FBAO maneuvers are necessary in this case, and rapid transport should be initiated to the closest appropriate facility. A pediatric tertiary care center with pediatric otolaryngology (ENT) and anesthesia support available is ideal.

If the patient is in respiratory failure or arrest, then FBAO maneuvers to remove or partially relieve the obstruction are necessary. In the conscious pediatric patient, provide abdominal thrusts per basic life support (BLS) guidelines. If the patient becomes unconscious, proceed to cardiopulmonary resuscitation (CPR). The only modification to CPR in the case of choking is that the airway should be quickly visually inspected before each set of breaths and any *visible* foreign body should be removed. Conscious infants are managed with alternating sets of five back blows between the shoulder blades followed by five chest thrusts similar in technique to CPR. If the infant becomes unconscious, proceed with CPR per BLS guidelines.

> **Never do blind finger sweeps in patients suspected of having an FBAO. This action is likely to seat the object farther in the airway. Only perform a finger sweep and attempt to remove an object if you can directly visualize it.**

For prehospital practitioners certified in advanced life support (ALS), visualization with laryngoscopy and removal of the object using Magill forceps may be appropriate, if allowed by local protocol. Care should be exercised not to traumatize the upper airway tissues during visualization and removal of a foreign object. Tissues in this region are highly vascularized, and any trauma is likely to cause significant bleeding, which may further complicate airway management strategies.

### Anaphylaxis

Anaphylaxis is a sudden onset, systemic disease process caused by the release of inflammatory mediators from cells within specific body tissues. Anaphylaxis can manifest with symptoms in multiple organ systems, including the respiratory, gastrointestinal, and circulatory tissues.

Anaphylaxis is most often the result of an exposure to a specific trigger. These triggers often include foods, medications, and insect bites or stings. It is common for individuals who experience anaphylaxis to have been previously exposed to the trigger in question without experiencing systemic effects. In some cases, they may have had extensive exposure to certain triggers, only to develop a serious reaction without warning. It is estimated that 37% to 85% of anaphylaxis is triggered by exposure to foods. **Table 2-4** lists common triggers.

Anaphylaxis should be suspected in patients with sudden onset of respiratory distress in proximity to exposure from a known trigger. When there is no known or suspected exposure, additional clues that anaphylaxis might be present include swelling of the lips and tongue (angioedema), tightness in the chest, inspiratory stridor, wheezing, nausea, vomiting, diarrhea, abdominal pain, tachycardia, and tachypnea.

The release of inflammatory mediators from mast cells and basophils can cause many symptoms, including

| **Table 2-4** Common Anaphylaxis Triggers | |
|---|---|
| Food and food additives | ▪ Peanuts |
| | ▪ Tree nuts |
| | ▪ Seeds |
| | ▪ Milk |
| | ▪ Eggs |
| | ▪ Shellfish |
| | ▪ Food coloring agents |
| Insects stings and bites | ▪ Ants |
| | ▪ Wasps |
| | ▪ Bees |
| Environmental | ▪ Natural rubber and latex |
| | ▪ Domestic animal dander (cat or dog) |
| Medications | ▪ Antibiotics (particularly sulfa and penicillin agents) |
| | ▪ Chemotherapy agents |
| | ▪ Monoclonal antibody therapeutic agents |

© Jones & Bartlett Learning.

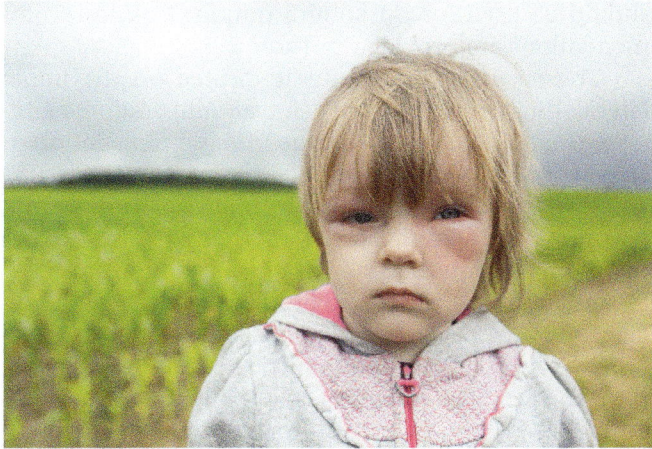

**Figure 2-5** A pediatric patient experiencing an allergic reaction.
© Vadim Ratnikov/Shutterstock.

hives, urticaria, pruritis, and swelling (**Figure 2-5**). These can also be clues that the patient is suffering from an allergic reaction with anaphylaxis.

When anaphylaxis is left untreated, it can proceed to respiratory failure and arrest. The same inflammatory mediators that cause airway compromise can also

**Table 2-5** Epinephrine Dosing for the Treatment of Anaphylaxis (Intramuscular Injection)

| Weight | Rapid Dosing or Autoinjector | Calculated Dosage |
|---|---|---|
| <10 kg (infants) | Rapid dosing and the use of autoinjectors not recommended in patients less than 10 kg | 0.01 mg/kg (0.01 mL/kg of 1 mg/mL concentration epinephrine) |
| 10 to 25 kg (infants and children) | 0.15 mg via autoinjector or drawn up into syringe | |
| >25 to 50 kg | 0.3 mg via autoinjector or drawn up into syringe | |
| >50 kg | 0.5 mg drawn up into syringe | Maximum single dose is 0.5 mg |

- Epinephrine concentration should be 1 mg/mL or 1:1,000.
- Maximum single dose is 0.5 mg
- Doses may be repeated at 5- to 15-minute intervals if clinically indicated.
- Autoinjectors are only available in 0.1 mg, 0.15 mg, and 0.3 mg prefilled syringes.

© Jones & Bartlett Learning.

cause circulatory collapse and lead to anaphylactic shock, a specific form of distributive shock. Anaphylaxis is discussed further in Lesson 4, *Shock*.

The immediate goal when treating anaphylaxis is to stop the progression of the allergic reaction. Intramuscular epinephrine should be administered without delay. This may be administered from an appropriately sized autoinjector or drawn up from a vial into a syringe. Epinephrine with a concentration of 1:1,000 should be used for IM administration. Dosing recommendations are provided in **Table 2-5**.

The vastus lateralis muscle located on the upper lateral thigh region is ideal for administration of intramuscular (IM) epinephrine. IM administration is considered more rapid and safer than intravenous (IV) administration due to reduced incidence of cardiac complications. IM administration also has better and more rapid distribution than subcutaneous administration.

In addition to IM epinephrine, supplemental oxygen should be provided if patients have evidence of hypoxia. Inhaled beta agonists such as albuterol can aid in relieving lower airway obstruction due to bronchoconstriction. Oral or IV corticosteroids such as methylprednisolone or prednisone can be administered to help mitigate prolonged inflammatory effects, but these will take 4 to 6 hours for the full effect to be seen and should not be used as first-line treatment in anaphylaxis with respiratory distress. Diphenhydramine or an oral $H_2$ blocker such as famotidine can aid in relieving hives and itching; however, these agents will not relieve acute airway swelling and should not be used as first-line treatment for respiratory distress.

See **Table 2-6** for a summary of anaphylaxis treatment.

**Table 2-6** Anaphylaxis Treatment Summary

| Agent | Effects |
|---|---|
| Epinephrine (intramuscular) | - Slows or stops progression of anaphylactic reaction<br>- Mitigates angioedema that causes upper airway swelling<br>- Relieves lower airway bronchoconstriction<br>- Causes peripheral vasoconstriction and reduces distributive hypoperfusion |
| Oxygen | - Mitigates hypoxia |
| Inhaled beta agonists | - Relieve bronchoconstriction in lower airways and reverse lower airway obstruction |
| Glucocorticoids | - Reduce systemic inflammation and mitigate inflammatory mediators released from mast cells and basophils |
| Histamine blockers ($H_1$ and $H_2$) | - Can aid in reducing itching and hives |

© Jones & Bartlett Learning.

## Upper Airway Infection

Upper airway infections are common in pediatric patients. Most children younger than 6 years will experience 6 to 8 "colds" per year, lasting approximately 14 days each. Viral illnesses account for many of these respiratory infections. As children grow older, the frequency and duration of cold symptoms decreases. While most these upper respiratory infections do not result in serious illness, occasionally they will become severe enough to warrant emergency medical evaluation and treatment.

### Croup

Croup is a narrowing of the upper airway caused by a respiratory infection (**Figure 2-6**). It is the most common infectious cause of upper airway obstruction in children aged 6 months to 6 years, and the majority of cases are caused by the parainfluenza virus. Croup may also be called laryngotracheobronchitis.

The most common sign of croup is a barking cough ("seal bark"), which may be accompanied by inspiratory stridor and fever. Hoarseness, decreased oral intake due to throat pain, tachypnea, and respiratory distress may be present, particularly when the patient is agitated. The signs and symptoms of croup are often exacerbated at night after the patient has gone to sleep. In some cases, once the patient has calmed, the symptoms may be largely improved by the time emergency medical services (EMS) arrives or the patient has arrived in the emergency department (ED). While an x-ray of the neck is not required for diagnosis of croup, if one is obtained, the classic "steeple sign" may be present, indicating significant narrowing of the upper airway (**Figure 2-7**). Croup is a clinical diagnosis that can be made by obtaining an accurate history and performing a thorough physical exam. No ancillary diagnostic testing is necessary as long as there is no concern for other causes present.

An accurate physical exam is critical in patients with possible croup. When inspiratory stridor is heard, it is important to remember that it likely represents narrowing of the upper airway. Inhaled beta agonists such as albuterol are *not* appropriate for the treatment of upper airway constriction and will likely only agitate the patient further, delay proper therapy, and increase tachycardia due to sympathomimetic effects.

Treatment for croup is largely supportive in nature. There is no curative treatment for croup, and the condition will resolve once the body has fought and cleared the virus. Initial treatment involves keeping the patient calm and avoiding unnecessary agitation. Vascular access should only be obtained if absolutely necessary as it can significantly increase agitation and push the patient from respiratory distress into respiratory failure or arrest.

Initial treatment for moderate to severe croup includes the use of nebulized epinephrine as a first-line agent to reduce respiratory distress. Nebulized epinephrine will decrease the irritation, swelling, and edema present in the upper airway tissues, thereby reducing upper airway resistance. Supplemental oxygen to maintain $SpO_2$ >94% can be administered as necessary.

Once respiratory distress has been treated with nebulized epinephrine and supplemental oxygen, IV

# Croup

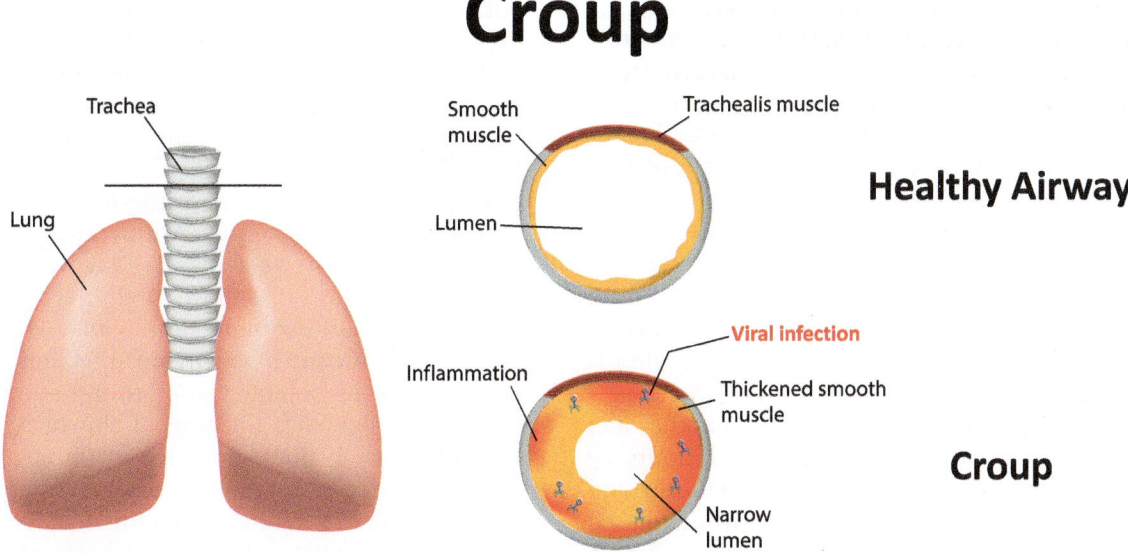

**Figure 2-6** The respiratory infection that leads to croup causes the upper airway to narrow significantly.

© joshya/Shutterstock.

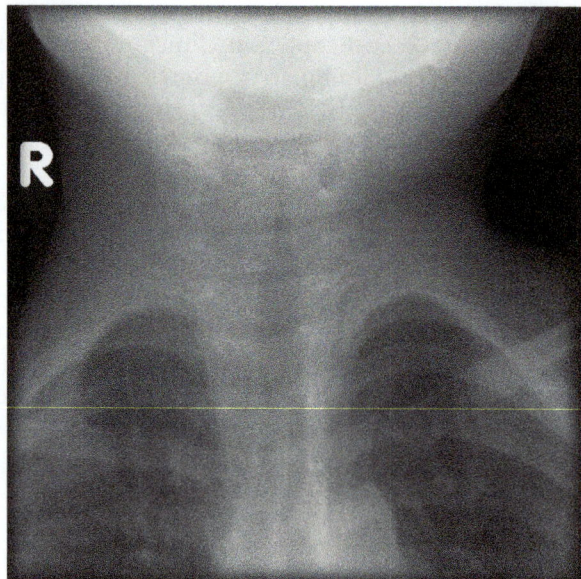

**Figure 2-7** Significant narrowing of the airway in patients with croup leads to the classic "steeple sign."

Case courtesy of Dr Michael Sargent, Radiopaedia.org, rID: 6086

## NEBULIZED EPINEPHRINE

Nebulized epinephrine comes in two forms: racemic epinephrine and L-epinephrine. Racemic epinephrine contains equal amounts of the D and L isomers of the epinephrine molecule. L-epinephrine is a mixture made of the L isomer exclusively. The decision regarding which mixture to use will be guided by local protocol and availability at your institution or service. Each mixture has similar clinical efficacy; however, dosing varies depending on which form is used.

or oral corticosteroids may be necessary to prevent the patient from relapsing. Dexamethasone is a steroid with an approximate duration of action of 48 to 72 hours. It may be administered IV, IM, or orally. It is often preferred in croup as it can be given as a single administration, and the virus is often cleared after 2 or 3 days. Prednisolone is an alternative to dexamethasone; however, it must be administered every 12 hours by mouth. Both steroids have similar clinical efficacy and the decision regarding which one to use will be based largely on local protocols.

Croup with impending respiratory failure should be considered an airway emergency, and these patients may deteriorate rapidly. Manage respiratory failure as you would normally, realizing that intubation would be extremely difficult due to significant airway swelling and edema. Intubation should be avoided if possible, and the most experienced practitioner should be the one to attempt any advanced airway maneuvers. Rapid transport to the nearest appropriate facility should proceed without delay. A pediatric tertiary care facility with anesthesia and ENT available is preferred.

## Retropharyngeal Abscess

The retropharyngeal space extends from the base of the skull to the posterior mediastinum. Infections in this area are dangerous for multiple reasons, including airway compromise due to swelling and inflammation, and extension of the infection into the mediastinum, leading to further cardiopulmonary compromise. The lymph nodes that drain the retropharyngeal space are more prominent in pediatric patients and begin to atrophy prior to puberty.

Retropharyngeal abscess is most commonly caused by a bacterial upper respiratory infection that has progressed to suppurative adenitis of one or more of the retropharyngeal lymph nodes. Dental procedures and traumatic intubation attempts can also lead to infection of the retropharyngeal space.

Patients with retropharyngeal abscess will typically have an ill or toxic appearance with fever. Drooling will often be present as swallowing can be very painful, and children will have poor control over their upper airway secretions. Due to the inflammation and swelling of the deep neck spaces, patients will often not want to move their neck. Palpation of the neck may reveal an area of significant tenderness. A muffled "hot potato" voice may be present due to pain and swelling of the upper airway structures. Chest pain may be present if there is extension of the infection into the mediastinum.

Treatment of retropharyngeal abscess in the prehospital environment involves close monitoring of airway status and avoiding unnecessary interventions that may lead to agitation. Antipyretics to reduce fever and provide some analgesia may be helpful if the patient is willing to swallow. Definitive treatment involves a course of systemic antibiotics. These patients are at high risk for bloodstream infection; blood cultures should be obtained prior to initiation of antibiotics when possible. Imaging of the neck should be performed to evaluate for airway impingement and assess the need for additional airway management. Advanced airway maneuvers should be performed at an institution with pediatric anesthesia and otolaryngology support whenever possible due to the critical nature of these airways.

## Epiglottitis

Epiglottitis is an upper airway infection specifically of the epiglottis and surrounding structures. This infection leads to severe edema and swelling of the epiglottic tissue and can progress to life-threatening upper airway obstruction if left untreated.

The signs and symptoms of epiglottitis are similar to retropharyngeal abscess and include respiratory distress, difficulty swallowing, drooling, stridor, decreased oral intake, fever, and toxic appearance. Patients will often assume a tripod or sniffing position with extension of the neck in an effort to take pressure off the epiglottis and reduce throat pain. This also maximizes the diameter of the upper airway and reduces inspiratory resistance. The "three Ds" of epiglottitis have commonly been described as dysphagia, drooling, and distress. These children are often toxic appearing.

Differentiation between epiglottitis and retropharyngeal abscess is difficult without imaging and often not clinically important in the prehospital setting as the same initial treatment can be safely applied to both. Retropharyngeal abscess signs and symptoms usually progress more slowly than epiglottitis. History that reveals absent or incomplete vaccination or unknown vaccination status should raise suspicion for epiglottitis, especially in patients younger than 6 years, for whom prevalence is highest. Additional risk factors include patients who are immunocompromised. Patients with asplenia or sickle cell disease have a higher risk of infection from encapsulated bacteria, including Hib.

The primary treatment for epiglottitis is reducing agitation and keeping the patient calm so as not to increase airway irritation. IV access should be obtained only if necessary, and these patients should be kept with a caregiver for comfort as much as possible. Nebulized epinephrine can help reduce swelling of the upper airway structures and may decrease airway resistance if tolerated by the patient. If these patients experience rapid deterioration in their respiratory status, airway management will be difficult due to the swelling and edema present in the upper airway structures. Rapid transport to a pediatric tertiary care center with pediatric anesthesia and ENT available is recommended.

## Bacterial Tracheitis

Bacterial tracheitis is an exudative infection of the tracheal tissues. In some cases, extension into the structures of the larynx and mainstem bronchi may be seen. It is often preceded by a viral infection, which leaves the tissues of the trachea susceptible to invasive infection by the normal flora that colonize the upper respiratory tract. Bacterial tracheitis can also be seen in patients who have a tracheostomy tube or who have been intubated for a prolonged period without adequate pulmonary toilet regimens. It is most commonly seen in the first 6 years of life; however, it may be seen in older children if predisposing factors such as airway placement or immunodeficiency exist.

The signs and symptoms of bacterial tracheitis are similar to other upper airway obstructive pathologies caused by infection. These signs include fever, stridor, respiratory distress, cough with exudative secretions, and hoarseness. In contrast to other upper airway infections discussed, drooling is less commonly seen with bacterial tracheitis as the tissues involved in swallowing are generally not infected and there is little discomfort associated with oral intake.

Prehospital treatment is largely supportive in nature. Oxygen and respiratory support should be provided for comfort if the patient will tolerate these interventions. Assessment should be performed to determine if advanced airway placement is necessary. As with all upper airway obstructions, airway management will likely be difficult and should be deferred to specialists whenever possible. Long-term management for bacterial tracheitis includes antibiotic therapy.

# Lower Respiratory Emergencies

When there is obstruction, infection, or dysfunction below the level of the glottis, the patient is considered to have a lower respiratory emergency. Effective assessment of work of breathing and breath sounds combined with a thorough history of the present illness can help the prehospital practitioner localize the cause of the respiratory emergency to the lower airway. Accurate localization of the respiratory emergency is important as there are medications and therapies that work well in the upper airway, yet these same therapies have little effect in the lower airway, and vice versa.

## Lower Airway Obstruction

Lower airway obstruction is caused by physical or anatomic blockage of the lower airways. The most common causes of lower airway obstruction are inflammation and bronchoconstriction caused by asthma. Other potential causes of lower airway obstruction are included in Table 2-3.

Lower airway obstruction is most often treated with agents and medications that relieve bronchoconstriction and reduce inflammation. When the cause is physical obstruction of the lower airway by an inhaled foreign object, the focus should be on airway optimization and rapid transport, as prehospital interventions are limited in these scenarios.

## Asthma

Asthma is one of the most common diseases of childhood requiring emergency care. It is the most common chronic medical condition in pediatric patients. It is estimated that 7.5% of pediatric patients currently carry a diagnosis of asthma, with the most significant disease burden seen in patients ages 12 to 17 years. While adolescents represent the highest percentage of pediatric patients with asthma, the most significant mortality is seen in Black males between the ages of 5 and 11. Socioeconomic status and access to adequate healthcare resources contribute significantly to the level of asthma control.

The pathophysiology of asthma is complex. The lower airway obstruction is caused by inflammation and bronchoconstriction, both of which are mediated by inflammatory mediators released by cells in the body in response to a trigger. Triggers are often environmental; however, other conditions such as viral illness, exercise, and stress can lead to the systemic response that precipitates an asthma attack.

Once the body has been triggered, the lower airways become inflamed and increased mucus production may be present. Additionally, the smooth muscle around the bronchi will constrict in a process known as bronchoconstriction. This sets up a process of progressive hyperinflation as air is drawn into the lungs, but due to obstruction of the lower airways caused by bronchoconstriction and inflammation, exhalation is more difficult. In response to this, patients will increase their respiratory rate to maintain adequate minute ventilation, further decreasing expiratory time and exacerbating the hyperinflation state. Hypercarbia and hypoxia ensue.

Early assessment of patients experiencing an asthma exacerbation will often reveal the classic elements of respiratory distress discussed in the Pediatric Assessment Triangle. Tachypnea, significant accessory muscle use, tripod positioning, and altered level of consciousness may be present. Auscultation of the lung fields may demonstrate expiratory wheezing early in the disease course; however, wheezing may be biphasic (present on inhalation and exhalation) or even absent (silent chest) later in disease progression. When lower airway obstruction has progressed to the point that the patient is refractory to initial therapies and respiratory failure has set in, the patient is experiencing an acute *severe* asthma attack, otherwise known as status asthmaticus.

Recognition of the asthma exacerbation is a critical step in management. Spending time chasing an incorrect alternative diagnosis may prove fatal for the patient if proper treatment is delayed. The patient should be given an inhaled bronchodilator such as albuterol immediately if lower airway obstruction secondary to asthma exacerbation is suspected. Bronchodilators may be mixed with inhaled anticholinergic medications such as ipratropium to relieve bronchoconstriction and aid in reducing lower airway congestion. Epinephrine may also be injected intramuscularly in severe exacerbations. Magnesium sulfate, a smooth muscle relaxant, has been shown to relieve bronchoconstriction in status asthmaticus. Intravenous corticosteroids should be administered early in the course of the disease; however, these are not fast acting, and will only aid in reducing inflammation approximately 4 to 6 hours after administration. It is important to administer corticosteroids early to treat refractory disease; however, prehospital practitioners should be aware that they do not treat acute bronchospasm.

Patients who are hypoxic should be provided with supplemental oxygen as needed to maintain appropriate oxygen saturations. Noninvasive respiratory support such as CPAP, BPAP, and high-flow nasal cannula (HFNC) may be used in appropriate situations to help with work of breathing. Practitioners should be aware that adding positive airway pressure to the acutely decompensating asthmatic may exacerbate the obstructive process and worsen disease if the bronchoconstriction has not been addressed appropriately.

## Reactive Airway Disease

Reactive airway disease is a common cause of lower airway obstruction in pediatric patients. The pathophysiology is identical to asthma, and the term *reactive airway disease* is often used to describe the patient's condition when they do not yet have a diagnosis of asthma, such as in young children, or when it is the patient's first or second episode of wheezing. Reactive airway disease should be treated in similar fashion to asthma, and the main point of identifying it as a stand-alone disease process in this text is to aid the reader in becoming familiar with terminology in case they encounter it clinically in the future. When taking a patient history, if the parents describe that the patient has been treated for reactive airway disease in the past, consider this in the same clinical context as you would asthma and act appropriately.

## Lower Airway Infection

Infections that occur in the lower airway are a significant cause of respiratory distress in pediatric patients. Although definitive treatment and recovery from the infection is curative, these patients often require respiratory support as they recover from whatever infection they have acquired. The airway inflammation, congestion, and in some cases constriction that result from the infection are the major causes of the respiratory distress. When these causative factors are mitigated, the patient's respiratory distress will often resolve and the infection can be managed appropriately.

## Bronchiolitis

Bronchiolitis is a condition in infants and children in which inflammation and congestion occur in the small lower airways (bronchioles), typically in response to a viral respiratory illness. The most common age group affected by this disease process is children younger than 24 months. Typically, children with bronchiolitis have viral upper respiratory symptoms initially, including congestion, cough, rhinorrhea, and fever. The viral process generally peaks on or around days 3 to 5, and lower airway involvement may be noticed during this time. Severity, prognosis, and recovery time are closely linked with age at time of onset. Infants younger than 6 months tend to have more severe disease and the course is generally more prolonged.

The list of viruses that can cause bronchiolitis is long; however, respiratory syncytial virus is the most common pathogen associated with this disease process. Other common causes include rhinovirus, parainfluenza, human metapneumovirus, influenza, and adenovirus.

Patients who become infected with one of the previously mentioned respiratory viruses will initially have upper respiratory symptoms. As the disease progresses, the epithelial cells of the lower airway become involved, and significant inflammation and congestion of the lower airways occurs. In children older than 2 years, airway clearance mechanisms such as coughing and sneezing, combined with anatomically larger airways due to normal growth and development, result in a condition that is generally self-limited and does not require medical intervention. Children younger than 2 years have smaller airways that are more prone to obstruction from congestion. Airway clearance in children younger than 2 years is generally poor and thick secretions are often present in bronchiolitis, setting up a situation in which significant respiratory distress can develop. Infants will often not be able to tolerate feeding due to significant nasal congestion and the inability to breathe through the nose to coordinate the suck, swallow, breathe cycle. They may become dehydrated due to low oral intake and increased insensible losses from tachypnea and fever.

Treatment for bronchiolitis largely involves supportive care. Aggressive suctioning of the upper airway is often necessary to clear the nares and allow for breathing through the nose. A few drops of saline into the nares prior to suctioning can aid in loosening thick secretions and make them easier to remove. While bulb suctioning may be effective, suctioning with a mechanical device may be required. Oxygen should be provided to maintain appropriate oxygen saturation when necessary. Oxygen should be humidified when possible, as nonhumidified oxygen will often dry secretions and cause them to be thicker and more difficult to clear. Routine use of hypertonic saline nebulizer treatments outside of the hospital setting is not recommended and may cause bronchospasm. The use of inhaled bronchodilators is generally not effective in patients with bronchiolitis. In situations where the practitioner is unsure whether the patient is experiencing an acute exacerbation of asthma, reactive airway disease with a viral trigger, or bronchiolitis, a trial of inhaled bronchodilator medication such as albuterol is not unreasonable while other interventions such as nasal suctioning and respiratory support are initiated in a synchronous fashion. When patients are highly responsive to bronchodilator therapy and show significant improvement after administration, it is likely that they are not experiencing bronchiolitis and are having an acute exacerbation of asthma or reactive airway disease. It should be noted, however, that the routine use of bronchodilators in patients with known bronchiolitis or instances when acute bronchospasm is not suspected is not recommended.

The use of high-flow nasal cannula devices, sometimes abbreviated as HFNC or HHBNC (heated, humidified blended nasal cannula) has become increasingly popular in the past few years as an adjunctive treatment to support respiratory effort and decrease work of breathing as patients recover from bronchiolitis. These devices use a modified nasal cannula system to deliver a titratable flow and oxygen concentration that can be adjusted to meet the individual patient's needs. The air that is delivered is heated and humidified, which aids in preventing obstruction due to thick, dry secretions. Increasing flow can be used to relieve some of the work of breathing that patients experience. Flow rates are generally adjusted between 1 and 2 L/kg of bodyweight, and the fraction of inspired oxygen ($FiO_2$) is adjusted as necessary to maintain desired oxygen saturation. The maximum flow rate, which varies by device and manufacturer, is generally around 40 L/min. Increasingly, these devices are being employed in the prehospital environment and may be available depending on the equipment and capabilities of the local EMS agencies. When patients exceed 2 L/kg of flow or 60% $FiO_2$, escalation to a more aggressive noninvasive respiratory support method such as CPAP or BiPAP is necessary. Patients who fail noninvasive support will have to be managed with invasive methods such as intubation.

## Pneumonia

When infection extends beyond the airways and involves the actual lung tissue (parenchyma), it is considered to be pneumonia (**Figure 2-8**). Pneumonia can be viral or bacterial. Pneumonia is the leading cause of death in pediatric patients younger than 5 years, with most deaths occurring in developing countries.

Patients with pneumonia will often have significant respiratory distress and hypoxia. Because pneumonia is caused by an infectious agent, fever will often be present, and the clinical progression of disease has likely been evolving over the previous 24 to 72 hours before the patient requires emergency care. In addition to the expected signs of respiratory distress, patients may also describe chest pain and significant tachycardia. On physical examination, crackles may be auscultated over the involved lung lobe, particularly in bacterial pneumonia. Viral pneumonias are often more diffuse, and crackles or coarse lung sounds may be heard throughout the chest.

Treatment for pneumonia is largely supportive in the prehospital environment. Supplemental oxygen should be provided to maintain appropriate oxygen saturation (94% or greater). Suctioning of the upper airway is appropriate if nasal congestion is present. Antipyretics such as acetaminophen or ibuprofen may improve tachycardia and tachypnea by reducing the

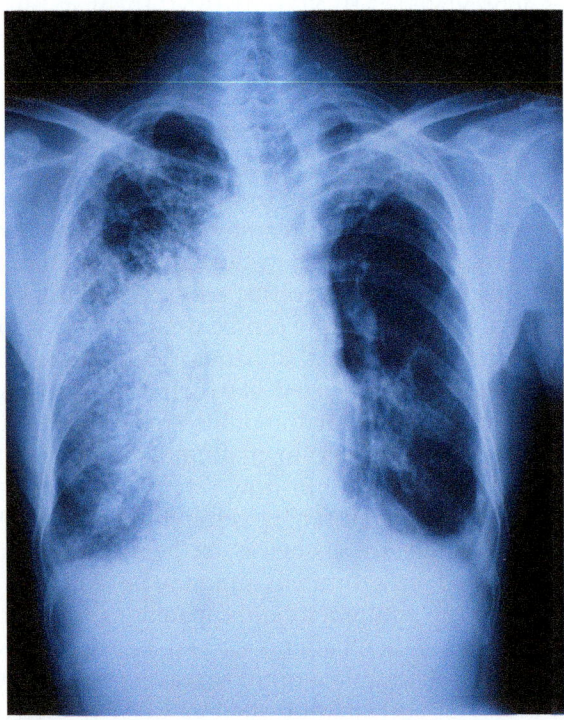

**Figure 2-8** Chest radiograph showing pulmonary infiltrates in the right lung of a patient with pneumonia.
© joloei/iStock/Getty Images Plus/Getty Images.

fever. Patients with pneumonia will have increased insensible fluid losses due to tachypnea and fever, and often their oral intake will be reduced. Intravenous fluid administration is often beneficial, and these patients may require fluid boluses if signs of dehydration are present.

Definitive care for pneumonia requires antibiotics when the cause is bacterial. Viral pneumonias require supportive care as the patient clears the virus.

## Pertussis

Pertussis is a lower respiratory infection caused by the *Bordatella pertussis* bacterium. There are many bacteria in the pertussis family, however *Bordatella* is the one most commonly associated with significant disease burden, and causes the disease commonly known as whooping cough or "100-day cough." The organism survives in respiratory secretions and is spread via droplet transmission. The overall incidence of pertussis has decreased by over 75% in the postvaccine era (since the 1940s); however, there has been a notable increase in the number of reported cases starting in the 1980s. Potential causes for this increase include: increased awareness, improved diagnostic capabilities, more accurate reporting, and waning immunity due to a number of factors. Additionally, pertussis bacteria, like all bacteria, are constantly evolving on a molecular level. Pertussis will often see a peak at regular intervals—approximately every 3 to 5 years. The last peak year was seen in 2012, with 48,277 cases reported. The last available data from 2018 indicates that over 15,000 cases were reported in that year.

Clinical illness from the pertussis bacteria follows a predictable three-stage progression (**Table 2-7**). The catarrhal stage is the first. Often patients will have absent or low-grade fever, coryza (inflamed mucous membranes around the nose), and a mild cough that will gradually become more severe. The catarrhal stage gives way to the paroxysmal stage after approximately 1 to 2 weeks. In the paroxysmal stage the cough becomes more severe and episodic. The coughing fits are rapid and often followed by significant inspiratory stridor, or a "whooping" noise. The secretions are thick and difficult to produce, especially in infants. Cyanosis and exhaustion will often follow coughing fits, as may posttussive emesis. The attacks become more frequent and severe, peaking approximately 2 weeks into the paroxysmal stage, and lingering for 2 to 3 weeks before gradually declining.

Once the coughing fits begin to decline, the patient is considered to be in the convalescent phase. There is gradual recovery and the coughing paroxysms become progressively less frequent. This phase will last approximately 3 weeks on average. The patient may appear to have fully recovered, although coughing paroxysms can

| Table 2-7 Progression and Signs of Pertussis | |
|---|---|
| **Stage** | **Clinical Features** |
| Stage 1:<br>Catarrhal<br>(1–2 weeks) | ▪ Coryza<br>▪ Absent or low-grade fever<br>▪ Mild, occasional cough, but not full-blown paroxysms<br>▪ History may indicate that the cough is becoming gradually more severe |
| Stage 2:<br>Paroxysmal<br>(3–5 weeks) | ▪ Coughing progresses to paroxysmal fits<br>▪ Coughing fits generally occur at night<br>▪ An average of 15 attacks in 24 hours may be seen during the peak of the illness course<br>▪ Thick mucus is present<br>▪ High-pitched inspiratory stridor (whooping) may be present at the end of coughing fits<br>▪ Cyanosis and apnea spells may be present<br>▪ Posttussive emesis<br>▪ Exhaustion and decreased level of consciousness associated with severe coughing fits |
| Stage 3:<br>Convalescent<br>(2–3 weeks) | ▪ Paroxysms decrease in frequency<br>▪ Gradual recovery is noted |

© Jones & Bartlett Learning.

recur with subsequent respiratory infections, as the airway remains highly reactive in the following months.

The clinical course of whooping cough is generally less severe in patients who have been vaccinated. Children born to mothers who have received a pertussis booster will have some immunity conferred to them through placental passage of antibodies and may have less severe disease if they become infected prior to being completely immunized.

The most serious disease complications generally occur in children younger than 12 months. Infants with pertussis will often experience significant episodes of apnea due to the respiratory infection. Secondary bacterial pneumonia is more likely after pertussis infection due to the compromised parenchyma of the lungs. In severe cases, children may have such severe coughing fits that rectal prolapse occurs. Pneumothorax, subdural hematoma, and refractory pulmonary hypertension have also been seen. Infection in patients with preexisting cardiac or pulmonary dysfunction adds significant additional risk to a patient who is already fragile.

The most effective treatment for pertussis is prevention through vaccination. Some patients may be incompletely vaccinated due to age or parental choice. Other patients who have been completely immunized may still be susceptible to contracting the disease due to host factors and incomplete immune response to the vaccine. The prehospital treatment for pertussis involves aggressive respiratory support measures such as supplemental oxygen and suctioning. Provide antipyretics for fever control when appropriate. Clinicians should be prepared to support patients who have episodes of apnea. Patients with severe respiratory distress may benefit from prone position ventilation. Definitive treatment involves antibiotic administration, specifically with a macrolide such as azithromycin. Antibiotics are most effective when initiated within 3 weeks of the infection beginning. Postexposure prophylaxis for close household contacts is often recommended and may include front-line healthcare workers if a high-risk exposure was encountered.

## CASE STUDY

### Case 1

#### Dispatch

You and your partner respond to a residence for an 11-month-old male with a fever and in respiratory distress (**Figure 2-9**). It is a cold winter evening. The outside air temperature is 20°F (−6.7°C).

#### Case Questions

▪ What are your initial concerns?
  ▪ The initial concern for this patient is respiratory distress with a fever, indicating that an infection is possible.

- Based on the dispatch information, what is the possible differential diagnosis for this patient?
  - Based on the dispatch information (fever and respiratory distress in a child younger than 1 year) and the time of year (winter with cold outside air temperature), the healthcare practitioner can begin to form a differential diagnosis for this patient, which should include the following:
    - Croup
    - Bronchiolitis
    - Pertussis
    - Epiglottitis
    - Tracheitis
    - Pneumonia

Scene assessment should include overall observations for safety. In addition to scene safety, observe the house for possible environmental conditions which could be exacerbating factors. Does the home smell like cigarette smoke? Is there an excessive amount of dust? Are there any pets present that could be causing an environmental allergen? Is the home carpeted, or are the floors a solid surface that may not contain as many allergens? Do you see any equipment or medications that may indicate the patient has a respiratory history, such as oxygen, nebulizer machines, or inhalers?

The observations you make while assessing the scene can help focus the history-taking process and narrow the differential diagnosis.

## Initial Observations

As you arrive at the front entrance of the home you are met by the mother, who appears anxious.

- Pediatric Assessment Triangle
  - Appearance
    - Restless
  - Work of breathing
    - **F**laring of the nares is present.
    - **R**etractions of the intercostal muscles noted.
    - **A**udible upper airway congestion is noted, no stridor or wheezing heard.
    - **P**ositioning appears comfortable in mother's lap.
  - Circulation
    - The skin appears warm and clammy.
    - There is no cyanosis present.

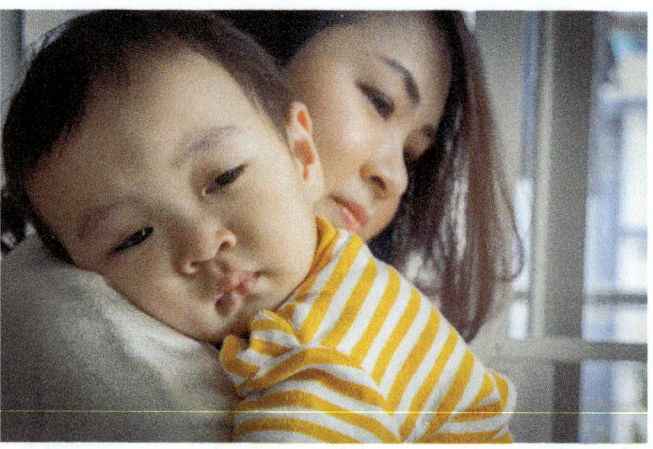

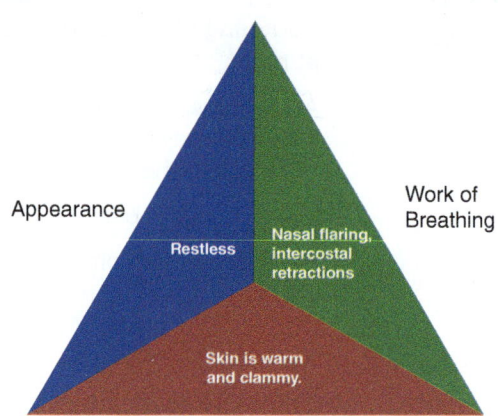

**Figure 2-9** The patient is an 11-month-old male with fever and respiratory distress.

A. © TimmyTimTim/Shutterstock B. Used with permission of the American Academy of Pediatrics, Pediatric Education for Prehospital Professionals, © American Academy of Pediatrics, 2000

The mother informs you that she went to the pediatrician 3 days ago and the patient tested positive for respiratory syncytial virus (RSV). She was given the following anticipatory guidance:

- Treat fever with antipyretics.
- Suction the nose frequently.
- Call 911 if the patient developed trouble breathing.

### Case Questions

- What additional precautions may be warranted based on these initial observations?
  - In addition to standard precautions, prehospital practitioners should have droplet protection on to help prevent infection.
  - Fever often leads to tachycardia and tachypnea. The increased respiratory rate associated with

fever can often be confused with respiratory distress. That is clearly not the case in this situation as the patient has additional signs of respiratory distress, including accessory muscle use and nasal flaring. In either case, the use of antipyretics for fever reduction may have the added benefit of reducing the respiratory rate associated with increased temperature.

- Bronchiolitis caused by RSV often peaks on days 3 to 5 of illness. The scenario presented here is quite common—patients will test positive and have relatively mild symptoms on day 1, and progress to significant respiratory distress requiring hospitalization between days 3 and 5 despite aggressive and appropriate care being provided at home. Parents should be reassured that they did nothing wrong by staying home, and they made the right decision to call 911 when they noted respiratory distress. It is appropriate to tell them that this condition often gets worse before it gets better, and some patients will require more aggressive treatment even when appropriate measures were taken by the pediatrician and parents at home.

- Based on your initial impression, is this patient "Quick" or "Not Quick"?

  - This patient is "Quick."

  - There is evidence of significant respiratory distress on the initial impression. The patient has nasal flaring and accessory muscle use. Although there is no evidence that the patient has circulatory compromise currently, he is restless, which is also an indicator of respiratory distress. He appears to be compensating, and there is no sign that circulation is compromised at this time.

- Have you identified respiratory distress, failure, or arrest?

  - The patient does not appear to have altered or decreased level of consciousness at this time and circulation is not compromised. Compensatory mechanisms appear to be intact, and this patient would best be classified as having respiratory distress.

## Primary Survey

The primary survey for this patient reveals the following:

- **X**—No bleeding is noted.
- **A**—Open, decreased patency due to copious amounts of clear nasal secretions.

- **B**—Respiratory rate is rapid. Nasal flaring and use of the intercostal muscles is noted. Expiratory wheezes are auscultated.
- **C**—Brachial pulses palpated and are noted to be strong and regular. Capillary refill is brisk. Skin is warm and the patient is noted to be diaphoretic.
- **D**—The patient is alert and appropriate. He appears to be restless. Glasgow Coma Scale (GCS) score is 15 (E4, V5, M6.)
- **E**—No evidence of injury or additional concerns noted on exposure.

### Case Questions

- Based on the findings noted in the primary survey, what would your initial interventions and treatment include?

  - Treatment should focus on supportive care that helps improve work of breathing.

  - It has been established that this patient is infected with RSV (positive test at primary care provider [PCP]). The most likely diagnosis at this time is bronchiolitis secondary to the RSV infection. The cause of the patient's respiratory distress is a combination of upper airway obstruction due to copious nasal secretions and lower airway inflammation and congestion secondary to the viral infection.

  - This patient should be suctioned to clear the upper airway of congestion. Blow-by oxygen can be applied to increase $FiO_2$ and treat hypoxia; however, if this is done without suctioning it will be less effective, as the patient's upper airway is congested with secretions.

- Are any life threats identified in this case?

  - Life threats include tachypnea, nasal flaring, and intercostal retractions.

Recognition of respiratory distress and addressing the cause before the patient progresses to respiratory failure and then arrest is of the utmost importance in pediatric respiratory emergencies. Circulatory collapse is most often caused by failure to address respiratory failure and arrest in this patient population.

## Suctioning

When should you suction your patient?

- Any time there is respiratory distress noted due to obstruction of the nares or upper airway from secretions, suctioning is generally appropriate.

How does nasal suctioning assist young children?

- Nasal suctioning helps to relieve respiratory distress in these patients by increasing the patency of the nares. Recall that decreases in the diameter of the airway increase resistance by a factor of four, so even a modest increase in airway diameter can lead to significantly decreased resistance and improved work of breathing.

- Infants younger than 6 months are especially susceptible to respiratory distress from obstructed nares. Recall that infants are generally considered to be obligate nose breathers prior to age 6 months. Obstruction of the nose increases the work of breathing and decreases an infant's ability to coordinate feeding. Breathing through the nose also humidifies and warms the incoming air. When patients breathe through their mouths, secretions will often become thicker as the air is not adequately warmed and humidified by the nasal turbinates.

What supplies are required for effective nasal suctioning?

- In general, a bulb syringe, normal saline, and a towel or tissue are all that is required to perform nasal suctioning (**Figure 2-10**).

- Depending on the local policy, suctioning may also be performed with a mechanical suctioning device. In this case, a flexible suction catheter appropriately sized for the patient will be necessary, in addition to sterile saline for lavage and irrigation.

What is the process for performing nasal suctioning?

- The patient should be placed supine on a flat surface. Patients will generally not be compliant with this, so it is important to have enough assistance to adequately and safely perform the procedure. Allow the parents or caregivers to help when possible.

- Placing the patient's arms above their head and pressing them to the sides of the patient's head can help maintain control of the arms and head at the same time and position the head midline for the procedure.

- Place 3 to 4 saline drops in the naris you plan to suction first. Allow 30 to 60 seconds for the saline to thin the nasal secretions.

- Expel the air from the bulb syringe and insert the tip into the naris. Release the bulb and allow it to go back to its inflated position, drawing air and secretions out of the nostril as it does so. Remove the tip from the nare and expel the suctioned contents onto the towel or tissue after each suctioning attempt.

- It may take multiple suction passes with the bulb syringe to clear the nare.

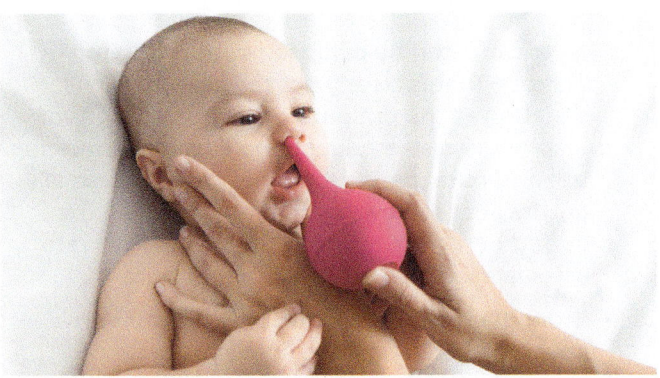

**Figure 2-10** A bulb syringe and normal saline can be used for effective nasal suctioning.
© Prostock-studio/Shutterstock.

- Use the same process on the opposite naris once the first naris has been cleared.

How often should you suction?

- Suction the nostrils until the airway has been adequately cleared and the nares are patent.

- Use caution with multiple aggressive suctioning attempts, as rebound inflammation of the tissues and bleeding of the nasal mucosa can occur.

## Detailed Assessment

### History Taking

After performing the initial interventions of nasal suctioning and applying blow-by oxygen, you begin to take additional history, which reveals the following:

**OPQRST:**

- **O**nset—Gradual, over the past 3 days
- **P**rovocation/palliation—None
- **Q**uality—N/A
- **R**adiation—None
- **S**everity—Unknown
- **T**iming—3 days

Pediatric patients should be continuously reevaluated throughout the encounter. They can decompensate rapidly and without warning.

Allowing the parent of caregiver to hold the child as much as possible to aid in compliance with the physical exam and treatment will be helpful. Toys and distraction devices such as phones or tablet devices may also be helpful.

**SAMPLER:**

- **S**igns/symptoms—Difficulty breathing, nasal flaring, accessory muscle use, copious amounts of nasal drainage, fever.

- **A**llergies—No known allergies to medications, foods, or the environment.

- **M**edications—Acetaminophen for fever, last given approximately 5 hours ago.

- **P**ast medical history—RSV-bronchiolitis diagnosed at PCP office 3 days ago.

- **L**ast oral intake—A few bites of cereal this afternoon. He became agitated while drinking milk from a bottle an hour ago and has not been able to eat or drink well for the past 24 hours.

- **E**vents leading up to the emergency—He has gotten progressively worse over the past 3 days. The mother contacted the pediatrician office and was advised to call EMS if the breathing got worse. Suctioning was not helping at home. Mother was not aware that she could use saline drops to help loosen nasal secretions.

- **R**isk factors—History of RSV-bronchiolitis diagnosis 3 days ago, age 11 months, copious nasal drainage.

## Vital Signs

As you were discussing the history, the patient was attached to the monitor and the following vital signs were obtained (**Figure 2-11**):

**Heart rate:**

- 150 beats/min

- The expected heart rate for a patient of this age is between 100 and 160 beats per minute. While it was initially in the normal range at 150 beats/min, note that it improved after suctioning and with blow-by oxygen. The patient's level of anxiety and distress was decreased when their work of breathing improved after intervention.

**SpO$_2$:**

- 92% on room air (RA)

- The patient is initially hypoxic but improves with nasal suctioning and supplemental oxygen. Target oxygen saturations in all pediatric patients are to maintain 94% or greater. This may be different in specific cases, such as patients with cardiac defects or chronic pulmonary disease. The patient's mother did not indicate that he has any history of congestive heart disease or chronic lung disease, so it is appropriate to target saturations greater than 94% in this case.

**End-tidal carbon dioxide (ETCO$_2$):**

- Unable to obtain due to patient noncompliance

**Respiratory rate:**

- 65 breaths/min

- The patient was initially tachypneic with a respiratory rate of 65 breaths/min; however, the rate improved with suctioning and oxygen. The expected respiratory rate in this patient is

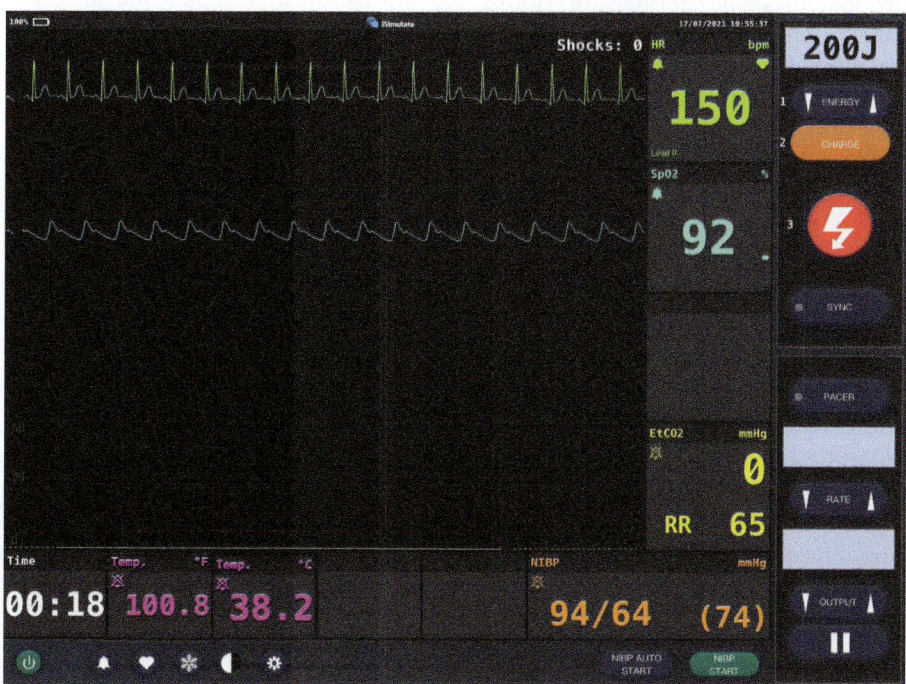

**Figure 2-11** Monitor screen of patient's vital signs.
Courtesy of iSimulate.

**Detailed Physical Exam**

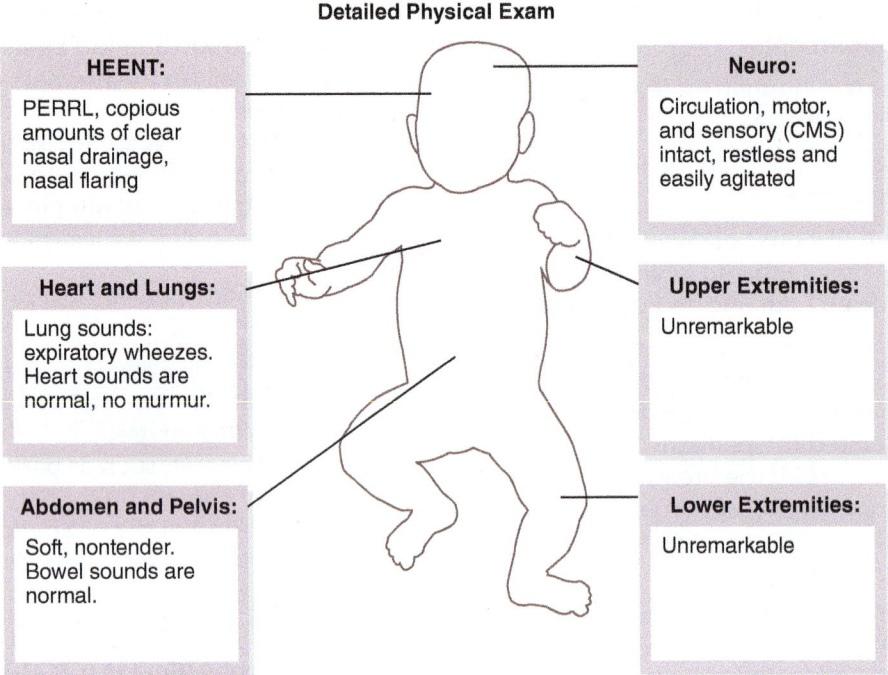

**HEENT:**

PERRL, copious amounts of clear nasal drainage, nasal flaring

**Heart and Lungs:**

Lung sounds: expiratory wheezes. Heart sounds are normal, no murmur.

**Abdomen and Pelvis:**

Soft, nontender. Bowel sounds are normal.

**Neuro:**

Circulation, motor, and sensory (CMS) intact, restless and easily agitated

**Upper Extremities:**

Unremarkable

**Lower Extremities:**

Unremarkable

**Figure 2-12** Detailed patient exam.

© Jones & Bartlett Learning.

30 to 60 breaths/min, and the tachypnea indicates he has a significant level of respiratory distress.

**Blood pressure:**

- 94/64 mm Hg
- The patient minimum systolic blood pressure should be above 60 mm Hg, which it is. This patient's blood pressure confirms what was identified on the initial impression—he is not experiencing any circulatory compromise at this time.

**Temperature:**

- 100.8°F (38.2°C)
- The patient is febrile, which is expected because he has a viral illness.

**Blood glucose:**

- 116 mg/dL
- A finger-stick glucose was obtained for this patient and showed 116 mg/dL, which is in the normal range. Infants with significantly increased work of breathing will often have decreased oral intake and may experience dehydration and hypoglycemia. It is important to obtain a blood glucose level in these patients.

This patient's initial vital signs indicate that he is in severe respiratory distress with tachypnea and hypoxia. Although it was not possible to obtain an ETCO$_2$ reading on this patient, ETCO$_2$ is not necessary to recognize the severity of respiratory distress.

Although the most likely diagnosis for this patient is bronchiolitis secondary to RSV infection, the possibility of superimposed bacterial pneumonia cannot be excluded without further evaluation and testing. Listening for focal lung sounds such as crackles or rhonchi isolated to a specific lobe of the lungs may help determine if pneumonia is more or less likely in this situation.

## Detailed Exam

Depending on the level of distress, a toe-to-head exam may be more effective in this patient given his age. In many cases the order and progression of the physical exam will be directed by what the patient will tolerate (**Figure 2-12**).

**HEENT:**

- **Head:** Unremarkable
- **Eyes:** Pupils equal, round, and reactive to light; no conjunctivitis or drainage noted
- **Ears:** Unremarkable
- **Nose:** Copious clear nasal secretions, nasal flaring present
- **Throat:** Clear, no exudates

**Chest, heart, and lungs:**

- **Pulses:** Brachial pulse easily palpated
- **Cardiac auscultation:** Regular rate and rhythm with no rub, gallop, or murmur noted

- Lung auscultation: Referred upper airway noises consistent with significant nasal congestion noted; diffuse rhonchi auscultated; expiratory wheezes
- Chest exam: Supraclavicular, intercostal, and subcostal retractions present

**Neurologic:**

- Neurovascular status intact; easily agitated

**Abdomen and pelvis:**

- Abdomen is soft and nontender; bowel sounds normal

**Extremities:**

- Upper and lower extremities unremarkable

**Back:**

- Unremarkable

## Treatment

Basic life support management of this patient would include close monitoring of the airway, suctioning of the nares to clear the secretions, supplemental oxygen (humidified if possible), and placing the patient in a position of comfort. Measures to decrease anxiety and agitation by keeping the patient with the caregiver as much as possible will also help.

Advanced life support care should include the previously mentioned measures, along with administration of appropriate medications, such as antipyretics.

More advanced forms of respiratory support such as HFNC or HHBNC could be employed if available and allowed by local protocols. Practitioners should always be prepared for the possibility of sudden deterioration and need for pharmacologically assisted intubation if necessary and allowed by local guidelines.

Initial treatment for this patient should not include the use of bronchodilators. This patient has congestion causing blockage of the lower airways and there is no element of bronchoconstriction present based on exam. Bronchodilators will not treat the congestion element of this patient's disease process, and they are likely to increase agitation, anxiety, and heart rate. Similarly, steroids and nebulized epinephrine are not indicated in this situation.

Nebulized hypertonic saline may be used in some institutions; however, routine use outside of the hospital setting is not recommended due to limited evidence of efficacy and risk of rebound bronchoconstriction.

## Ongoing Management

Patients with bronchiolitis often need repeated suctioning as secretions continue to build up in between clearance attempts. This patient is at high risk of deterioration and part of the ongoing management should include having positive-pressure ventilation and intubation equipment prepared and ready should he begin to decompensate.

After suctioning the patient, humidified oxygen was applied and the patient became much less agitated and restless. The patient's pulse came down to 130 beats/min and respirations decreased to 30 breaths/min, with significant improvement in the work of breathing noted. An appropriate dose of oral acetaminophen was administered, and the patient appeared more comfortable.

### Case Questions

- What is the most appropriate treatment destination and why?

  - The transport destination for this patient will be based largely on how he responds to initial treatment and what resources are available within the transport range of the local EMS service. This patient will likely require hospital admission and observation for continued supportive care as he recovers from the viral infection. If imminent respiratory failure and arrest are noted, it is appropriate to transport to the closest ED to take advantage of additional staffing and resources. If the patient appears stable for transport to a further destination, it is appropriate to bypass facilities in favor of a pediatric tertiary care center where the patient can be admitted and observed by specialized pediatric practitioners. This decision will also be impacted by the capabilities of the transporting service and the comfort of the transporting practitioner, in addition to local protocols and input from online medical direction.

- Can you safely transport this patient in your ambulance?

  - Safe transport of this patient can be accomplished by utilizing a commercially made device built to be attached to the ambulance stretcher. Another option would be to utilize the patient's own car seat and secure it into the captain's chair in the transport compartment. It is never appropriate to transport a pediatric patient in the lap of a caregiver or improperly secured to the ambulance stretcher.

- Will you allow mother and father to ride in the ambulance?

  - Parents and caregivers should be allowed to ride in the ambulance when it is safe to do so. Based on local policy and protocol, a family member allowed to ride in the transport compartment may be able to participate in patient care and calm the patient. In some cases, the safest place for the parent to ride may be up front, depending on the configuration of the ambulance. If possible, allow the caregiver to talk to the patient. This may aid in calming him.

The father provided you with the patient's car seat, which was properly secured in the patient compartment for transport. The mother was able to ride with the crew to the hospital and talked to the patient throughout the transport to decrease agitation and calm the patient.

The patient continued to be stable during transport and required no further interventions. The general

ED 15 minutes away was bypassed in favor of the large academic pediatric hospital 25 minutes away, as the patient was stable and appeared to respond well to suctioning, humidified oxygen, and acetaminophen administration. Online medical control was contacted and agreed with the transport destination and had no further recommendations for interventions.

## CASE WRAP-UP

Diagnosis: RSV-bronchiolitis

At the hospital, a chest x-ray was obtained and demonstrated increased interstitial markings and increased chest wall excursion. The patient was continued on humidified oxygen and required additional

suctioning. IV access was obtained and a normal saline bolus of 20 mL/kg was administered. The patient was admitted for continued supportive care and discharged after making a full recovery in approximately 7 days.

## CASE TAKEAWAY POINTS

RSV is the most common cause of viral bronchiolitis in pediatrics. Parainfluenza, influenza, and adenovirus are other common viral causes, often associated with less severe disease. Bronchiolitis commonly affects patients younger than 2 years and is more likely to cause severe

disease in patients younger than 6 months with history of prematurity, chronic lung disease, or cardiac pathology. Care for bronchiolitis is supportive in nature and includes suctioning, oxygen as needed, and respiratory support.

## CASE STUDY

## Case 2

### Dispatch

You and your partner respond to a local school for a 12-year-old female in respiratory distress. It is a warm, spring afternoon. The air temperature is 72°F (22.2°C).

### Case Questions

- What are your initial concerns?
  - The initial concern in this case is for a 12-year-old female experiencing respiratory distress. It is a spring afternoon, which means it is outside of the typical viral respiratory season. No fever was reported initially; however, this should be confirmed on physical exam.
- Based on the dispatch information, what is the possible differential diagnosis for this patient?
  - The differential diagnoses for respiratory distress in this age group include:
    - Asthma
    - Hyperventilation (anxiety or panic attack)
    - Foreign body obstruction
    - Cystic fibrosis

- Pneumonia
- Anaphylaxis
- Disordered control of breathing secondary to seizure or other neurologic disorder

Scene-specific considerations for this case include the fact that the patient is at school and the parents are likely not present. There will most likely be a school nurse present who may be able to assist with additional history for the patient. The patient may have medications, such as an emergency inhaler or EpiPen available in the school clinic.

### Initial Observations

As you arrive at the front entrance of the school, an administrative assistant leads you to the nurse's office where the patient is seated on an exam table (**Figure 2-13**).

- Pediatric Assessment Triangle
  - Appearance
    - Fatigued
    - Appropriately interacting with emergency personnel
  - Work of breathing
    - **F**laring of the nostrils is present.

The principal comes into the office and informs everyone that the mother has been contacted and is already on the way to the ED in anticipation that her daughter will be transported there.

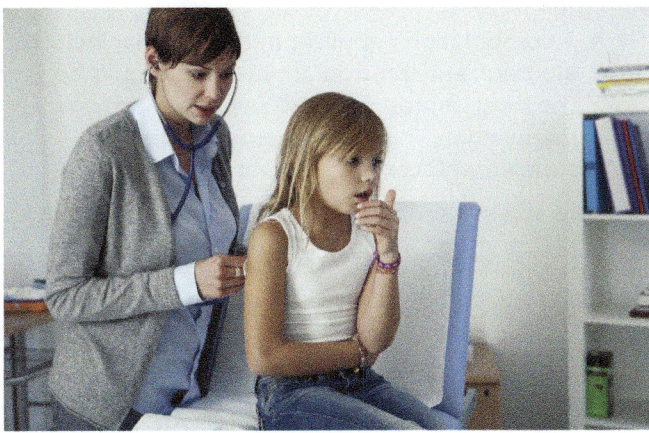

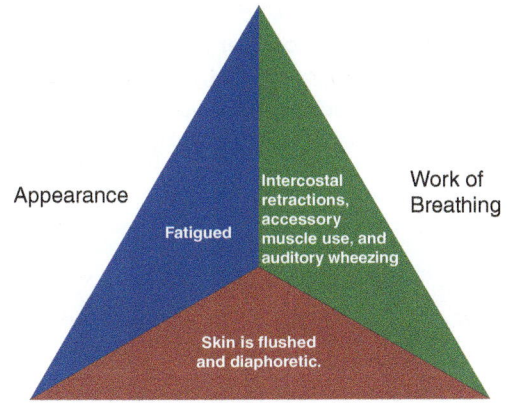

**Figure 2-13** The patient is a 12-year-old girl in respiratory distress.

© Image Point Fr/Shutterstock; Used with permission of the American Academy of Pediatrics, Pediatric Education for Prehospital Professionals, © American Academy of Pediatrics, 2000.

- **R**etractions of the intercostal muscles noted along with significant accessory muscle use.
- **A**udible expiratory wheezes are heard.
- **P**ositioning—patient is in a tripod position.
  - Circulation
    - The skin is flushed and diaphoretic.

According to the nurse, the patient came into the office after recess due to respiratory distress. She has received four puffs of her emergency inhaler without relief.

The nurse has the patient's medical file available and informs you that the patient was diagnosed with asthma at age 3 years. She has missed multiple days of school in the past due to asthma exacerbations, and she has been hospitalized on more than one occasion. She regularly has to come to the nurse's office for her quick-relief inhaler, especially in the spring. The patient normally responds well to using her inhaler; however, the nurse became concerned when she noted no improvement after albuterol administration, prompting her to call 911.

## Case Questions

- Based on your initial impression, is this patient "Quick" or "Not Quick"?
  - This patient is "Quick."
  - Based on the history provided by the school nurse, this patient appears to have poorly controlled severe persistent asthma. This determination was made based on the fact that she regularly has to use her rescue inhaler, misses multiple days of school due to asthma exacerbations, and has been hospitalized previously. The patient is not responding to her rescue inhaler as she normally does, which means she may be in status asthmaticus. This is a medical emergency with significant risk for decompensation and respiratory failure.
- Have you identified respiratory distress, failure, or arrest?
  - Currently the patient is in respiratory distress. Her level of consciousness is not altered, and she has intact circulatory status. She is compensating well, however rapid intervention is necessary to prevent her from progressing to respiratory failure, as on initial exam she is already appearing fatigued.

## Primary Survey

The primary survey for this patient reveals the following:

- **X**—No bleeding is noted.
- **A**—Open and patent.
- **B**—Respirations are rapid and shallow with intercostal retractions and accessory muscle use noted. Auditory wheezing is present. The patient is unable to complete a full sentence without stopping to catch her breath.
- **C**—Radial pulses palpated and are noted to be strong and regular. Capillary refill is brisk. Skin is flushed and the patient is noted to be diaphoretic.
- **D**—The patient is alert and appropriate. She appears to be fatigued. GCS is 15 (E4, V5, M6).
- **E**—No evidence of injury or additional concerns noted on exposure. She is sitting in a tripod position on the exam table.

## Case Questions

- Are there any life threats noted on the primary survey?
  - This patient has evidence of severe respiratory distress on the primary survey. The fatigued appearance, tachypnea, significant use of accessory muscles, audible wheezes, and inability to complete a full sentence are extremely concerning findings.
- Based on the findings noted in the primary survey, what would your initial interventions and treatment include?
  - Initial treatment for this patient should be focused on reversing bronchospasm and bronchoconstriction along with providing supplemental oxygen and respiratory support as appropriate.
- A combination nebulizer treatment that includes albuterol and ipratropium bromide would be the most appropriate first-line pharmacologic intervention. This can be aerosolized using supplemental oxygen to treat any hypoxia.
- IV access should be established in this patient in preparation for administration of IV medications if necessary. A fluid bolus is indicated if the patient has signs of dehydration.

## Determining the Severity of Asthma

Table 2-8 describes the different severity levels of asthma that can be encountered in the prehospital setting. Asthma severity can rapidly progress from mild to severe if undertreated. Aggressive management is necessary to prevent patients from progressing in severity.

**Table 2-8** Asthma Severity

| | Signs and Symptoms | Treatment |
|---|---|---|
| Mild | - Difficulty breathing during activity, well controlled | - Commonly treated at home<br>- Quick relief from short-acting beta-agonists<br>- May receive oral corticosteroids |
| Moderate | - Difficulty breathing interrupting or restricting activities<br>- Symptoms may last 1–2 days after treatment begins | - Often requires treatment in the emergency department<br>- Obtains relief from multiple doses of short-acting beta-agonists<br>- Receives oral corticosteroids |
| Severe | - Difficulty breathing when at rest<br>- Trouble with speaking<br>- Symptoms may last >3 days after treatment begins | - Often requires treatment in the emergency department with potential hospitalization<br>- Partial relief from multiple doses of short-acting beta-agonists<br>- Receives oral corticosteroids<br>- Adjunctive therapies are beneficial |
| Life threatening | - Unable to speak due to severity of difficulty breathing<br>- Diaphoretic | - Requires treatment in the emergency department with hospitalization<br>- Potential ICU admission<br>- Minimal to no relief from multiple doses of short-acting beta-agonists<br>- Receives IV corticosteroids<br>- Adjunctive therapies are beneficial |

Although the signs and symptoms present are good initial indicators of severity, they are subjective and may vary in description from practitioner to practitioner. Objective measures of asthma severity include the use of waveform capnography, oxygen saturation monitoring, and blood gas interpretation.

## End-Tidal $CO_2$

The use of $ETCO_2$ (also known waveform capnography, quantitative waveform capnography) to determine the characteristics of gas exchange in various respiratory disease processes is widely utilized in the prehospital setting.

Multiple devices are used to measure exhaled $CO_2$. Patients who do not have an advanced airway in place will most commonly utilize an $ETCO_2$ monitor that is integrated within a nasal cannula (**Figure 2-14**).

## Capnography Interpretation

In addition to evaluating the respiratory rate, the waveform capnograph will also depict the partial pressure of exhaled carbon dioxide ($ETCO_2$). The calculated normal value for $ETCO_2$ is 38 mm Hg, and 35 to 45 mm Hg is considered the physiologic normal range. The body's ability to off-load carbon dioxide via the respiratory system is a function of both circulation and minute ventilation. In the presence of intact circulatory status, the body's ability to off-load carbon dioxide is primarily driven by the minute ventilation. Changes in tidal volume and respiratory rate have a dramatic and instantaneous, breath-to-breath effect on the exhaled carbon dioxide detected by the $ETCO_2$ detector.

In conditions where minute ventilation is decreased (apnea, bradypnea, airway obstruction, bronchoconstriction) the ability to breathe off carbon dioxide is decreased. As a result, carbon dioxide builds up in the lungs, and this is reflected by increasing $ETCO_2$ levels. Conversely, in conditions where the minute ventilation is increased, the amount of carbon dioxide being "breathed off" by the lungs is also increased and will be reflected in lower $ETCO_2$ readings detected by the $ETCO_2$ probe.

> A patient with asthma with an increasing $ETCO_2$ is becoming hypercarbic. The presence of hypercarbia and hypoxia is a sign that the asthmatic patient is in crashing respiratory failure and at risk of impending respiratory arrest.

The discussion of capnography would be incomplete if we did not address both the partial pressure of carbon dioxide (discussed earlier) and the interpretation of the $ETCO_2$ waveform itself (**Figure 2-15**).

The $ETCO_2$ waveform has four phases. In Figure 2-15B, the four phases can be seen in greater detail.

- Phase 1:
  - Points A to B.
  - End of patient inhalation.
  - No $ETCO_2$ detected as the air passing by the $ETCO_2$ detector (inhaled atmospheric air) does not contain a detectable amount of carbon dioxide.
- Phase 2:
  - Points B to C.
  - Beginning of exhalation.
  - There is a sharp rise in the carbon dioxide detected by the $ETCO_2$ probe, as a rush of air with detectable carbon dioxide passes by the sensor.
  - Point C represents the alpha angle. The inside angle of this corner of the waveform should be close to 90 degrees in patients without significant airway dysfunction.

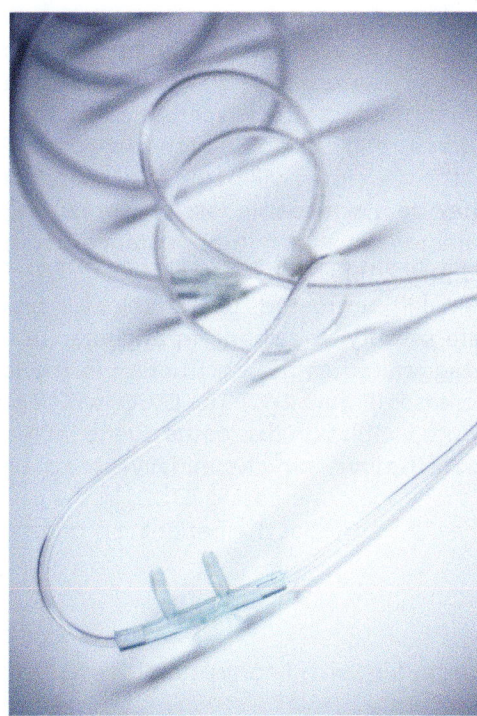

**Figure 2-14** Nasal cannula can be integrated with an $ETCO_2$ monitor to measure exhaled $CO_2$

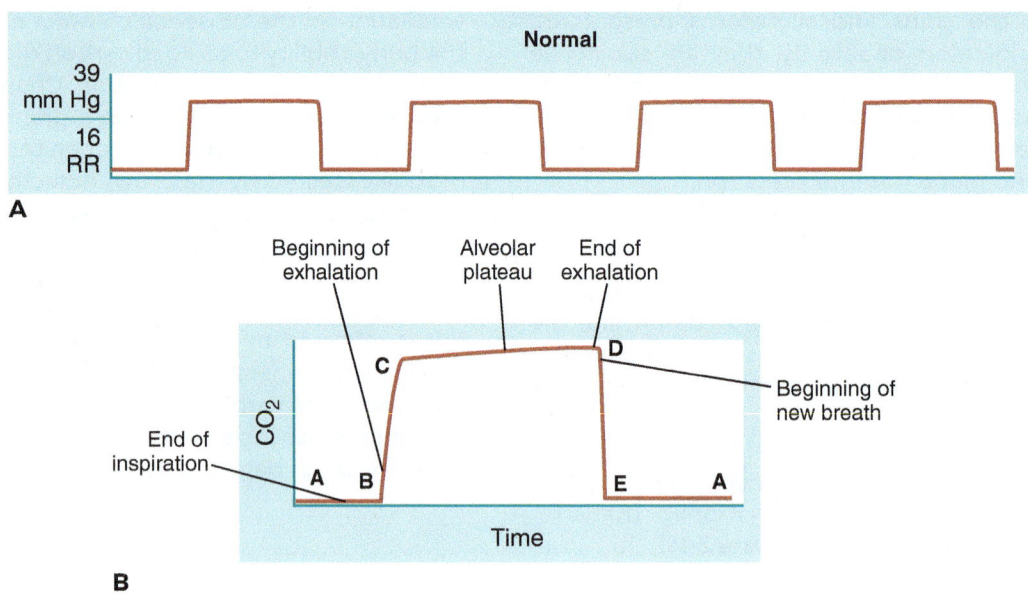

**Figure 2-15** **A.** Normal waveform. **B.** The four phases of the waveform.

© Jones & Bartlett Learning.

- As obstruction and ventilation:perfusion mismatch in various areas of the lungs increases, so does the alpha angle, leading to an upsloping phase 2 to 3, which is beginning to resemble a shark fin.
- Phase 3:
  - Points C to D.
  - Alveolar plateau.
  - When the ventilation and perfusion of the alveoli are uniform and there is no obstruction or other dysfunction present, this should essentially be a flat "plateau" representing consistent and stable exhalation of carbon dioxide during the entire expiratory phase.
  - Lower airway obstruction will result in a "loss of plateau" causing phase 2 and 3 to blend together, into an upward sloping curve, shark fin appearance.
- Phase 4:
  - Points D to E.
  - Initiation of inspiration.
  - There is a sudden drop in detectable carbon dioxide as the air rushing past the detector (atmospheric air) has no detectable carbon dioxide.
  - In situations where there is lower airway obstruction, the angle at point D may become more obtuse, further exaggerating the shark fin appearance of the waveform and indicating increased severity of airway obstruction.

## Waveform Capnography and Asthma

There are some waveform capnography findings that are specific for lower airway obstruction. The pediatric emergency practitioner should be familiar with these findings as they can herald respiratory failure and arrest.

During a mild asthma attack, the patient will be tachypneic, however the lower airway obstruction is not severe enough to appreciably effect tidal volumes, and the respiratory system for managing exhaled carbon dioxide remains intact. This is seen as a decreased $ETCO_2$ partial pressure (hypocarbia) with tachypnea. Phases 2 and 3 of the waveform will begin to blend together and there may be a noticeable loss of plateau in phase 3. The characteristic shark fin appearance begins to develop (**Figure 2-16**).

When left untreated, the attack will progress to moderate severity. The shark fin appearance becomes more exaggerated as the obstruction in the lower airways increases (**Figure 2-17**). The $ETCO_2$ will begin to rise, and minute ventilation decreases due to increasing obstruction of the lower airways. Initially these patients may be very tachypneic. Increasing $ETCO_2$ in the presence of tachypnea is a sign that the patient is progressing from

**Hypercarbia with tachypnea is respiratory failure.**

**Hypercarbia with decreasing respiratory rate is respiratory failure progressing to respiratory arrest.**

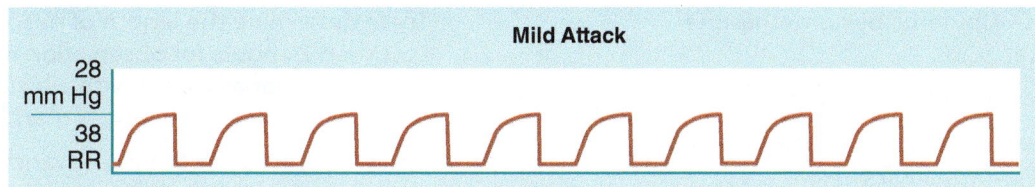

**Figure 2-16** During a mild asthma attack the lower airway obstruction is not severe enough to appreciably effect tidal volumes.

© Jones & Bartlett Learning.

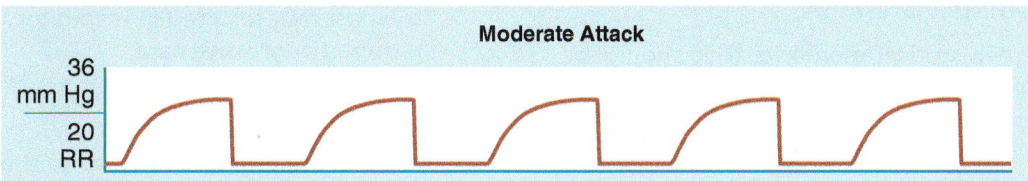

**Figure 2-17** In an asthma attack of moderate severity, the shark fin appearance becomes more exaggerated due to increased obstruction in the lower airways.

© Jones & Bartlett Learning.

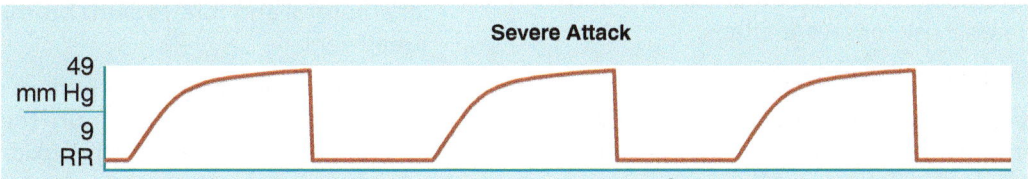

**Figure 2-18** A severe asthma attack is indicated by increasing $ETCO_2$ in the presence of tachypnea.

© Jones & Bartlett Learning.

moderate to severe attack. Hypercarbia with tachypnea indicates respiratory failure and when left untreated can progress to respiratory arrest rapidly.

When the patient is left untreated or the attack becomes so severe that it begins to progress to respiratory arrest, there will be a decrease in respiratory rate while $ETCO_2$ remains high. The shark fin appearance of the waveform will become even more exaggerated (**Figure 2-18**). The respiratory rate will continue to slow until respiratory arrest ensues.

## Detailed Assessment

### History Taking

As your partner prepares a nebulizer treatment of albuterol and ipratropium bromide for the patient, you obtain more history:

**OPQRST:**

- **O**nset—Sudden onset shortness of breath while running on the playground.

- **P**rovocation/palliation—Physical activity provoked the attack, her respiratory distress is worse when lying down.

- **Q**uality—She is in moderate discomfort.

- **R**adiation—None.

- **S**everity—No pain.

- **T**iming—Approximately 30 minutes.

This is a classic presentation of asthma exacerbation provoked by physical activity and refractory to rescue inhaler use. The history excludes pneumonia and other infectious causes as they would be more chronic in onset and there was no fever noted in the primary survey.

**SAMPLER:**

- **S**igns/symptoms—Difficulty breathing, supraclavicular and intercostal accessory muscle use noted, audible wheezes, unable to speak in full sentences

- **A**llergies—No known allergies

- **M**edications—Albuterol, beclomethasone dipropionate
- **P**ast medical history—Asthma and bronchitis
- **L**ast oral intake—Lunch in the cafeteria about 90 minutes prior to EMS arrival
- **E**vents leading up to the emergency—Playing on the playground; received 4 puffs of albuterol inhaler approximately 1 hour ago; returned to nurse's station approximately 30 minutes ago when breathing became more difficult
- **R**isk factors—History of asthma

There are a few critical elements that should be obtained in a pediatric asthma history. These elements can indicate the severity of the patient's asthma, the level of control, and risk for decompensation. The elements include the following:

- Frequency of emergency inhaler use (increased use means poor asthma control)
- Impact on activities of daily living
  - Children who frequently miss school due to asthma have poor control over their asthma and are at increased risk for severe attack.
- Prior hospitalizations for asthma
  - Children with a prior hospitalization for asthma have a demonstrated history of poorly controlled severe asthma.

- Try to determine the length of hospitalization. Less than 24 hours for observation is more reassuring that a patient with a history of multiple hospital stays longer than 24 hours.
- Prior asthma attack requiring advanced airway insertion
  - Patients who have previously required the insertion of an advanced airway for management of their asthma are at significant risk for severe attack. A history of intubation means that they have had an asthma attack in the past that resulted in respiratory arrest and required aggressive care.

## Vital Signs

As you were discussing the history, the patient was attached to the monitor and the following vital signs were obtained (**Figure 2-19**):

**Heart rate:**

- 123 beats/min.
  - Increases to 138 beats/min with administration of albuterol and ipratropium bromide nebulizer treatment
- The expected heart rate for a patient of this age is between 70 and 120 beats/min. The increase in heart rate reflects that she is hypoxic, agitated, and in distress.

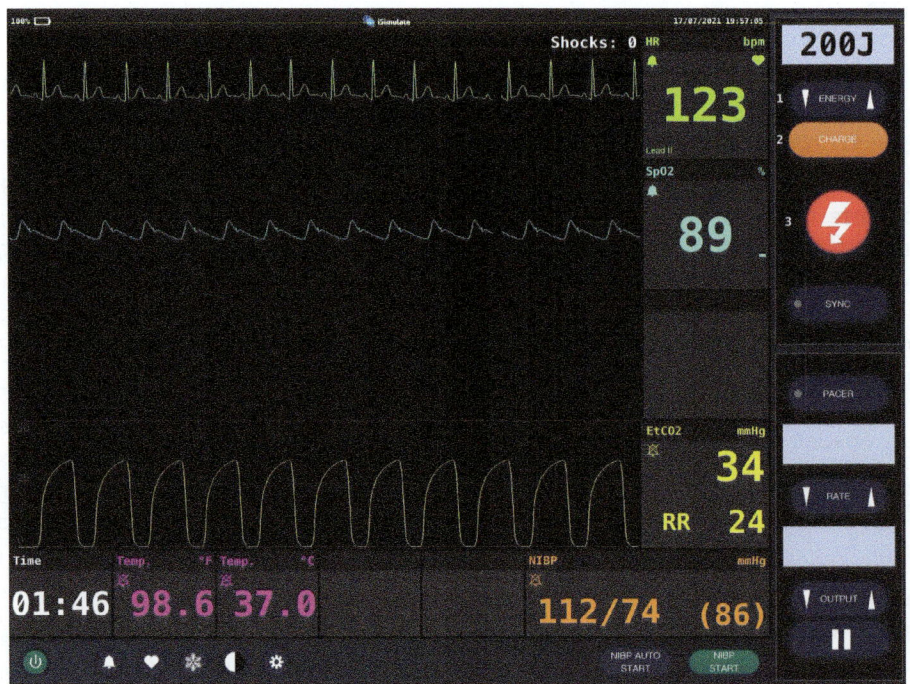

**Figure 2-19** Vital signs monitor.
Courtesy of iSimulate.

- The increase in heart rate with administration of the nebulizer treatment does not necessarily reflect worsening clinical status. When inhaled beta agonists are administered, an increase in heart rate should be expected as an effect of beta receptor stimulation. If the respiratory status appears to be improving, then the rise in heart rate is likely due to beta stimulation.

- If the heart rate in increasing with evidence of poor perfusion and worsening respiratory status, this is an ominous sign and represents a need to escalate therapy.

**SpO$_2$:**

- 89% RA.

  - Increases to 94% with nebulized albuterol and ipratropium bromide and oxygen administration.

- This patient is initially hypoxic. She appears to respond well to the nebulizer and oxygen administration with an increase in SpO$_2$.

- In some cases, the amount of detectable wheezing that is heard will *increase* after bronchodilator administration. This is because more air is moving through the lower airways after the bronchoconstriction is relieved, and more air movement results in increased lower airway sounds. In some cases, increased wheezing with better ventilation is evidence that treatments are effective.

**ETCO$_2$:**

- 34 mm Hg.

- This patient is tachypneic with a slightly lower than normal ETCO$_2$ reading. This indicates that the lower airways are still ventilating well enough to "breathe off" carbon dioxide. It is important to consider whether the level of exhaled carbon dioxide is appropriate for the patient's respiratory rate.

- The waveform demonstrates a "loss of plateau" between phases 2 and 3, indicating that there is lower airway obstruction present.

**Respiratory rate:**

- 24 breaths/min.

- Respiratory rate improves to 20 breaths/min after administration of nebulizer treatment.

- The patient is tachypneic for her age, although the tachypnea does not appear to be severe.

**Blood pressure:**

- 112/74 mm Hg

- The expected systolic blood pressure in this patient should be 80 to 110 mm Hg.

- This patient appears to be mildly hypertensive. This could be due to anxiety and distress.

- There does not appear to be any signs of hemodynamic compromise based on the heart rate and blood pressure.

- Blood pressure may increase modestly with inhaled beta-agonist administration.

- It is important to keep a close eye on blood pressure as you escalate asthma treatment. In severe status asthmaticus, magnesium sulfate (a smooth muscle relaxer) may be used to help relieve bronchoconstriction. This medication will also cause smooth muscle relaxation of the peripheral vasculature and can lead to decrease in blood pressure. Hypotension is often a contraindication to administration of magnesium sulfate, and patients may need an IV fluid bolus to increase blood pressure and cardiac preload prior to administration of this medication in emergency situations.

**Temperature:**

- 98.6°F (37.0°C).

- The patient is afebrile. As mentioned earlier, this is a pertinent negative, and decreases the likelihood that the patient's respiratory distress is secondary to a lung infection.

**Blood glucose:**

- 104 mg/dL.

- A finger-stick glucose was obtained for this patient and showed 104 mg/dL, which is in the normal range.

- Certain asthma therapies will have the effect of increasing blood glucose levels. Albuterol is a beta agonist and at very high concentrations can theoretically raise the serum blood glucose concentration. IV steroids such as methylprednisolone and dexamethasone will also cause transient elevations in blood glucose.

The vital signs and physical exam indicate that this patient is having a moderate asthma attack. Based on the level of tachypnea present, the expected ETCO$_2$ is lower than what is observed, indicating that lower airway obstruction is severe enough to cause decreased minute ventilation despite tachypnea. The patient is also hypoxic, indicating that lower airway obstruction is decreasing alveolar gas exchange to the point of decreasing blood oxygen concentration. In addition to this, the physical exam shows significant accessory muscle use, inability to speak in full sentences,

**Detailed Physical Exam**

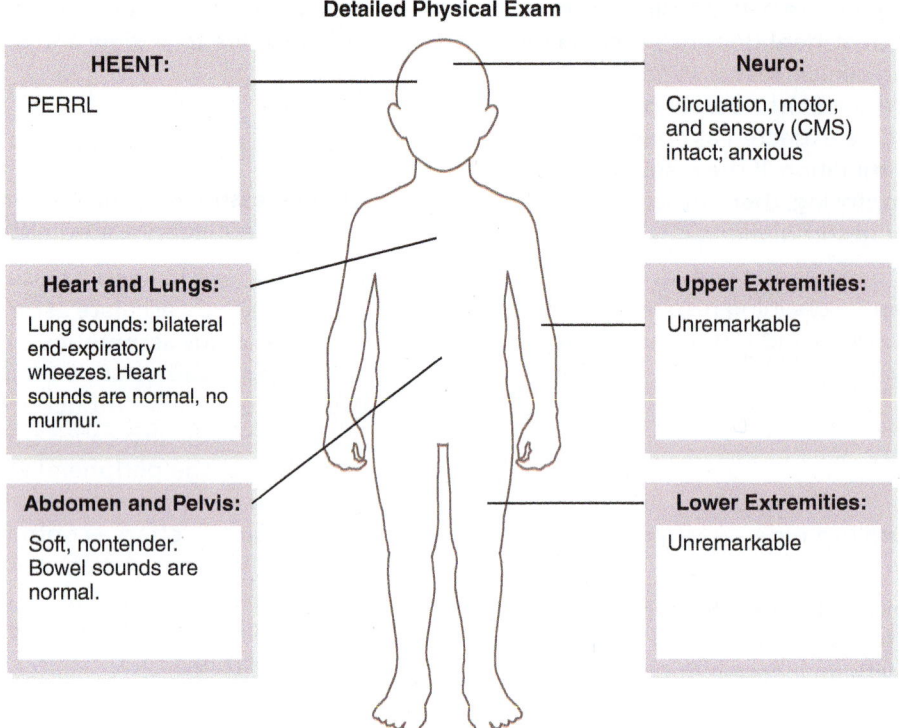

**Figure 2-20** Detailed patient exam.
© Jones & Bartlett Learning.

and diffuse audible wheezing. If left untreated, this patient could rapidly progress to severe attack and respiratory arrest.

## Detailed Exam

As your partner continues to provide the nebulizer treatment and obtain IV access, you begin your exam (**Figure 2-20**).

**HEENT:**

- **H**ead: Unremarkable
- **E**yes: Pupils equal, round, and reactive to light; no conjunctivitis or drainage noted
- **E**ars: Unremarkable
- **N**ose: Unremarkable
- **T**hroat: Clear, no exudates

**Chest, heart, and lungs:**

- Pulses: Radial pulse easily palpated
- Cardiac auscultation: Tachycardic rate and regular rhythm with no rub, gallop, or murmur noted
- Lung auscultation: Tachypnea with diffuse expiratory wheezes noted
- Chest exam: supraclavicular and intercostal accessory muscle use noted

**Neurologic:**

- Neurovascular status intact; no evidence of decreased level of consciousness

**Abdomen and pelvis:**

- Abdomen is soft and nontender; bowel sounds normal

**Extremities:**

- Upper and lower extremities unremarkable

**Back:**

- Unremarkable

## Treatment

Treatment goals for this patient should focus on reversing the bronchoconstriction and correcting hypoxia. Basic life support measures include administration of oxygen and nebulized albuterol and ipratropium bromide if permitted by protocol. Placing the patient in a position of comfort to aid in decreasing distress and anxiety will also be helpful.

In addition to the BLS interventions, IV access should be obtained in this patient. Increased insensible losses from elevated respiratory rate can lead to dehydration and an IV fluid bolus might be required. IV access is also necessary for medication administration. Refractory status asthmaticus (not responding to initial inhaled bronchodilator therapy) will often require administration of magnesium sulfate to aid in smooth muscle relaxation around the bronchioles. IV corticosteroids such as methylprednisolone or dexamethasone have been shown to decrease hospital length of stay and overall severity, however these are not fast-acting interventions. The effects of IV steroids in asthma are often not seen for at least 4 to 6 hours after administration. Although early administration of IV steroids is important, it should not delay the administration of medications or interventions that are faster acting and provide more immediate relief. The administration of intramuscular epinephrine can also be considered in severe asthma exacerbations.

Patients who continue to be refractory to initial interventions may require escalating respiratory support. BiPAP or CPAP support can aid in decreasing work of breathing while giving medication interventions time to work. These interventions must be balanced with the patient's ability to tolerate them, however. In some cases, the patient may be so distressed by the feeling of the positive airway pressure device on their face that they are not able to interface well with the ventilator and the intervention runs the risk of pushing them from severe distress into respiratory failure. It should also be noted that asthma is a disorder of lower airway obstruction, which leads to difficulty in exhalation. Positive-pressure methods of noninvasive ventilatory support will often increase difficulty with exhalation initially, which can increase the severity of respiratory distress. When used properly by experienced practitioners, noninvasive ventilatory support is a valuable adjunctive treatment in asthma management that can delay or eliminate the need for advanced airway placement.

Ketamine has been discussed in the literature with mixed results. The pharmacologic properties of ketamine lead to catecholamine release when administered, leading to bronchodilation. The routine use of ketamine outside of the hospital setting for the management of asthma varies by jurisdiction and local policy. However, if advanced airway placement becomes necessary, ketamine is a reasonable choice for sedation prior to airway insertion due to the previously mentioned bronchodilator properties. The choice to use ketamine in patients with severe asthma is a nuanced one that should be made with your organization's medical director.

## Pediatric Intubation

Pediatric intubation is a high-risk, low-frequency occurrence. The decision to intubate a pediatric patient should never be taken lightly. Due to the complex interplay of tachypnea, hyperinflation with decreased tidal volumes, and baseline hypoxia combined with hypercarbia, intubation of asthmatic patients requires precise ventilatory management that cannot be achieved through ventilation with a bag-valve mask or with most prehospital transport ventilators. Additionally, chronically hyperinflated patients will have altered hemodynamic parameters affecting pressures to both the right and left hearts. The sudden transition from negative-pressure breathing and the associated cardiopulmonary relationship to positive-pressure breathing and its known effects on cardiac function increases the risk of sudden circulatory collapse during and after invasive airway placement. Some of these factors also exist when using noninvasive positive-pressure ventilatory techniques, particularly when higher than normal pressures are utilized. For all of these reasons, intubation of the pediatric patient, especially when asthma is the cause of respiratory failure, should be avoided if at all possible until the patient is at a definitive care destination with additional resources such as respiratory therapy, mechanical ventilators, and physicians experienced in pediatric critical care.

It should be noted that intubation alone does not make ventilation easier for asthmatic patients, it only provides a direct route for air to enter the trachea. The bronchoconstriction and lower airway obstruction will still exist after intubation if left untreated.

Pediatric patients who are hypoxic and hypercarbic at the initiation of advanced airway placement have dramatically decreased compensatory reserve and are prone to rapid evolution of hypoxia and potential hypoxic brain injury, bradycardia, and cardiac arrest. Cardiac arrest management in the asthmatic patient is extremely difficult.

**Advanced airway placement by inexperienced practitioners has a high likelihood of resulting in failed intubation attempt in pediatric patients. Even when pediatric patients are successfully intubated, the complicated physiologic interplay between the cardiac and pulmonary systems is difficult to manage outside of the pediatric critical care environment.**

## Pediatric Intubation Considerations

Younger pediatric patients often need a towel roll placed behind their shoulder blades to better align the airway axis and increase visualization of the trachea. Ramping or elevation of the head of the bed may also aid in visualization.

The larynx of the pediatric airway is more superior and anterior. This will also complicate visualization.

In some cases, during the visualization attempt, the entire trachea may unintentionally be elevated with the distal end of the laryngoscope, allowing only the esophagus to be viewed. It may be reasonable if no tracheal structures are visible to retreat with the distal end of the laryngoscope blade, watching for the trachea to drop into view once the blade has been pulled back far enough.

Insertion of the endotracheal tube to an excessive depth leading to right mainstem intubation is common in pediatric patients, even by experienced practitioners. In the absence of radiographic assessment of tube placement, lung sounds should be assessed frequently, and any decrease or asymmetry in chest wall movement should be examined with careful attention to the possibility of mainstem intubation. Careful retraction of the tube with gentle tension may be all that is necessary to appropriately position the endotracheal tube. The risk of barotrauma from mainstem intubation is high.

Confirmation of endotracheal tube placement should be made by direct visualization of the tube passing the vocal cords and detection of $ETCO_2$ on quantitative waveform capnography. In the healthcare setting, an x-ray should be obtained to ensure that tube depth is appropriate and mainstem intubation has not occurred.

Ensure that pediatric patients are ventilated at an age-appropriate rate and avoid hypo- or hyperventilation. In asthmatic patients in particular, an increased expiratory time may be necessary to allow for full exhalation of the hyperinflated lungs. Be vigilant to recognize and avoid auto-PEEP and breath stacking, especially when using assist control ventilator modes.

## Ongoing Management

IV access was initiated, and the patient was given methylprednisolone. An additional albuterol nebulizer treatment was given during transport. The patient's respiratory distress improved; however, diffuse wheezing was still heard. The hypoxia improved with oxygen administration and the nebulizer treatments. Medical control was contacted and the decision was made to transport the patient to the university pediatric hospital 15 minutes away. The mother was contacted and updated on the patient's status. No further deterioration was noted during transport.

### Case Questions

- What is the most appropriate treatment destination and why?

  - The decision was made to take this patient to a pediatric-specific care center due to the potential for respiratory failure. The availability of physicians trained in pediatric emergency medicine and critical care is a consideration, as they possess the knowledge and skills to best manage the decompensating pediatric asthma patient.

- Can you safely transport this patient in your ambulance?

  - The patient was restrained to the stretcher safely.

## CASE WRAP-UP

Diagnosis: Asthma exacerbation

At the hospital the patient continued to have diffuse wheezing. Additional nebulizer treatments and IV methyl prednisone were administered. The patient's respiratory rate and oxygen levels improved in the ED. She was discharged with instructions to follow-up with her PCP, who referred her to a pulmonologist. The patient was seen by a pediatric pulmonologist and her home asthma medications were adjusted to better manage her asthma and hopefully avoid future exacerbations.

## CASE TAKEAWAY POINTS

Asthma is one of the most frequently encountered chronic diseases in pediatric patients. It is the third leading cause of pediatric hospitalization in the United States. Asthma exacerbation is the primary reason why many pediatric patients seek emergency care. Rapid intervention by prehospital EMS crews can dramatically alter the course of hospitalization and shorten the length of stay. Initiating effective therapy with minimal delay can avoid unnecessary and unsafe intubation of pediatric asthma patients in the field. The actions taken by prehospital medical professionals have a major impact on long-term asthma care, mortality, and morbidity.

## LESSON WRAP-UP

Respiratory emergencies remain the leading cause for parents to seek care for their children in the ED. Although most respiratory emergencies are mild and respond well to supportive care and anticipatory guidance, some will be life-threatening and require aggressive intervention and airway management. Respiratory emergencies are scary for all parties involved, including the patient, the family, and the healthcare practitioners.

Focusing on family-centered care and confidently managing the emergency will go a long way to decreasing the fear and anxiety that is present.

The ability to differentiate between respiratory distress, failure, and arrest is vital and begins as soon as you make visual contact with the patient. Prompt recognition and intervention in respiratory emergencies can make the difference between life and death.

## REFERENCES

American Heart Association. Part 4: pediatric basic and advanced life support. 2020 American Heart Association Guidelines for cardiopulmonary resuscitation and emergency cardiovascular care. https://cpr.heart.org/en/resuscitation-science/cpr-and-ecc-guidelines/pediatric-basic-and-advanced-life-support

Asmar BI. Bacteriology of retropharyngeal abscess in children. *Pediatr Infect Dis J.* 1990 Aug;9(8):595-597.

Campbell RL, Kelso JM. Anaphylaxis: emergency management. UpToDate. https://www.uptodate.com/contents/anaphylaxis-emergency-treatment?search=anaphylaxis&topicRef=106778&source=see_link#H26

Centers for Disease Control and Prevention. Most recent national asthma data. Last reviewed March 30, 2021. Accessed October 7, 2021. https://www.cdc.gov/asthma/most_recent_national_asthma_data.htm

Centers for Disease Control and Prevention. Pertussis (whooping cough). Last reviewed November 18, 2019. Accessed December 5, 2020. https://www.cdc.gov/pertussis/index.html

Centers for Disease Control and Prevention. Table 1: recommended child and adolescent immunization schedule for ages 18 years and younger, United States, 2021. Last reviewed February 2, 2021. Accessed October 7, 2021. https://www.cdc.gov/vaccines/schedules/hcp/imz/child-adolescent.html

Choi J, Lee GL. Common pediatric respiratory emergencies. *Emerg Med Clin North America.* 2012;30(2):529-563.

Cutrera R, Baraldi E, Indinnimeo L, et al. Management of acute respiratory diseases in the pediatric population: the role of oral corticosteroids. *Ital J Pediatr.* 2017;43(1):31. doi:10.1186/s13052-017-0348-x

Dinakar C. Anaphylaxis in children: current understanding and key issues in diagnosis and treatment. *Curr Allergy Asthma Rep.* 2012;12(6):641-649. doi:10.1007/s11882-012-0284-1

Dodson H, Cook J. Foreign body airway obstruction. In: StatPearls [Internet]. Treasure Island, FL: StatPearls Publishing; 2021. Updated July 26, 2021. https://www.ncbi.nlm.nih.gov/books/NBK553186/

Ebeledike C, Ahmad T. Pediatric pneumonia. In: StatPearls [Internet]. Treasure Island, FL: StatPearls Publishing; 2021. Updated August 12, 2021. https://www.ncbi.nlm.nih.gov/books/NBK536940/

Erickson EN, Bhakta RT, Mendez MD. Pediatric bronchiolitis. In: StatPearls [Internet]. Treasure Island, FL: StatPearls Publishing; 2021. Updated July 22, 2021. https://www.ncbi.nlm.nih.gov/books/NBK519506/

Goldstein NA, Hammersclag MR. Peritonsillar, retropharyngeal, and parapharyngeal abscesses. In: Feigin RD, Cherry JD, Demmler-Harrison GJ, Kaplan SL, eds. *Textbook of Pediatric Infectious Diseases.* 6th ed. Philadelphia, PA: Saunders, 2009: 177.

Hansen M, Meckler G, Lambert W, Dickinson C, Dickinson K, Guise JM. Paramedic assessment and treatment of upper airway obstruction in pediatric patients: an exploratory analysis by the Children's Safety Initiative-Emergency Medical Services. *Am J Emerg Med.* 2016;34(3):599-601. doi:10.1016/j.ajem.2015.12.082

Harless J, Ramaiah R, Bhananker SM. Pediatric airway management. *Int J Crit Illn Inj Sci.* 2014;4(1):65-70. doi:10.4103/2229-5151.128015

Heikkinen T, Järvinen A. The common cold. *Lancet.* 2003 Jan 4; 361(9351):51-59. doi:10.1016/S0140-6736(03)12162-9

McClay JE, Murray AD, Booth T. Intravenous antibiotic therapy for deep neck abscesses defined by computed tomography. *Arch Otolaryngol Head Neck Surg.* 2003 Nov;129(11):1207-12. doi:10.1001/archotol.129.11.1207

McDermott KW (IBM Watson Health), Stocks C (AHRQ), Freeman WJ (AHRQ). Overview of Pediatric Emergency Department Visits, 2015. HCUP Statistical Brief #242. August 2018. Rockville, MD: Agency for Healthcare Research and Quality. https://www.hcup-us.ahrq.gov/reports/statbriefs/sb242-Pediatric-ED-Visits2015.pdf

Milési C, Boubal M, Jacquot A, et al. High-flow nasal cannula: recommendations for daily practice in pediatrics. *Ann Intensive Care.* 2014;4:29. doi:10.1186/s13613-014-0029-5

Page NC, Bauer EM, Lieu JE. Clinical features and treatment of retropharyngeal abscess in children. *Otolaryngol Head Neck Surg.* 2008 Mar;138(3):300-306. doi:10.1016/j.otohns.2007.11.033

Pappas DE, Hendley JO, Hayden FG, Winther B. Symptom profile of common colds in school-aged children. *Pediatr Infect Dis J.* 2008 Jan;27(1):8-11. doi:10.1097/INF.0b013e31814847d9

Ralston SL, Lieberthal AS, Meissner HC, et al.; American Academy of Pediatrics. Clinical practice guideline: the diagnosis, management, and prevention of bronchiolitis. *Pediatrics.* 2014 Nov;134(5):e1474-502. doi:10.1542/peds.2014-2742

Richards AM. Pediatric respiratory emergencies. *Emerg Med Clin North Am.* 2016 Feb;34(1):77-96. doi:10.1016/j.emc.2015.08.006

Sicherer SH, Simons ER, Section on Allergy and Immunology. Epinephrine for first-aid management of anaphylaxis. *Pediatrics.* 2017 March;13(3):e20164006. doi:10.1542/peds.2016-4006

Tebruegge M, Curtis N. Infections related to the upper and middle airways. In: Long SS, Pickering LK, Prober CG, eds. *Principles and Practice of Pediatric Infectious Diseases*. 3rd ed. New York: Elsevier Saunders; 2012:205.

Thompson M, Vodicka TA, Blair PS, et al.; TARGET Programme Team. Duration of symptoms of respiratory tract infections in children: systematic review. *BMJ*. 2013 Dec 11;347:f7027. doi:10.1136/bmj.f7027. Erratum in: *BMJ*. 2014;347:f7575.

Turner TL, Kopp BT, Paul G, Landgrave LC, Hayes D Jr, Thompson R. Respiratory syncytial virus: current and emerging treatment options. *Clinicoecon Outcomes Res*. 2014;6:217-225. doi:10.2147/CEOR.S60710

Ungkanont K, Yellon RF, Weissman JL, Casselbrant ML, González-Valdepeña H, Bluestone CD. Head and neck space infections in infants and children. *Otolaryngol Head Neck Surg*. 1995 Mar;112(3):375-382. doi:10.1016/s0194-5998(95)70270-9

Wald ER. Retropharyngeal infections in children. UpToDate. Reviewed September 2021. https://www.uptodate.com/contents/retropharyngeal-infections-in-children

World Health Organization. Pertussis vaccines: WHO position paper—August 2015. *Wkly Epidemiol Rec*. 2015 August 28;35(90):433-460.

# CHAPTER 3

# Trauma

## LESSON OBJECTIVES

- Discuss the kinematics of pediatric trauma.
- Review the trauma triad of death.
- Identify the common types of injuries and their treatments.
- Discuss the management of pediatric trauma patients using the Pediatric Assessment Triangle and XABCDE approach.

## Introduction

Unintentional injury remains a leading cause of death in pediatric patients older than 1 year. Although there are myriad types of unintentional injury, the leading causes of death for pediatric patients throughout the years have consistently included drowning, motor vehicle crashes (MVCs), burns, and homicide. Males are almost twice as likely to die from unintentional injury than females.

It is estimated that 9.2 million children visit the emergency department (ED) annually due to unintentional injury (**Figure 3-1**). Injuries due to falls were the leading cause of nonfatal injury in pediatrics. Rates of nonfatal injury due to burns or falls were highest in children ages 4 and younger, whereas MVC-related and poisoning injuries were highest among adolescents (**Figure 3-2**).

It is possible to prevent many unintentional injuries. Even with advances in trauma care, prevention of unintentional injury remains the best method for reducing mortality and morbidity. EMS, fire, and first responder organizations are uniquely positioned in the community to take an active role in injury prevention, education, and response. As mentioned previously, historical data has identified the top causes of unintentional injury and death in pediatric patients. This allows local public safety organizations to institute community initiatives to educate citizens on the leading causes of death and how to prevent them. Specific areas of focus for local public safety organizations should include the following:

- Water safety awareness and swimming education
- The dangers of cosleeping and the importance of proper safe sleep practices in newborns and infants
- The proper use of vehicle restraint systems and proper installation of child safety seats appropriate for the height, weight, and age of the child
- Fire safety education
- Suicide awareness and prevention

Although eliminating unintentional injury completely is unlikely, reducing the burden of mortality and morbidity due to trauma and unintentional injury is possible. The responsibility for this rests with local public safety organizations and the community.

## Kinematics of Pediatric Trauma

Pediatric patients experience traumatic forces in different ways than adults. This is because anatomically they have different proportions, and psychologically, they may react in different ways than adults when experiencing a traumatic injury.

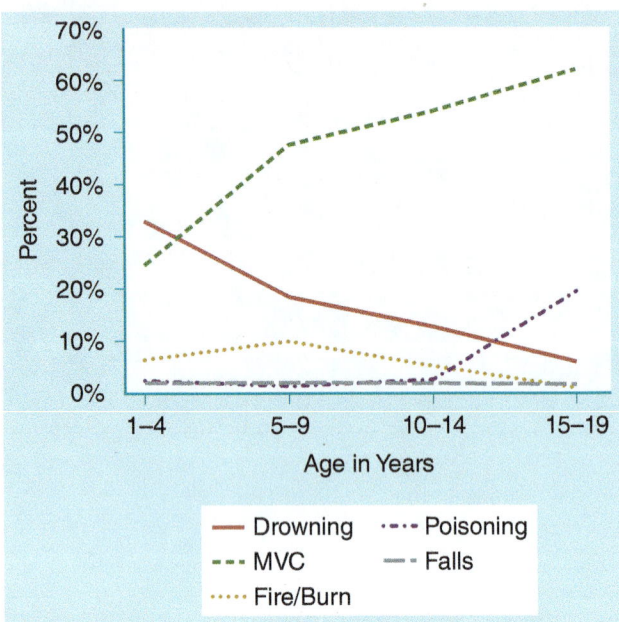

**Figure 3-1** Selected causes as percentages of total unintentional injury fatalities among children ages 1 to 19 years, 2019.

Data from Centers for Disease Control and Prevention. Leading causes of death reports, 2000–2019. WISQARS. https://wisqars.cdc .gov/fatal-leading.

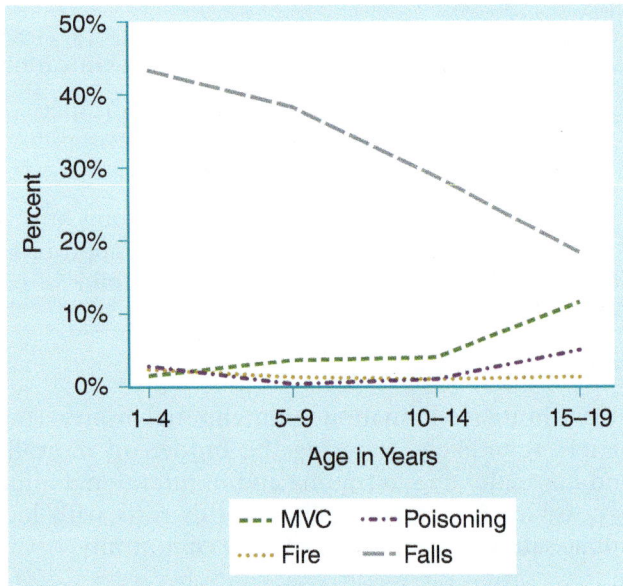

**Figure 3-2** Selected causes as percentages of total unintentional nonfatal injuries among children ages 1 to 19 years, 2019.

Data from Centers for Disease Control and Prevention. Leading causes of nonfatal injury reports, 2000–2019. WISQARS. https:// wisqars.cdc.gov/nonfatal-leading.

The smaller frame of pediatric patients results in less area for traumatic forces to dissipate over, and the forces experienced from traumatic blows are concentrated on a much smaller region. Pediatric patients also have less muscle mass and adipose tissue than adults, and their skeletons offer less protection to the internal organs than the fully ossified adult skeleton does. This results in more severe internal organ and tissue damage than seen in adults, with less visible outward signs of those injuries.

## Seat Belts and Motor Vehicle Crashes

It is estimated that 59% of child safety seats in the United States are improperly installed. Another study indicated than when infant car seats were utilized, only 5% of parents were able to install these devices properly without mistakes. When fatal injuries are suffered by children in motor vehicle crashes, up to 43% of them were improperly restrained. States with more stringent safety restraint laws and enforcement in general have lower fatality rates from motor vehicle crashes. When seat belts or child safety restraint systems such as car seats or boosters are improperly used, the risk for multisystem trauma is increased. Injuries to the head, neck, face, chest, abdomen, and lower spine may be exacerbated by improper use of safety restraint systems.

> **Child safety restraint systems are most effective when used properly and installed correctly. Incorrect usage may result in additional or more severe injury.**

## Falls

Pediatric fall injuries may differ from the typical patterns seen in adults. Compared to adults, pediatric patients have larger heads in proportion to their bodies. This gives them a higher center of gravity and makes falling headfirst much more likely. The likelihood of headfirst falls decreases over time as the pediatric patient's body becomes more proportional in adolescence and adulthood. Falls from a low height, less than the height of the patient, tend to result in upper extremity trauma or injuries to the face and neck. This is due to the patient trying to brace with outstretched arms or falling headfirst into objects. Falls from a medium height may result in more significant head and neck injuries, along with lower extremity trauma. When the height involved is significant, multisystem trauma is more likely. Head, neck, upper and lower extremity, and pelvic injuries are likely to be encountered. Internal organ damage resulting from the secondary impact of organs against bony structures also occurs.

## Bicycle Collision Injuries

A survey in 2019 asking parents how often their children wear proper protective equipment while riding a bicycle indicated that nearly 20% of children in that group never wore head protection while riding a bicycle. The statistics for helmet usage while riding a skateboard, scooter, or roller skating were similarly low. This is despite significant evidence that injury can be prevented or drastically reduced when protective equipment is used while riding bicycles, scooters, roller skates, and other wheeled toys.

When children are not wearing proper protective equipment, head, neck, face, and upper extremity injuries are likely to be encountered after a bicycle accident. When proper protective equipment is used, injuries to the head, neck and face may still be encountered, but will likely be less severe. Injuries to the upper extremities will likely be the more severe injuries encountered when personal protective equipment is used while playing with wheeled toys.

Frontal impacts on bicycles are often associated with a specific pattern of injury. Intra-abdominal injuries, particularly to the spleen and liver, are often encountered as a result of the abdomen striking the handlebars during the "up and over" sequence of events that happens with a head-on bicycle collision. Straddle injuries to the perineum and genitalia can result in significant injury. Labial tears, testicular fractures, and injuries to the penile shaft are all possible when the forces encountered during a straddle injury are significant. A complete examination, including the genitourinary system, is recommended when a straddle injury is suspected.

## The Trauma Triad of Death

Decades of research into trauma has consistently demonstrated that mortality and morbidity from traumatic injuries can be reduced by paying specific attention to three elements that are collectively referred to as the "trauma triad of death" (**Figure 3-3**):

- Hypothermia
- Acidosis
- Coagulopathy

Patient outcomes are improved when these three processes are mitigated. Patients have poorer prognosis, increased mortality and morbidity, and increased length of hospitalization when these three elements are not managed effectively.

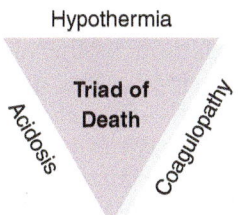

**Figure 3-3** The trauma triad of death.
© Jones & Bartlett Learning.

## Hypothermia

Unintentional hypothermia in the trauma patient may result from a number of factors. Patient exposure to assess and treat injuries, failure to cover patients after exposure for examination, and administration of large volumes of unwarmed fluids all contribute to decreased body temperatures. The environment in which the trauma occurs may also contribute to hypothermia.

Low temperatures directly impact the activity of platelets and the enzyme reactions necessary for effective clotting to occur. The more significant the hypothermia, the less effective the body's clotting mechanisms become. In addition, shivering to generate body heat increases metabolism and may worsen acidosis due to anaerobic energy production present with hypoperfusion encountered in trauma victims. This combination may further exacerbate coagulopathy.

> **Children are especially susceptible to excessive heat loss and hypothermia due to the increased body surface area in proportion to their weight when compared to adults.**

## Acidosis

The metabolic and enzymatic reactions that the human body carries out to sustain life require a tightly controlled biologic environment. The pH of the internal environment is a critical factor in allowing these reactions to proceed. When hypoperfusion is encountered at the tissue level, cells begin to transition to anaerobic respiration. This method of energy production is less effective and produces lactic acid as a byproduct. As lactic acid builds up, the body's buffer system becomes overwhelmed causing metabolic acidosis. Acidic conditions are not optimal for enzymatic reactions to proceed, and the ability to effectively clot is impacted significantly. Coagulopathy ensues.

Acidosis can also be exacerbated by overzealous administration of chloride-containing isotonic crystalloids, which results in a hyperchloremic metabolic acidosis in addition to the already underlying ischemic metabolic acidosis. The normal plasma concentration of chloride is maintained between 96 and 106 mEq/L (some labs may have a slight variance in established normal chloride range). Normal saline (0.9% NaCl) contains 154 mEq/L of both sodium and chloride. Even though the solution is isotonic, it contains a concentration of both sodium and chloride that is above normal serum values. Significant elevations in serum chloride concentration are possible when patients receive large amounts of fluid for volume resuscitation. Careful consideration should be given to the choice of isotonic crystalloid used for volume resuscitation.

## Coagulopathy

Coagulopathy is the final common pathway for the previously mentioned elements of the trauma triad. When patients are profoundly acidotic and hypothermic, underlying coagulopathy is significantly exacerbated. Trauma patients are already susceptible to coagulopathy due to consumption of clotting factors in response to bleeding and loss of plasma clotting factors with exsanguination. Additionally, aggressive fluid resuscitation with isotonic crystalloids may further dilute remaining clotting factors and contribute to poor clotting ability. Endothelial damage as a direct result of trauma is also a contributing factor.

When possible, a fluid strategy that balances isotonic crystalloid administration with aggressive administration of proportional amounts of blood products (packed red blood cells [pRBCs], fresh frozen plasma [FFP], and platelets) is preferred over isotonic crystalloid administration alone for volume resuscitation. Local institution policy and guidelines should be considered when pursuing these strategies. Local emergency medical services (EMS) agencies should partner with regional trauma centers and gain an understanding of what massive transfusion protocol and fluid resuscitation strategy is used in the ED so that EMS agency protocols can be integrated with initial hospital management.

Mitigating the effects of hypothermia and acidosis will aid in gaining control of runaway coagulopathy that can be seen in trauma patients.

## Managing the Triad

Aggressive hemorrhage control and management of airway, breathing, and circulation (XABC) are all key factors in mitigating the trauma triad of death. Controlling hemorrhage will decrease clotting factor loss and consumption—this is the reason why addressing exsanguination comes before airway, breathing, and circulation. It will also decrease the amount of fluid necessary to achieve adequate volume resuscitation.

Controlling hypothermia will make clotting more effective and aid in controlling hemorrhage and microvascular complications. Patient should not be left exposed any longer than is necessary to assess, examine, and treat an area. Warmed fluids should be administered whenever possible. The use of warm blankets and other heat-sparing devices such as circulating warm air or fluid blankets is also helpful to maintain normothermia.

Controlling acidosis will increase the effectiveness of the enzymatic reactions necessary for clotting. Ensuring that patients are given supplemental oxygen when necessary is important. Adequately managing the airway with both basic and advanced techniques

> **Damage control resuscitation (DCR) is an overall approach, rather than any single specific intervention. The aim is to keep the patient alive by managing all three aspects of the trauma triad of death.**

### TRANEXAMIC ACID (TXA)

**TXA is a drug that inhibits the body's natural process of clot breakdown (fibrinolysis). Although this medication is not approved for management of hemorrhage associated with trauma, the off-label use of TXA for the treatment and prevention of trauma-associated hemorrhage is becoming more common.**

**It is important to note that TXA does not promote clot formation, and it does not directly address any of the three elements of the trauma triad. Whereas coagulopathy may be indirectly addressed to a small extent by administering TXA, in the absence of coagulation factors necessary for clot formation, coagulopathy is likely to persist despite TXA administration. TXA administration is currently controversial in pediatrics, because limited data is available regarding its use.**

**In pediatric trauma patients with major trauma, hemodynamic instability, or significant risk for ongoing severe blood loss, TXA should be considered and administration guided by local protocols or in consultation with medical control.**

is another important component of mitigating hypoxia that may lead to acidosis. Special attention should be paid to respiratory rate in patients with advanced airways to avoid under- and overventilation. Close attention should be paid to fluid choice for volume resuscitation, and avoidance of iatrogenic acidosis should be targeted as a goal of initial management.

# Types of Injuries

Multiple injuries may be encountered in the pediatric patient. Trauma may be isolated (only one area injured) or multisystem (multiple different injuries to multiple different systems). In either case, it is important to consider the mechanism of injury (MOI), kinematics, and symptoms described by the patient to form a clinical suspicion of what types of injuries are present. Although many injuries may be obvious, keep in mind that some traumatic injuries may be subtle (such as seat belt marks, handlebar marks, etc.), and the effects of these injuries may not be appreciated until the child has significant morbidity or mortality.

## Hemorrhage

Bleeding can be divided into two types: internal and external. External bleeding may be easily seen, although in some cases it is only detected during a thorough physical exam. Internal bleeding is more difficult to diagnose, and it generally requires the practitioner to maintain a high index of suspicion, obtain an accurate history, and perform a careful physical exam. Knowing the mechanism of injury and other details will also help determine how significant the concern for internal bleeding should be.

### External Hemorrhage

External bleeding can be divided into three subtypes (**Figure 3-4**):

- Capillary
- Venous
- Arterial

Capillary bleeding occurs when the injury is superficial. The bleeding is slow and easily controlled. This type of bleeding responds well to direct pressure and will often stop spontaneously as the blood clots. A simple wound dressing is sometimes necessary to control capillary bleeding if the injury is extensive (e.g., large areas of road rash).

Venous bleeding occurs when the injury causes damage to venous structures below the dermis. Veins are low-pressure vessels and hemostasis can often be achieved with direct pressure and wound dressings.

## Types Of External Bleeding

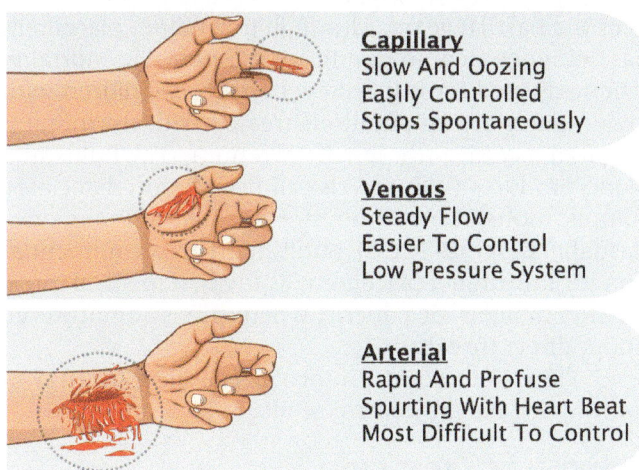

**Capillary**
Slow And Oozing
Easily Controlled
Stops Spontaneously

**Venous**
Steady Flow
Easier To Control
Low Pressure System

**Arterial**
Rapid And Profuse
Spurting With Heart Beat
Most Difficult To Control

**Figure 3-4** The three types of external bleeding are capillary, venous, and arterial.
© N.Vinoth Narasingam/Shutterstock.

The flow will often be steady, and blood may be darker when veins are involved. The blood flow in veins is passive; spurting or pulsatile flow is not seen with venous bleeding.

Arterial bleeding is the most difficult to control. Blood will usually be bright red and the flow will be pulsatile or spurting. The pressure in arteries is high and blood can be projected many feet away. This is the most difficult type of bleeding to control and will often require direct pressure.

In some cases, the trauma is so severe or is in a location in which it is not possible to stop the bleeding with direct pressure or a tourniquet. This is referred to as "junctional" hemorrhage and occurs at sites where the extremities connect to the torso. These injuries are often related to blasts, explosions, and heavy machinery accidents. The forces encountered are significant and the trauma often involves multiple systems. Controlling hemorrhage at sites of junctional bleeding is extremely difficult and these injuries carry a high rate of mortality and morbidity. Specially designed tourniquets for use at sites of junctional bleeding (junctional tourniquets) are available. Additional training and familiarization with these products is required before deploying them in the field. Discuss this with your organization's leadership and follow local policy and protocol when managing junctional hemorrhage.

### Tourniquets

Tourniquets are often associated with the control of arterial bleeding. It is important to note that tourniquet application is appropriate in any situation where bleeding is not controlled with the initial intervention of direct pressure, regardless of the suspected source (capillary, venous, or arterial). The early use of tourniquets for bleeding control in civilian EMS has been gaining favor over the past 10 years. Although tourniquet placement has demonstrated no significant difference in mortality when adjusted for Injury Severity Score, children with lower extremity amputations treated with tourniquets required significantly less intravenous (IV) fluids and blood products (reduced risk of transfusion-associated complications). The Committee on Tactical Emergency Casualty Care (C-TECC) published the recommendation for tourniquet placement as the first medical intervention in pediatric patients when care is administered under direct threat.

Follow your local protocols regarding the use of tourniquets for the control of bleeding.

### Hemostatic Dressings

The U.S. Food and Drug Administration has approved multiple forms of gauze impregnated with hemostatic agents to aid in hemorrhage control (**Figure 3-5**). These dressing require packing of the wound, which may not be allowed by protocol in many jurisdictions. It is important to read and understand the directions for the proper use of these dressings prior to deploying them in the field.

## Internal Hemorrhage

Internal hemorrhage is not readily visible on visual examination of the patient. The medical practitioner must develop a suspicion for internal bleeding based on the history, examination, and mechanism of injury. Pediatric patients are highly susceptible to internal organ damage (because of the organs' anatomic position and less adipose tissue) and bleeding because their bones are less rigid.

Any patient with signs of hemodynamic compromise in the setting of trauma should be presumed to have

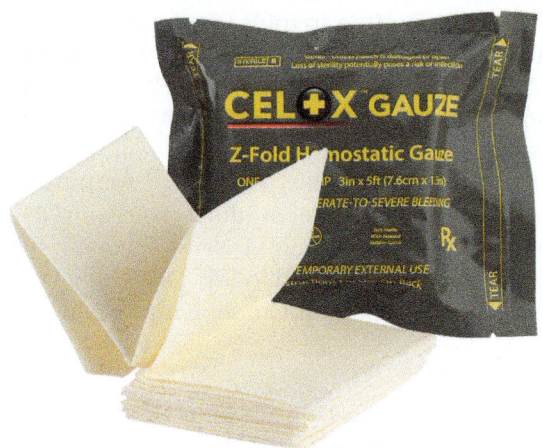

**Figure 3-5** Hemostatic gauze can aid in hemorrhage control.

internal bleeding until proven otherwise. Clues that internal bleeding may be present include tachycardia, tachypnea, delayed capillary refill, hypotension, and altered mental status. Hypotension is a late finding and signals that the patient is in extremis. Hypotensive patients are in circulatory failure and at high risk for cardiac arrest.

Internal hemorrhage is not managed in the field. The primary goals for prehospital treatment of internal hemorrhage are rapid recognition that the patient may have internal bleeding, initiation of transport without delay, and optimization of oxygenation and perfusion while en route to a destination with adequate surgical services to definitively care for the patient. Internal hemorrhage requires aggressive support and may require surgical intervention by physicians with specialized training in pediatric trauma and critical care. Take this into consideration when determining how and where you will transport the pediatric trauma patient with suspected internal bleeding.

> **Bleeding control is an essential task in trauma management. External bleeding should be controlled immediately when it is encountered. Internal bleeding may be subtle and cannot be controlled in the field. This type of bleeding requires rapid transport to a hospital with the specialized staff and services necessary to provide initial surgical care and medical stabilization for these patients.**

## Airway Injuries

The management of airway injuries is critical to ensure adequate ventilation and oxygenation of the pediatric patient. Direct trauma to the anterior neck, which is rare in pediatric patients, may result in airway obstruction.

Children running with objects in their mouth may fall and cause disruption to the tissues in the retropharyngeal space. This scenario is seen with objects such

> **A thorough history of trauma in the hours and days preceding the patient's presentation to emergency services is important. Direct trauma to the neck or interior of the oral cavity may result in airway obstruction. Early intervention for any airway obstruction is essential to ensure oxygenation and ventilation of the child.**

as popsicle sticks, pens or pencils, and other toys or objects that are long with a rigid tip. As the patient falls forward, the object is forced into the back of the throat as the front end strikes a hard surface. This results in tissue damage and bleeding. Hemorrhage in this area can cause further airway compromise.

Injuries in which a cable or other thin and rigid object encounters the face or neck with great force, commonly termed "clothesline" injuries, may be associated with tracheal or esophageal disruption.

Internal decapitation is also possible when the forces applied to the neck are sufficient. This has been seen in cases of children riding on the front of motorcycles or ATVs at high speed and coming into contact with cables that support telephone poles or laundry lines.

Burn injuries to the upper airway are especially severe and can progress rapidly to respiratory failure and arrest. Any patient injured in relation to a fire or smoke with singed nasal or oral mucosa should be assumed to have an upper airway burn. Early recognition in awake and alert patients and transfer to a pediatric burn center is essential. Patients with significant compromise may require video/direct laryngoscopy for placement of an endotracheal tube, which may be challenging based on the amount of edema.

Management of most airway injuries centers on early recognition. If the child is at risk for spinal injury based on the mechanism of injury or physical exam findings, spinal motion restriction should be utilized with airway management. In cases of minor airway trauma, minimally invasive treatments such as positioning, suctioning, and simple airway adjunct placement (oropharyngeal airway [OPA]/nasopharyngeal airway [NPA]) may be all that is needed to maintain adequate oxygenation and ventilation.

In cases in which the injury is more severe, advanced airway placement using a supraglottic airway (SGA) device may be required. Supraglottic devices have the advantage of allowing blind insertion, and they can be used to quickly establish a patent airway. SGA or bag-valve mask (BVM) will be effective in the majority of children requiring effective oxygenation and ventilation.

In cases where injury has caused foreign body airway obstruction (due to teeth or other objects), the use of an SGA device may not be possible. When significant swelling is present, SGA placement may cause further damage or fail to seat properly and establish a patent airway. This can be seen in burn cases or situations in which the patient has ingested a caustic substance.

Securing the airway with an endotracheal tube may be necessary in cases for which simple maneuvers are not successful, BVM is unable to support effective oxygenation and ventilation, an SGA is not appropriate, and the patient is at risk for respiratory failure leading to arrest. Carefully consider the nature of the injury and examine the patient for signs that airway disruption has occurred (tracheal asymmetry, subcutaneous emphysema, swelling around the neck). Be prepared for blood and foreign bodies (such as teeth) in the airway. Expect that the anatomy may be disrupted, and landmarks used for airway visualization may be displaced or obstructed. Airway management should be delegated to the most experienced person on scene and tools such as video or fiberoptic laryngoscopy should be used when available. Have a backup plan, such as a surgical airway, ready to go and discuss the progression of the procedure.

## AIRWAY MANAGEMENT

**Securing the airway in a severe trauma case is stressful, and the scene will likely be chaotic. It is appropriate to call a "time out" to focus the team and discuss the procedure briefly before proceeding. All team members should have a clear understanding of what actions will be taken during the procedure and what actions will be taken if the attempt fails. Basic airway maneuvers will be effective in most patients. Spinal immobilization should be maintained for any child with a concern for concomitant spinal injury. Bag-valve mask will be effective in the majority of children with ineffective oxygenation and ventilation. When ineffective, SGA or endotracheal intubation will be necessary.**

When advanced airway placement has failed, medical practitioners should be familiar with their "crash airway" algorithm for failed or impossible intubation. This algorithm should include surgical airway options such as needle or surgical cricothyroidotomy. The discussion about what will be done if the "impossible airway" is encountered should occur before the advanced airway attempt proceeds and preparations should be in place. When necessary, online medical control should be contacted.

## Chest Injuries

Chest injuries encompass both bony injuries and internal injuries. In children, a pneumothorax, hemothorax, or internal pulmonary injury may be present, even without evidence of external trauma, such as rib fractures or flail segments.

Understanding the negative-pressure physiology involved in respiration is important for the management of a pneumothorax or a tension pneumothorax. Normally, the pressure within the thoracic cavity is in balance with the pressure in the atmosphere. As the patient begins to breathe, negative pressure is generated in the chest and air from the atmosphere fills the lungs, bringing the pressures back into balance. Negative pressure in the chest during inspiration also causes increased right-sided venous return to the heart and momentarily increases preload. When the lining of the chest is disrupted, air will begin to occupy space inside the chest, outside of the lungs (pneumothorax). This compresses the lungs on the affected side and, if it continues to grow, it will begin to compress the mediastinal structures such as the great vessels and the heart. The negative pressure generated during inspiration leads to more air outside of the lungs, further compressing the thoracic and mediastinal structures. Right-sided preload that is normally generated during inspiration is eliminated and the passive preload of the heart generated by venous return is constricted. This leads to isolated right-sided heart failure that will quickly progress to left-sided heart failure if left untreated.

> **The key to treating a pneumothorax that causes respiratory and circulatory compromise is to reestablish the pressure gradient between the external atmosphere and the thoracic cavity. This is accomplished initially with urgent needle decompression. Definitive management requires chest tube placement.**

## Closed Pneumothorax

A closed pneumothorax occurs when the parenchyma of the lungs and pleura are disrupted, allowing air to escape into the thoracic cavity. Common causes of traumatic closed pneumothorax are listed in **Table 3-1**. This type of injury can happen spontaneously (no identifiable injury or cause) or traumatically. In cases of chest trauma, blunt force with sufficient energy anywhere on the ribcage can cause pneumothorax. Fractured ribs can also disrupt the tissues internally and lead to closed pneumothorax. A major risk factor for this condition is smoking (traditional and electronic cigarettes).

Patients with closed pneumothorax may have symptoms immediately after the injury, or the condition may present with progressively worsening symptoms over the course of minutes to hours following the injury. The most common symptoms include dyspnea,

| **Table 3-1** Common Traumatic Causes of Closed Pneumothorax |
| --- |
| Motor vehicle crash |
| ▪ Side impact |
| ▪ Head on with chest impacting the steering wheel |
| ▪ Ejection |
| ▪ Improperly restrained in car seat |
| Auto versus pedestrian injuries |
| Sports injuries |
| ▪ Fast moving objects such as baseballs or hockey pucks into the chest |
| ▪ Blunt trauma from baseball bats or hockey sticks |
| ▪ Player on player impact in football, soccer, lacrosse, or hockey |
| ▪ Falls from heights, which may be seen in gymnastics |
| Assault with blunt force trauma |

© Jones & Bartlett Learning.

low oxygen saturation, chest pain, and tachycardia. Exam findings include diminished breath sounds over the affected side and tracheal deviation (late finding). As the pneumothorax progresses and compresses the structures of the chest (tension pneumothorax), jugular venous distention, diminished perfusion, hypotension, and altered level of consciousness will occur. These are late findings.

Treatment for a closed tension pneumothorax includes immediate needle decompression of the affected side. This is usually done with a large-bore needle with a catheter inserted at the recommended site of the 4th or 5th intercostal midaxillary line. (The 2nd intercostal space, midclavicular line remains an optional site for pediatric patients; however, practitioners should use the site with which they are most familiar). An immediate rush of air may be heard, signaling you are in the correct area. The patient should experience immediate relief. A one-way valve or stopcock should be applied to the end of the catheter to allow for intermittent venting of the chest as air will continue to accumulate due to the underlying injury. Patients should be placed on high-flow oxygen via nonrebreather or have their ventilations assisted as appropriate. Use caution and avoid overinflation or high airway pressures during ventilation as these may exacerbate the underlying injury.

When performing needle decompression, it is important to insert the needle over the top of the inferior rib, as opposed to under the bottom of the superior rib. Each rib has a neurovascular bundle that follows a course along the inferior aspect of the bone and is protected by a small recess. When a needle is inserted under the rib, this neurovascular bundle is at increased risk of injury.

## Open Pneumothorax

When penetrating trauma to the chest disrupts the pleura, air from the atmosphere can rush into the thoracic cavity as negative pressure is developed in the chest during inspiration. Exhalation in the lungs is almost completely passive under normal physiologic conditions and relies primarily on the elastic recoil of lung tissues. This allows air to accumulate within the pleural space with each breath. Active exhalation is not effective in these cases as the air will simply enter back into the opening during subsequent inhalations. As air accumulates, it will begin to place pressure on the mediastinal structures, including the heart, trachea, and great vessels. This leads to decreased preload and reduced end diastolic volume within the left ventricle. The final outcome of these factors is obstructive shock and hemodynamic collapse.

Immediate treatment for open pneumothorax includes placing an occlusive dressing on the wound. It is important to note that the occlusive dressing should only be sealed on three sides. The fourth side should remain open in order to allow air to escape. The open side of the occlusive dressing should rest flat against the skin so that during active exhalation it allows air to escape, and during inhalation it seals to the chest and prevents air from entering.

### TENSION PNEUMOTHORAX

Pneumothorax, whether open or closed, has the potential to become a tension pneumothorax that shifts the mediastinal structures within the chest. When these structures are shifted, their points of attachment within the chest cavity are pulled tight. This leads to a buildup of tension on these structures and their

chest cavity attachments. When tension is present in the context of pneumothorax, obstructive shock develops. Once signs of obstructive shock and hemodynamic collapse are present, the term *tension pneumothorax* is used to describe the injury. Rapid recognition of this condition and using this term appropriately when giving a patient report alerts the receiving staff to the severity of the situation and allows them to prepare for a patient who is likely suffering from shock as a result of their injury.

## Hemopneumothorax

In certain cases of blunt or penetrating trauma, blood can accumulate in the pleural space in addition to air. This happens when blood vessels within the chest are injured and significant bleeding occurs. The result is called a hemopneumothorax. The clinical presentation of hemopneumothorax is similar to pneumothorax. Shortness of breath, respiratory distress, decreased oxygen saturation, and signs of obstructive shock may be present. Physical examination of the chest may reveal dullness to percussion, as opposed to a standard pneumothorax which has a tympanic response to percussion.

The treatment for this condition is similar to pneumothorax. When decompression is performed in the ED, there may be a large rush of blood in addition to

An alternative to needle decompression is finger thoracostomy. This procedure allows the medical practitioner to palpate the pleural space and lung parenchyma while decompressing the chest. This tactile feedback can also be used to judge how effective the decompression attempt was. It should be noted that this technique causes an open pneumothorax by definition and the practitioner should be prepared to manage this appropriately (occlusive dressing). In some cases, this technique may be more effective than needle decompression. Local policies and protocols should always be followed and performing this procedure requires extensive additional education and training.

air. When large amounts of blood are present, it is important to consider that hypovolemic shock may be present from a significant blood loss.

## Head Injuries

Traumatic brain injury (TBI) is the leading cause of mortality and morbidity in pediatric trauma. Pediatric patients have a proportionally larger head in relation to the rest of their body up until around age 6 years. The pediatric skull is relatively thin and not fully ossified, providing incomplete protection in cases of head trauma.

The leading causes of head injury in pediatric patients fall into three categories: falls, motor vehicle crashes, and nonaccidental trauma (NAT; injuries of abuse). Patients younger than 2 years are particularly susceptible to head injuries secondary to child abuse.

## Concussion

Concussion is often used to describe a diagnosis of mild TBI; however, it may be more accurate to use the term *concussion* to describe the clinical manifestations that are present after a mild TBI has occurred.

Concussion can be caused by any activity where a direct blow to the head, face, or neck has occurred. Any high-impact activity that causes blows to other parts of the body that are then transmitted to the head can also cause a concussion. Children and adolescents playing high-impact contact sports such as football, soccer, lacrosse, hockey, and/or wrestling are at increased risk of suffering concussion. Falls and other accidents not related to sports can also cause concussion.

It is estimated that 1.1 to 1.9 million sports-related concussions occur in individuals younger than 18 years in the United States every year. The rate of concussion reporting has increased over the last two decades as initiatives to increase recognition and treatment of concussion have grown. Most athletic programs are required to have return-to-play guidelines for athletes who may have sustained a mild TBI. These guidelines may necessitate that athletes who have specific symptoms, such as loss of consciousness, amnesia, or altered level of consciousness, be transported to a hospital for further evaluation.

The cause of concussion is related to shearing forces on the neural structures of the brain. These forces are most likely to be encountered with injuries involving rotational forces; however, any blow to the head can result in shearing of neural structures.

Concerning signs in concussion patients include seizure or loss of consciousness at the time of impact, amnesia, repetitive questioning, nausea, vomiting, altered mental status, or significant mechanism of injury.

The treatment for concussion requires a long-term, interdisciplinary approach, with a gradual return to activity prescribed by a physician specializing in concussion injuries. Treatment in the prehospital environment includes thorough assessment and examination for additional injuries; maintaining airway, breathing, and circulation; and frequent reassessment of mental status to quickly identify any alteration in mental status. Rapid transport to a hospital capable of caring for pediatric patients with TBI is also important.

## Intracranial Hemorrhage

There are four primary types of intracranial bleeds to consider (**Figure 3-6**). The injuries are named based on the location where bleeding is present:

- Epidural hematoma
  - The bleeding occurs between the dura and the skull (epi—"upon or over," dura—the outermost lining of the brain). This bleeding may occur with relatively minor trauma to the head. This trauma disrupts blood vessels (primarily arteries) running under the skull, and blood accumulates rapidly between the skull and dura.
  - Epidural hematoma injuries may produce a brief loss of consciousness following the injury. Following the loss of consciousness, a "lucid interval" may occur, where the patient appears to return to neurologic baseline. This lucid interval varies in length but is followed by acute deterioration in mental status as the injury progresses.

- Subdural hematoma
  - The bleeding occurs below the dura and above the arachnoid mater (sub—"under or below," dural—the outermost lining of the brain). This type of bleeding often results from rapid acceleration and deceleration of the brain.

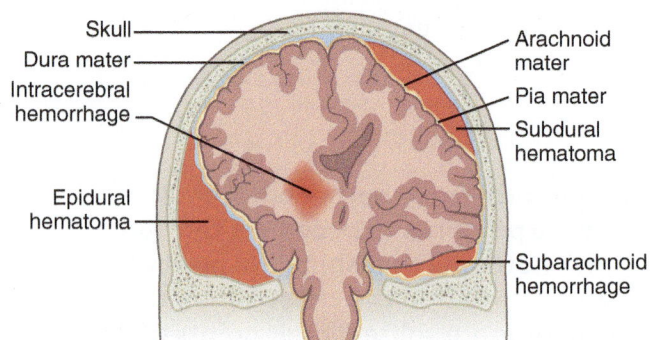

**Figure 3-6** The four primary types of intracranial bleeds: intracerebral hemorrhage, epidural hematoma, subdural hematoma, and subarachnoid hemorrhage.

© Jones & Bartlett Learning.

This rapid movement causes the bridging veins to shear with diffuse bleeding into the subdural space. This bleeding varies in intensity. The pediatric brain occupies nearly the entire volume of the skull (as opposed to elderly patients who have brain atrophy and volume loss) and even modest amounts of blood in the subdural space can cause increased intracranial pressure (ICP).

- This injury is pathognomonic for abuse when seen in children younger than 2 years without an explained mechanism of significant trauma (automobile accident, fall from height, etc.) or known bleeding disorder.

- Bulging fontanelles, emesis, and inconsolability are all signs that a subdural bleed may be present.

- Subarachnoid hemorrhage

  - The bleeding occurs below the arachnoid mater, but outside of the actual brain tissue (parenchyma).

  - Subarachnoid hemorrhage can be present in cases of abusive and accidental head trauma. Underlying medical conditions can also lead to spontaneous subarachnoid hemorrhage.

  - When the bleed occurs spontaneously due to ruptured aneurysm, a "thunderclap" headache, or "worst headache of my life" may be described. These headaches are often associated with pain out of proportion to the clinical exam, completely debilitating the patient. Signs of meningismus (stiff neck, photophobia, phonophobia) may be present.

  - The most significant risk factor for spontaneous (nontraumatic) subarachnoid hemorrhage is a family history. Connective tissue disorders such as Ehlers-Danlos, elevated blood pressure, sympathomimetic drug use, and cigarette smoking are also known to increase the risk of spontaneous subarachnoid hemorrhage.

- Intracerebral hemorrhage

  - This bleeding occurs within the actual brain tissue (parenchyma). Sometimes these bleeds are referred to as intraparenchymal hemorrhages. Significant head trauma can cause this type of injury, along with numerous underlying medical conditions and nontraumatic causes.

  - This injury may involve smaller vessels inside the brain and presents with a slow insidious process that is similar to stroke in adults.

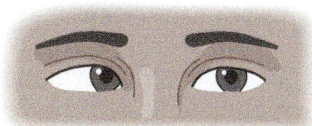

**Figure 3-7** Left CN VI palsy. Note how the patient's left eye fails to gaze laterally (abduct) due to failure of CN VI signaling to the lateral rectus muscle. The right eye is able to gaze medially (toward the nasal bridge) as the medial rectus muscle is controlled by CN III, which remains intact until much later during herniation syndromes.
© Jones & Bartlett Learning.

## Herniation and Cushing Reflex

When TBI leads to significantly elevated ICP, herniation of the brain through the foramen magnum is possible. As the pressure increases within the cranial vault, the brain tissue will be compressed to the point that it is pushed through the large opening at the base of the skull.

Headache and visual disturbance may be early signs of increased ICP. Cranial nerve (CN) VI (abducens) is highly susceptible to compression and CN VI palsy may be seen as herniation progresses (**Figure 3-7**).

As ICP increases, a triad of symptoms known as the Cushing reflex may be seen. Decreased cerebral perfusion leads to peripheral vasoconstriction and increased blood pressure. This dramatic rise in blood pressure is detected by baroceptors in the carotid bodies and a reflex bradycardia occurs in an effort to mitigate the hypertension. As herniation progresses, the respiratory centers in the brain are compressed, leading to altered respiratory patterns.

> **The Cushing reflex is a set of three findings:**
> - **Increased blood pressure**
> - **Decreased heart rate**
> - **Altered respiratory pattern**
>
> It is a late finding of herniation, and immediate steps to decrease ICP should be taken.

## Management

Resuscitation for TBI should be focused on optimizing ventilation, oxygenation, and perfusion in order to minimize further brain injury and prevent secondary brain injury. Hypotension is universally associated with worse outcomes.

Elevated ICP can be managed with osmotic diuretics such as mannitol. Hypertonic saline (3%) is also commonly used in the acute management of elevated ICP.

When signs of impending herniation are evident, controlled hyperventilation may be necessary. These signs include the following:

- Asymmetric or fixed and dilated pupils
- Extensor (decerebrate) posturing
- Acute neurologic deterioration (decrease by 2 or more points in Glasgow Coma Scale [GCS] score with initial score of <8)

End-tidal carbon dioxide ($ETCO_2$) should be used whenever possible, and targeted hyperventilation to achieve an $ETCO_2$ of 30 to 35 mm Hg has been shown to acutely decrease ICP while awaiting initiation of more definitive therapies such as osmotic diuresis, hypertonic saline administration, or surgery.

Recognizing that a TBI might be present is essential to management. Transport to a tertiary pediatric trauma center that has physicians trained in neurosurgery and trauma is essential to decreasing mortality and morbidity in these patients.

## Fractures

Fractures make up approximately 20% of pediatric traumatic injuries. Prior to the end of puberty, pediatric growth plates remain open and provide a weak point that is vulnerable to fracture when forces are applied. Pediatric tendons also tend to be stronger in comparison to the bones, making fracture more likely than sprain or strain when compared to similar mechanisms of injury seen in adult patients.

Common pediatric fracture sites include the following:

- Distal forearm
  - Fracture of the distal forearm accounts for approximately 25% of all pediatric fractures. These fractures occur when the patient falls forward or backward onto an outstretched arm. The distal ends of the radius and ulna are susceptible to injury. Patients with diminished grip strength, pain with squeezing, bruising, point tenderness, or pain with pronation/supination in the setting of recent fall or trauma may have a distal forearm fracture.
- Clavicle
  - The pectoral girdle is supported anteriorly by the clavicles. These bones are relatively thin and shaped like an "S" with narrow medial and lateral ends, making them susceptible to injury. Contact sports, falls, and MVCs are common causes of clavicle fractures. Signs that this fracture may be present include tenderness to palpation, obvious angulation or deformity, dropping of the shoulder, or pain reported by the patient. This injury accounts for approximately 11% of pediatric fractures.
- Distal humerus
  - Fractures in this location account for approximately 5% of pediatric fractures. This injury occurs when the patient falls back onto their elbow or an outstretched arm with sufficient force to break the humerus superior to the condyle, resulting in a supracondylar fracture. This area is particularly susceptible to fracture as it is one of the narrowest portions of the humerus. Patients will be reluctant to use the arm. Significant swelling on the posterior portion of the elbow may be present along with tenderness to palpation. This type of fracture may require surgical fixation.

Suspicion of a fracture cannot be made on mechanism of injury alone. Although significant mechanism of injury may raise the likelihood that a fracture is present, pediatric patients are susceptible to broken bones even when the forces applied are minimal. In some cases, the manner in which the force is applied contributes more to the fracture occurring than the magnitude of the force itself. Obvious angulation or deformity combined with recent trauma indicate that the extremity is fractured. More subtle clues include reluctance to use the extremity (cradling of the arm or refusal to bear weight), tenderness to palpation, bruising or discoloration, crepitus, and swelling. Fractures may be present despite the absence of all of these signs, and any concern warrants evaluation by a physician and imaging if appropriate.

The primary prehospital treatment for a fractured extremity is pain control and splinting. Continuous reassessment of neurovascular function and sensation distal to the fracture site is necessary to ensure that circulatory and sensory function remain intact. Transport to a facility with specialized pediatric orthopedic capabilities is important for definitive management.

## Burns

Approximately 25% of all burn injuries are in children younger than 16 years. The majority of these injuries occur in pediatric patients younger than 5 years. Child abuse, scalding liquids, and house fires are common sources of burn injury in pediatric patients. Electrical injury and chemical exposure may cause burn injuries that are severe and do not present in standard or expected ways.

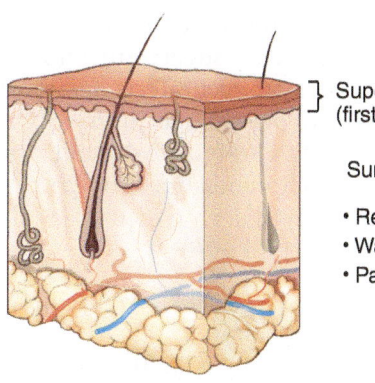

**Figure 3-8** A superficial burn involves only the epidermis. A mild sunburn is an example of a superficial burn.

© National Association of Emergency Medical Technicians (NAEMT).

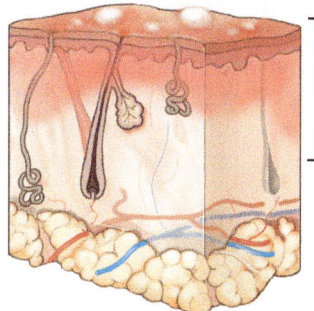

**Figure 3-9** A partial-thickness burn extends beyond the epidermis to portions of the underlying dermis. A scald injury is a common cause of a superficial burn.

© National Association of Emergency Medical Technicians (NAEMT).

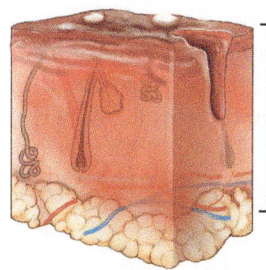

**Figure 3-10** Full-thickness burn.

© National Association of Emergency Medical Technicians (NAEMT).

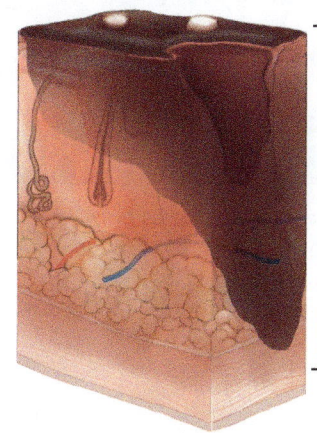

**Figure 3-11** Fourth-degree burn.

© National Association of Emergency Medical Technicians (NAEMT).

## Superficial Burns

Superficial burns involve only the epidermis (**Figure 3-8**). They are red and tend to be very painful as the nerve fibers are not damaged and sensory function is intact. Momentary contact with a hot surface or a mild sunburn are common causes of superficial burns.

## Partial-Thickness Burns

These burn injuries involve the epidermis and portions of the underlying dermis (**Figure 3-9**). Blisters, weeping, and peeling of the skin are usually present. Severe sunburns, momentary scald injuries from brief submersion or spilled hot liquids, and extended contact with hot surfaces are common causes of partial-thickness burns.

## Full Thickness and Subdermal Burns

When contact with a hot surface is prolonged, such as when a patient is entrapped or pinned under a hot object or next to a heat source, the burn may extend into the deepest layers of the dermis, leading to a full-thickness burn (**Figure 3-10** and **Figure 3-11**). If the

**Children may pull on the handles of pots or pans, leading to hot liquids spilling onto them. This exposure is different than submersion, although both injury types can be severe. Spilling hot beverages can also lead to scald injury. It is important to get as much history as possible and document your findings, as burn injuries may be the result of abuse.**

heat source is not removed and burning continues, layers of tissue below the dermis, such as muscle, fat, and fascia, may become involved—this is called a subdermal burn (**Figure 3-12**). Sources of these severe burn injuries include prolonged exposure to a heat source while entrapped, open flame or flammable liquid injury, and prolonged immersion in hot liquids.

## Burn Assessment

Assessing the airway of the burn patient is critical. Singed nose hairs, black sputum, or a burned oropharynx indicate that the patient is at high risk for airway compromise. Aggressive management of the airway takes priority in these situations. Burns to the chest and back can also compromise the patient's ability

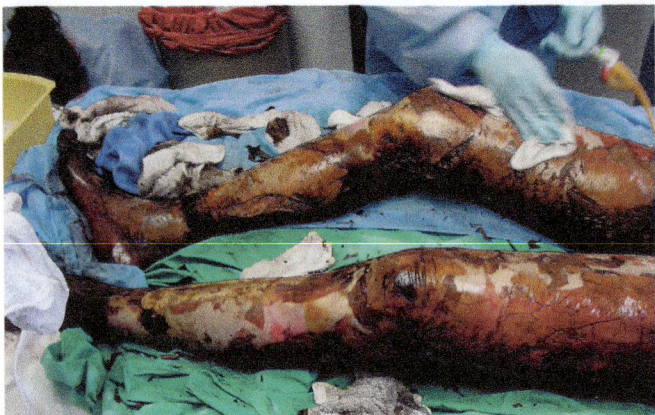

**Figure 3-12** Example of deep, full-thickness burn with charring of the skin and visible thrombosis of blood vessels.
Courtesy of Dr. Jeffrey Guy.

to breathe, as it will be painful to take full breaths and skin tightening may occur with severe burn injuries.

It is important to get an accurate estimate of the body surface area (BSA) percentage injured by each type of burn. The "rule of 9s" (**Figure 3-13**) and "rule of palms" may be used to help with this. The percentage of each area that has suffered each type of burn should be reported separately (**Figure 3-14**).

## Treatment

Scene safety and getting the patient to a safe area for treatment are the initial priorities in burn injuries. Stop the burning process by removing or eliminating the heat source if necessary. Clothing should be removed before it adheres to the patient. Carefully remove jewelry (it may still be hot to the touch) before swelling puts the patient at risk for strangulation of an extremity. Use nonadherent, dry, sterile dressings and cover the patient with a burn sheet if available. Burn patients will have trouble with thermoregulation and are at significant risk for hypothermia. Control the temperature

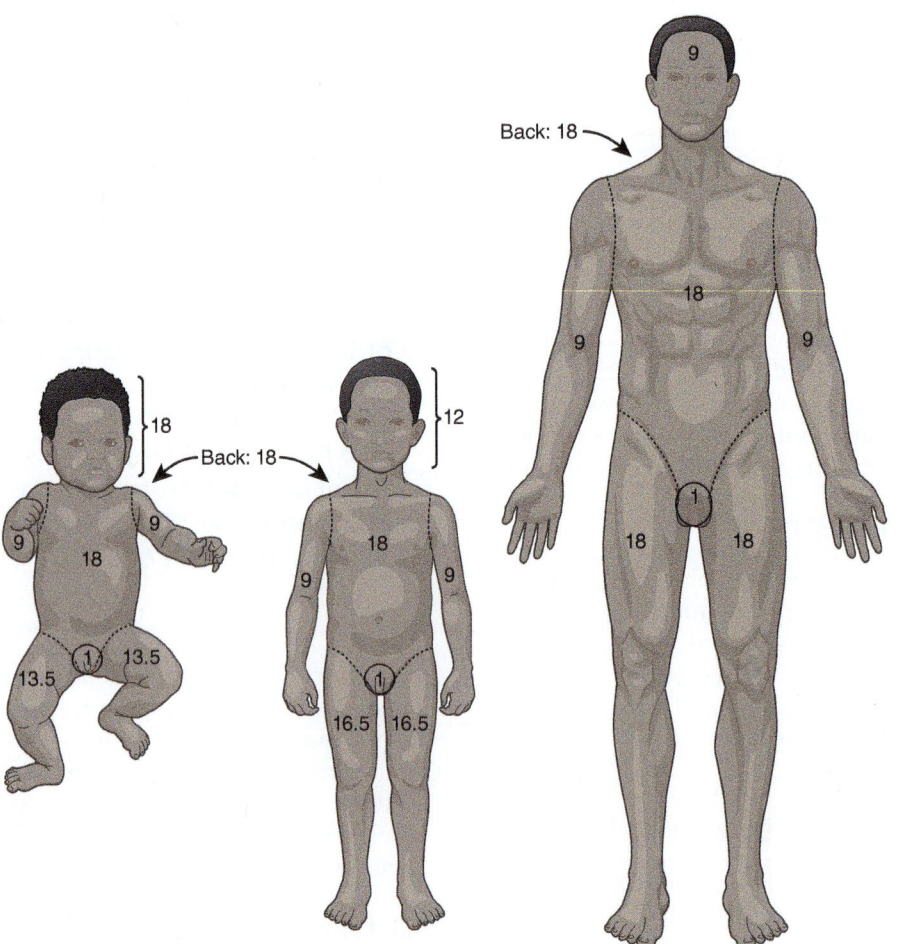

**Figure 3-13** Rule of nines.
© Jones & Bartlett Learning.

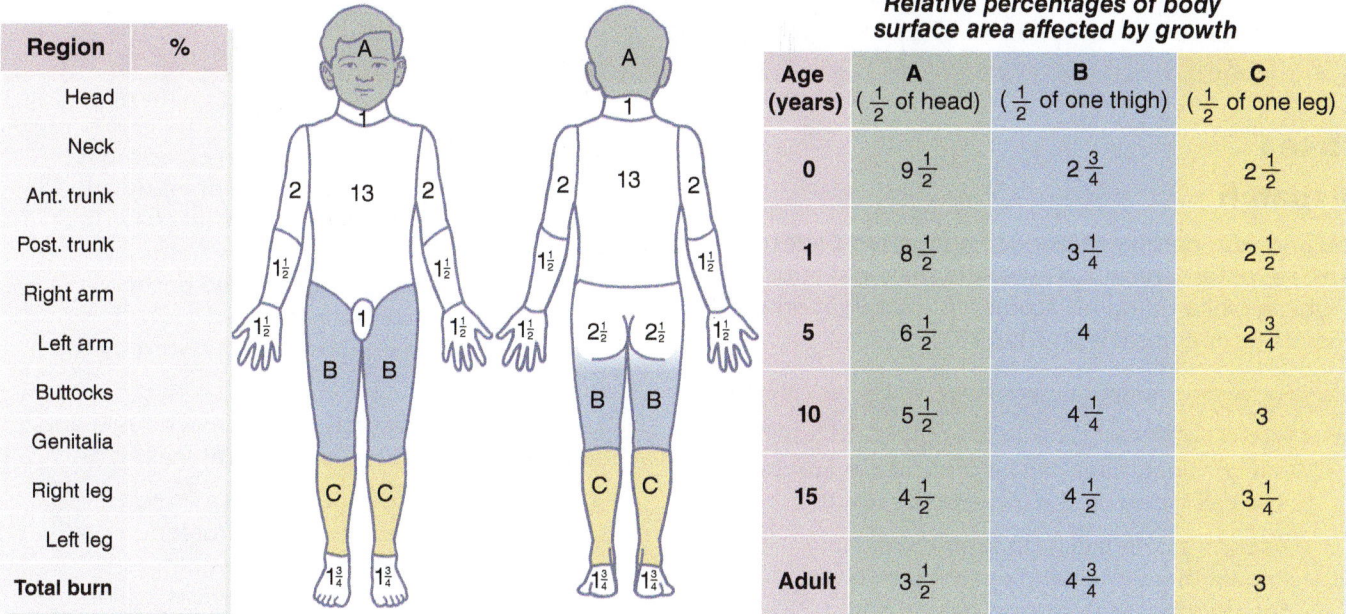

| Region | % |
|---|---|
| Head | |
| Neck | |
| Ant. trunk | |
| Post. trunk | |
| Right arm | |
| Left arm | |
| Buttocks | |
| Genitalia | |
| Right leg | |
| Left leg | |
| **Total burn** | |

**Relative percentages of body surface area affected by growth**

| Age (years) | A ($\frac{1}{2}$ of head) | B ($\frac{1}{2}$ of one thigh) | C ($\frac{1}{2}$ of one leg) |
|---|---|---|---|
| 0 | $9\frac{1}{2}$ | $2\frac{3}{4}$ | $2\frac{1}{2}$ |
| 1 | $8\frac{1}{2}$ | $3\frac{1}{4}$ | $2\frac{1}{2}$ |
| 5 | $6\frac{1}{2}$ | 4 | $2\frac{3}{4}$ |
| 10 | $5\frac{1}{2}$ | $4\frac{1}{4}$ | 3 |
| 15 | $4\frac{1}{2}$ | $4\frac{1}{2}$ | $3\frac{1}{4}$ |
| Adult | $3\frac{1}{2}$ | $4\frac{3}{4}$ | 3 |

**Figure 3-14** The Lund-Browder chart is useful for estimation of the total body surface area (TBSA) that has been burned.

Modified from Lund, C. C., and Browder, N. C. Surg. Gynecol. Obstet. 1944; 79:352-358.

## CALCULATING FLUID NEEDS USING THE PARKLAND FORMULA

Using the Parkland burn formula to calculate the fluid requirement in a burn patient is an important skill. The formula and an example of how to use it for a burn patient follow:

24-hour fluid total = 4 mL/kg × body weight in kg × %TBSA burned

Half of the 24-hour fluid total should be administered in the first 8 hours.

Example:

An 8-year-old patient weighing 32 kg has suffered full-thickness burns over 30% of his body after pot of hot oil spilled onto him in the kitchen. How much fluid should he receive in the next 24 hours? How much of that fluid should be administered within the first 8 hours?

4 mL/kg × 32 kg × 30% TBSA = 3,840 mL of fluid in the next 24 hours

3,840 mL / 2 = 1,920 mL to be administered in the first 8 hours following the injury

of the environment and use blankets on the burn dressing if necessary to help the patient maintain body heat.

Fluid resuscitation to account for increased insensible losses is critical in the first 24 hours following a burn injury. The Parkland burn formula is one notable guide to help direct initial fluid administration.

Pediatric patients will have lower glucose reserves and an increased metabolic demand following a burn injury, leaving them at risk for hypoglycemia. Patients smaller than 20 kg should receive 5%

dextrose in lactated Ringer's solution as a resuscitation fluid. Lactated Ringer's solution is preferred to normal saline because it can mitigate the effects of hyperchloremic metabolic acidosis that are seen when large volumes of 0.9% normal saline are administered.

Pain management is critical in managing burn injuries. Fentanyl is a good option for pain control. Morphine can also be used if the patient's blood pressure and respiratory rate are sufficient.

# CASE STUDY

## Case 1

### Dispatch

You and your partner respond to a reported pedestrian versus a motor vehicle. A 10-year-old male was struck by a vehicle while riding his scooter in his neighborhood. Outside temperature is 84°F (28.9°C).

### Case Questions

- What considerations can be discussed en route to the call based on the dispatch information?
  - As soon as this call is dispatched and it is known that a pediatric patient is involved, the responding personnel should begin thinking of appropriate transport destinations for pediatric multisystem trauma. Discuss appropriate destinations with your partner. Consider the distance and transport times to these destinations based on traffic and other factors. Remember that transport destination, method, and the decision to initiate rapid transport should be made early in the case and with minimal delay.

- What are your initial concerns about scene safety?
  - The initial concerns in this case primarily involve scene safety and size-up. Traffic control will be an issue. Take care to position the responding apparatus appropriately to provide cover for responding personnel as they work. It is also important to position transport units in such a way that they can easily exit the scene and not get blocked in. In some cases where automobiles have struck pedestrians, particularly children, a crowd can gather and may become agitated. Having police backup to help control bystanders and allow responders to work with minimal distraction or interruption is helpful.
  - Ensuring that fire and rescue backup is on the way, if not part of the initial response, is also important. Fire apparatus can provide good cover for EMS operations and protect the scene from inattentive drivers. Rescue operations may be necessary if the patient is pinned beneath a vehicle or requires some sort of extrication.

- Assess the scene carefully as you approach and identify the mechanism of injury and the different injury patterns that may be encountered based on the nature of the accident, size and speed of the vehicles, and surfaces involved. Note if any protective equipment was worn by the patient.

- What personal protective equipment (PPE) and equipment should be used on this call?
  - PPE for this case should involve standard precautions, eye and splash protection at a minimum. Basic trauma equipment, including bleeding control devices, splints, basic and advanced airway tools, and spinal immobilization devices, should be taken to the patient's side.

### Initial Observations

As you arrive on scene you note that it is a quiet residential street with minimal traffic. You position the ambulance to protect the scene. As you and your partner are gathering equipment, the father of the patient and the driver of the vehicle come rushing to the ambulance. They look panicked and keep repeating, "He's bleeding so much! He's losing a lot of blood!" You approach the patient and see a 10-year-old male lying supine on the ground, crying loudly, with a large pool of blood around his right leg (**Figure 3-15**).

- Pediatric Assessment Triangle
  - Appearance
    - Alert and restless
  - Work of breathing
    - The patient has rapid, shallow, and equal respirations.
    - **F**laring not present
    - **R**etractions not present
    - **A**udible airway noises—no abnormal sounds noted on initial observation
    - **P**ositioning—the patient does not appear to be tripoding or otherwise positioning his airway
  - Circulation
    - Skin pale and diaphoretic

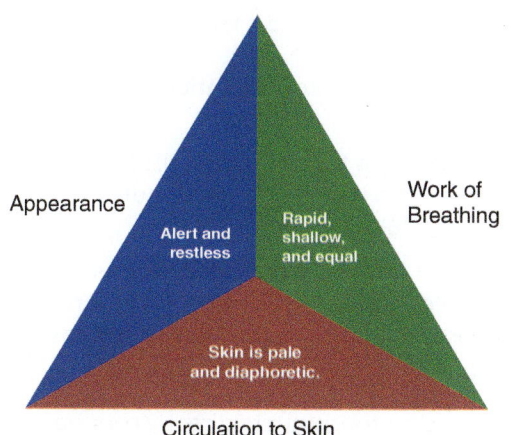

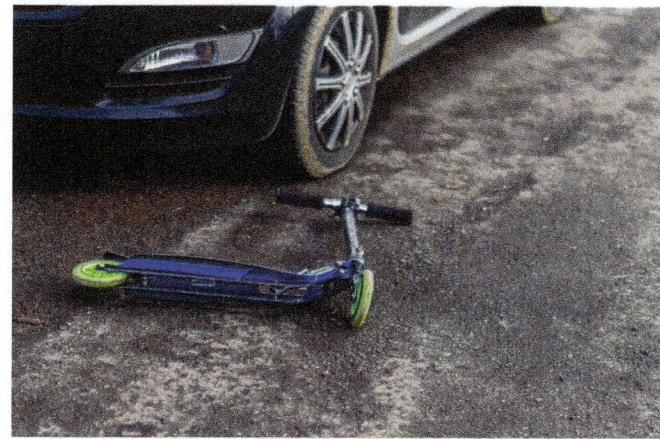

**Figure 3-15** The patient is a 10-year-old male who was struck by a motor vehicle.

Used with permission of the American Academy of Pediatrics, Pediatric Education for Prehospital Professionals, © American Academy of Pediatrics, 2000; © Animaflora PicsStock/Shutterstock

## Case Questions

- Based on your initial impression, is this patient "Quick" or "Not Quick"?

  - This patient is "Quick."

  - The pale and diaphoretic skin indicates that the patient has some element of hypoperfusion he is trying to compensate for. In the setting of large blood loss from the right leg, the presentation is compelling for evolving hypovolemic shock.

  - The rapid, shallow breathing is an indication that the patient is compensating for blood loss and decreased oxygen delivery to the peripheral tissues by increasing minute ventilation.

- Have you identified any possible red flags?

  - The major red flags in this case are obvious blood loss and poor perfusion.

## Primary Survey

The primary survey for this patient reveals the following:

**X**—Pulsatile bleeding from a right open femur fracture.

**A**—Open, screaming in pain.

**B**—Respiratory rate is estimated to be about 30 breaths/min with rapid and shallow respirations.

**C**—Radial pulses are weak and thready. Capillary refill time is delayed. The patient's skin is pale, diaphoretic, and clammy.

**D**—Alert and restless; GCS score is 15 (E4, V5, M6).

**E**—The patient is lying supine on the pavement. Bruising is noted on the abdomen. There are multiple abrasions and lacerations from road rash.

## Case Questions

- Based on the findings noted in the primary survey, what would your initial interventions and treatment include?

  - Treatment should focus on identifying and controlling immediately life-threatening conditions.

  - Bleeding control should be the initial priority. The patient's respiratory distress is a result of hypoperfusion due to blood volume loss. The decision on how to best control this bleeding will vary based on available resources and local protocol. Dressing a wound over an open fracture will be painful and possibly ineffective. Medications for pain control might not be an option if the patient's blood pressure is decreased. A tourniquet may be the best option for reliable bleeding control in the most rapid fashion.

  - Based on the mechanism of injury, spinal motion restriction will be required for this patient. He will be unable to reliably articulate if he has head, neck, or back pain due to the distracting leg injury.

  - Treatment for shock should be initiated in tandem with bleeding control when possible.

This would include placing the patient on high-flow oxygen via nonrebreather or assisting ventilations if respiratory effort is inadequate.

- IV access should be initiated with two large-bore IVs if possible. IV fluid boluses of isotonic crystalloids should be given. A pediatric fluid bolus is 20 mL/kg. The patient may require multiple boluses to maintain adequate perfusion. If a patient requires more than 40 to 60 mL/kg, let the receiving hospital know, as blood products may be needed.

- Any additional assessment or treatment on non–life-threatening injuries should take place once immediately life-threatening injuries have been addressed.

## Tourniquet Use

When should a tourniquet be used?

- Any time there is arterial or heavy venous bleeding that is not controlled by application of a pressure bandage, applying a tourniquet is appropriate. If applying a pressure dressing is not practical or the bleeding is so severe that immediate and reliable control is necessary to prevent the loss of life or limb, moving straight to tourniquet use prior to attempting a pressure dressing is reasonable.

- Amputations of an extremity will typically require immediate tourniquet application to control bleeding.

- In any case where signs of shock or other life threats are present secondary to heavy bleeding and a limited number of practitioners are available, immediate application of a tourniquet may be necessary. This would include mass-casualty incidents or other large-scale disasters.

When should a tourniquet not be used?

- When bleeding is minor and it can be controlled with pressure dressings or other readily available means, application of a tourniquet is not necessary.

- Junctional trauma at the neck, axillae, or groin may not be amenable to tourniquet application. Packing or direct control of bleeding may be preferred in these situations. Specially designed junctional tourniquets are available for trauma

in these locations and may be available in some systems.

What additional considerations are there for tourniquet use?

- Windlass-style tourniquets must be cinched tight prior to tightening the windlass device (**Figure 3-16**).

- When properly applied, distal pulses should not be palpable. Application of a second tourniquet may be necessary to achieve this in some cases.

- Do not use tourniquets over joints or bulky clothing.

- Avoid using tourniquets directly over fractures.

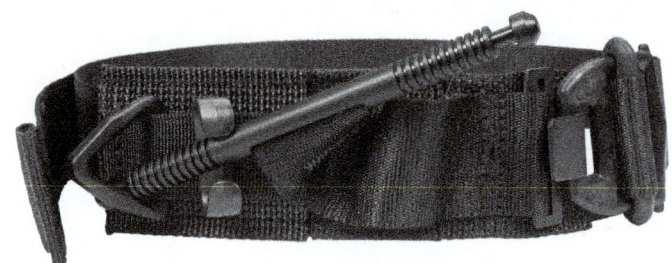

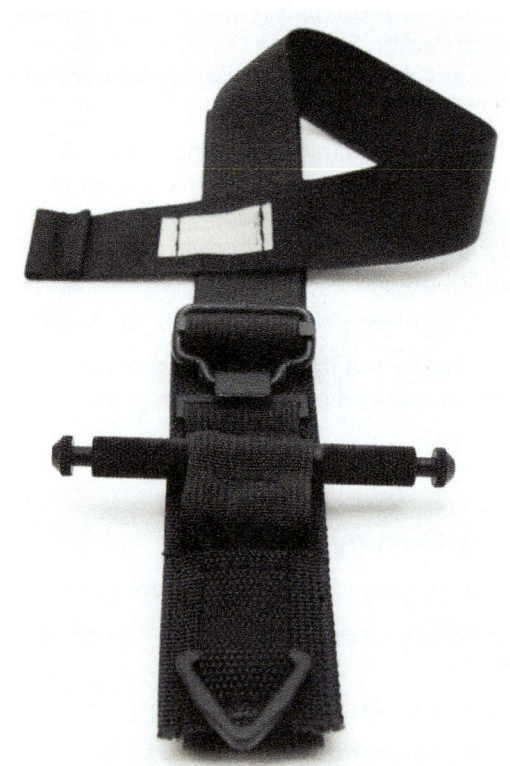

**Figure 3-16** Many tourniquets have a windlass device to tighten the tourniquet.

- Once a tourniquet has been applied, it should not be released until it has been assessed by a physician at the receiving facility.
  - Releasing a tourniquet after application could potentially lead to ongoing bleeding or microthrombi and toxic metabolites entering the circulation.
- Tourniquet application will likely be very painful and medications for analgesia may be necessary. This must be balanced with the potential blood pressure effects seen with certain analgesic medications.

Most of the literature for tourniquet use is focused on previously healthy adult soldiers in war zones, and large-scale trials in pediatric patients to demonstrate efficacy and safety are limited for obvious reasons. There are, however, multiple individual case reports of tourniquets being used effectively in pediatric patients (**Figure 3-17**). The Pediatric Trauma Society has issued guidance in support of tourniquet use for children with severe uncontrolled extremity hemorrhage.

Some tourniquets may be too large for effective application in smaller children. Always follow the manufacturer's guidelines for limb circumference and patient size and weight. Sufficient pressure must be applied (exceeding systolic blood pressure) in order to stop blood flow to the site of injury. Remember that the end goal is to stop exsanguinating hemorrhage and maintain perfusion to vital organs and tissues. Meeting this goal provides the best chances for survival in pediatric trauma.

## Detailed Assessment

### History Taking

After taking measures to control bleeding and provide respiratory support, you begin to take additional history, which reveals the following:

**OPQRST:**

- **O**nset—Immediately after being struck by a car

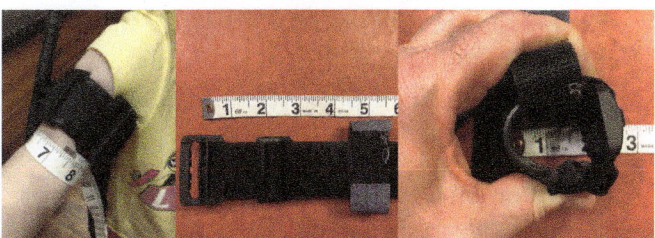

**Figure 3-17** The picture shows a 6-year-old female with tourniquet, the tourniquet length in inches, and the smallest circumference that can be achieved with tourniquet fully cinched.

Courtesy of Jonathan Willoughby.

- **P**rovocation/palliation—Movement
- **Q**uality—Sharp
- **R**adiation—None
- **S**everity—10/10
- **T**iming—Injury occurred approximately 5 minutes ago.

**SAMPLER:**

- **S**igns/symptoms—Obvious open fracture of the right femur. The bleeding has been controlled with a tourniquet. There is significant bruising to the abdomen. Multiple abrasions and lacerations are noted with no active bleeding.
- **A**llergies—No known allergies to medications, foods, or the environment
- **M**edications—None
- **P**ast medical history—None
- **L**ast oral intake—Pizza and a juice box approximately 1 hour ago
- **E**vents leading up to the emergency—The patient was riding his scooter when he crossed the street and was struck by a car traveling approximately 25 mph.
- **R**isk factors—None

## Case Questions

- Why do trauma patients require continuous reevaluation?
  - Pediatric trauma patients can decompensate rapidly. They tend to compensate well initially, and then rapidly deteriorate, as opposed to a more gradual deterioration that may be seen in adults. There may also be other injuries that were not obvious on the primary survey, which may begin to evolve and declare themselves during the call.
- What additional measures could be taken to help calm this patient?
  - Allowing the patient's family member to ride with him in the patient compartment when safe and allowed by policy can help to calm the patient. Providing guidance for breathing control and distraction with videos or games on a phone or other mobile device may also be helpful. Pharmacologic pain control and anxiolysis may be necessary but should be used with caution as it can negatively impact blood pressure and reparatory effort.

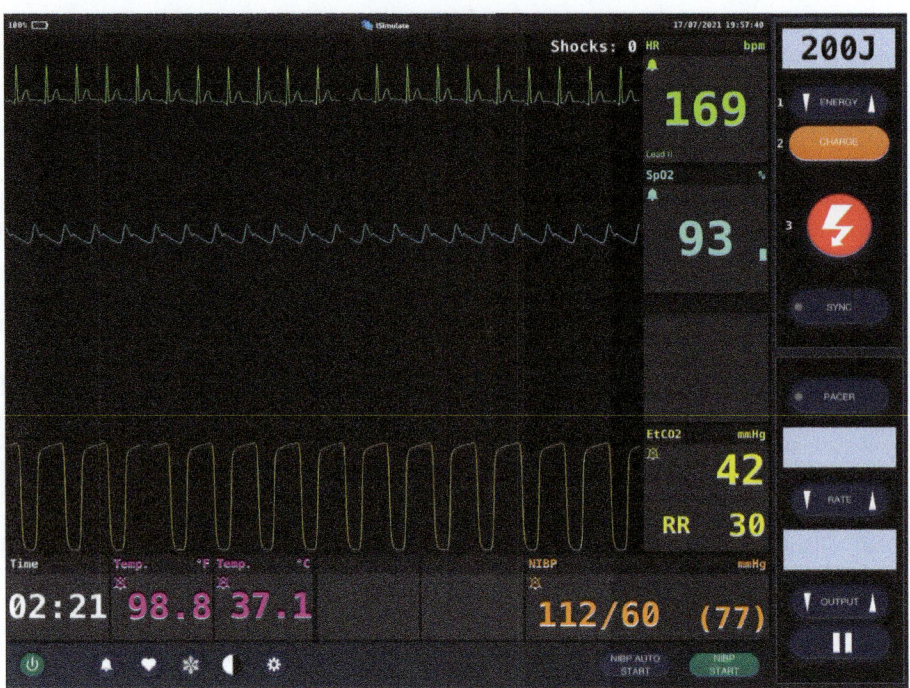

**Figure 3-18** Monitor display of patient's vital signs.
Courtesy of iSimulate.

## Vital Signs

As you were discussing the history, the patient was attached to the monitor and the following vital signs were obtained (**Figure 3-18**):

**Heart rate:**

- 169 beats/min
- The expected heart rate for a patient of this age is 60 to 100 beats/min. This patient is clearly increasing his cardiac output in an attempt to compensate for decreased peripheral perfusion and hypovolemia due to blood loss.

**SpO$_2$:**

- 93% on room air (RA). Improves with oxygen via nonrebreather.
- Providing supplemental oxygen to this patient is important to help mitigate the effects of hypoperfusion to the peripheral tissues. While avoiding peripheral tissue hypoxia is important, it must be balanced with the goal of limiting hyperoxia and the free radical damage that comes with it. Remember that goal oxygen saturations are 94% to 99%. If the patient is persistently saturating at 100%, it may be necessary to wean the supplemental oxygen or deescalate to a more appropriate delivery device (switch to nasal cannula).

- SpO$_2$ monitoring may be difficult when extremity perfusion is altered due to the body's physiologic response and compensatory mechanisms for shock. Always consider the complete clinical picture.

**ETCO$_2$:**

- 42 mm Hg

**Respiratory rate:**

- 30 breaths/min
- The patient is tachypneic and increasing his minute ventilation in an effort to increase oxygenation to the peripheral tissues in the face of decreased peripheral perfusion.
- Tachypneic patients may also have underlying abdominal injury that decreases the inhaled tidal volume with each breath due to pain or compression of the thoracic cavity from blood accumulation.
- If the patient is tachypneic with breaths that have decreased volume, consider the cause of the diminished tidal volume. Always carefully assess the abdomen and determine if abdominal injury is playing a role in the patient's respiratory distress.

**Blood pressure:**

- 112/60 mm Hg
- The patient's blood pressure is appropriate at this time, indicating that he is in compensated shock.

The delayed capillary refill, and cool, clammy, and diaphoretic skin reinforce this assessment.

- Blood pressure alone is not an indicator of shock, and this patient's entire clinical picture of normal blood pressure in the face of decreased peripheral perfusion is an ominous sign. Even though compensation is adequate currently, rapid deterioration is possible once the patient's compensatory mechanisms are exhausted.

- While permissive hypotension has been discussed as a management strategy in adult trauma victims, there is no literature to support the use of this strategy in pediatric patients. Pediatric patients do not tolerate drops in blood pressure like adults do, and rapid hemodynamic collapse is likely if blood pressures are allowed to linger below established normal values when shock is present.

- Recognition that this patient is at risk for impending hemodynamic collapse is the first step toward preventing rapid deterioration. Immediate intervention must be taken as this is a life-threatening finding.

**Temperature:**

- 98.8°F (37.1°C)

- Hypothermia is a part of the trauma triad of death, and maintaining normal body temperature is important in this patient.

- Warm blankets and warmed IV fluids may be necessary to maintain normal body temperature.

**Blood glucose:**

- 104 mg/dL (5.8 mmol/L)

- Patients who are stressed will have a catecholamine release that can raise the blood glucose level precipitously.

**Weight:**

- 35 kg

- It is important to quickly think about what weight-based medications and dosages you may need for this patient if they decompensate. It may be reasonable to quickly jot down or calculate code dosages of medications if time permits.

- The appropriate volume for a 20 mL/kg bolus for this patient is 700 mL.

This is a previously healthy 10-year-old male who was struck by a vehicle traveling approximately 25 mph, resulting in an open femur fracture of the right leg and large-volume blood loss. He is alert and oriented at this time and in significant pain. His airway is open and intact, and he has signs of respiratory distress—possibly due to pain, although trauma to the thoracic or abdominal cavity is not excluded at this time. The patient is exhibiting signs of compensated hypovolemic shock and is at high risk for rapid deterioration.

The bleeding has been controlled by a tourniquet to the right extremity and the patient is on oxygen via nonrebreather. He should be immobilized and rapid transport should be initiated, with a detailed exam and continuous reassessment en route to the appropriate transport destination.

## Detailed Exam

**HEENT:**

- **H**ead: Minor abrasions present. No major trauma or injuries noted.

- **E**yes: Pupils are equal, round, reactive to light (PERRL).

- **E**ars: Unremarkable, no drainage or fluid noted

- **N**ose: Unremarkable, no drainage or fluid noted

- **T**hroat: Unremarkable

**Chest, heart, and lungs (Figure 3-19):**

- Pulses: Peripheral pulses are palpable. They are rapid and thready. The patient is tachycardic.

- Cardiac auscultation: Regular rate and rhythm with no rub, gallop, or murmur noted.

- Lung auscultation: The lungs are clear to auscultation bilaterally. Breath sounds are equal.

- Chest exam: Chest wall movement is symmetric. There is no injury noted to the chest on visual inspection.

**Neurologic:**

- Distal pulses are absent in the right lower extremity secondary to tourniquet application.

- Neurovascular status in the remaining extremities is intact.

- The patient's level of consciousness is appropriate; he does not appear to have an altered level of consciousness.

**Abdomen and pelvis:**

- Bruising, rigidity, distention, and diffuse tenderness to palpation are noted on the abdomen.

- The pelvis is stable.

**Extremities:**

- Upper extremities: Minor abrasions and lacerations noted. No active bleeding. Radial pulses palpated bilaterally. Noted to be rapid and weak.

**Detailed Physical Exam**

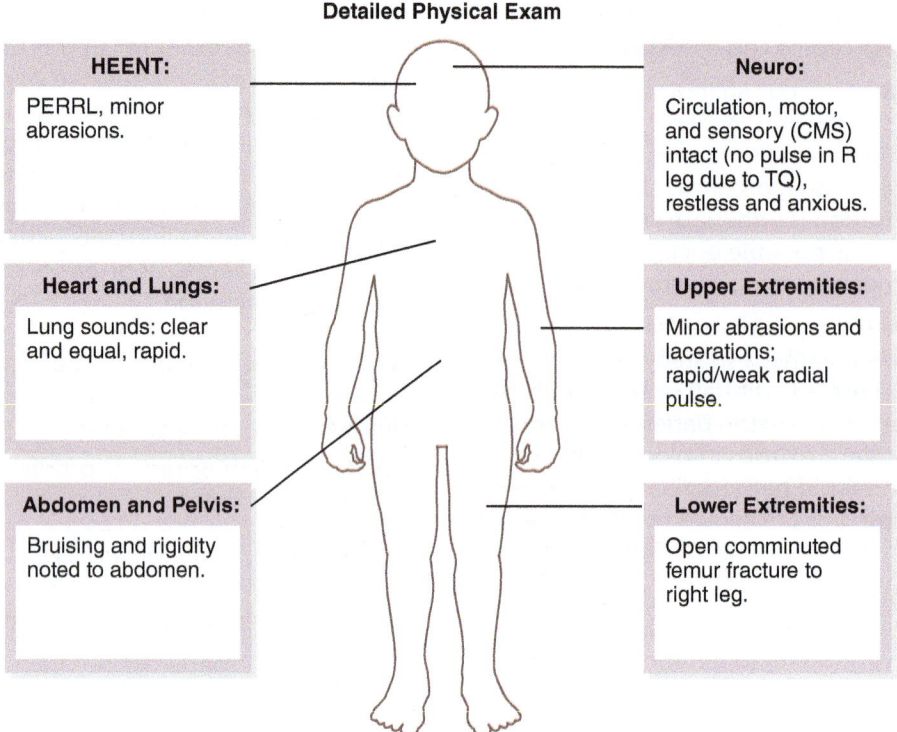

**HEENT:**

PERRL, minor abrasions.

**Heart and Lungs:**

Lung sounds: clear and equal, rapid.

**Abdomen and Pelvis:**

Bruising and rigidity noted to abdomen.

**Neuro:**

Circulation, motor, and sensory (CMS) intact (no pulse in R leg due to TQ), restless and anxious.

**Upper Extremities:**

Minor abrasions and lacerations; rapid/weak radial pulse.

**Lower Extremities:**

Open comminuted femur fracture to right leg.

**Figure 3-19** Detailed patient exam.
© Jones & Bartlett Learning.

- Lower extremities: Left lower extremity unremarkable with intact neurovascular status; right lower extremity noted to have open comminuted femur fracture. Pulsatile bleeding has been controlled with tourniquet application. No palpable distal pulses.

**Back:**

- Multiple abrasions, lacerations, and bruises consistent with road rash. No active bleeding.

## Treatment

Treatment for this patient is centered on hemorrhage control, respiratory support, circulatory support, and rapid transport to the closest appropriate facility. Depending on the circumstances, air medical transport may be the most appropriate means of transportation. Many air medical and critical care transport programs carry whole blood products for trauma patients.

The right lower extremity injury with active arterial bleeding should be managed immediately as it is encountered, with pressure dressing or tourniquet as appropriate for your protocol and scope of practice. Supplemental oxygen was provided via nonrebreather with improvement in oxygen saturation noted.

The bruising, rigidity, distention, and tenderness (peritoneal signs) all point to significant intra-abdominal bleeding. This may also be contributing to the patient's respiratory distress. Pelvic fractures are rare in children but increase in frequency as the child gets older. Any patient with pelvic instability should have a binder placed, whether they are hemodynamically stable or not.

This patient should receive IV fluid resuscitation due to the signs of poor perfusion and tachycardia. Initial boluses should be 20 mL/kg of an isotonic crystalloid solution, such as lactated Ringer's or normal saline. Response to fluids can be gauged clinically. This patient's blood pressure is already within normal range, so the clinical parameters to monitor for improvement would be tachycardia, tachypnea, and distal perfusion to the extremities. If the patient's pulse begins to normalize, the capillary refill time falls to less than 2 seconds, and the tachypnea improves, it is likely that fluid resuscitation is working.

Fluids should be warmed whenever possible to help mitigate any temperature drop that can be seen with administration of fluids that are less than physiologic body temperature. If patients are not responsive to crystalloids, then whole blood products may be necessary. If you feel that blood products may be necessary or the patient is not responding to crystalloid administration, inform the receiving facility so that these resources can be available on arrival.

Pain management for this patient should be approached with caution. Although pain management is important, careful consideration should be given to the impact narcotic medications can have on hemodynamic and respiratory status. Consider ketamine if part of local protocols.

## Tranexamic Acid

Tranexamic acid (TXA) is a drug that has been used to aid in bleeding control since the 1960s. In the last two decades it has seen increased use in prehospital treatment of trauma patients with refractory hemorrhage.

To understand how TXA works, a brief overview of how clotting occurs is necessary. When a patient sustains an injury that damages the skin, soft tissue, or blood vessels, collagen and other proteins are exposed. This initiates a cascade of protein activation known as coagulation. The final common pathway for both the intrinsic and extrinsic coagulation processes is fibrin cross-linking. As platelets and red blood cells clump together, forming a plug to stop blood loss, it does not form a stable complex. Hundreds of thousands of individual protein molecules called fibrin are deposited into this clump of platelets and RBCs. The individual molecules of fibrin are charged in such a way that when they are close to each other, they align and link together, similar to magnetic beads. This process, known as fibrin deposition and cross-linking, creates a lattice of fibrin throughout the clump of platelets and RBCs. This lattice stabilizes the clot and helps fix it into position so it can stop blood loss.

The body is in a constant state of clot formation and clot breakdown. As soon as clot formation begins, the process of breaking down that clot is also initiated. This is accomplished in large part by a substance called tissue plasminogen activating factor. You may have heard of this before by its more common name, tPA. This substance has been synthesized and is often administered to patients with ischemic stroke or acute coronary syndrome (myocardial infarction). tPA leads to plasminogen activation, which lyses the fibrin cross-links—a process called fibrinolysis. This leads to clot destabilization and breakdown. Clot destabilization and breakdown are desired effects when the patient is having a stroke or myocardial infarction; however, when there is massive hemorrhage, clot breakdown is not desired.

Tranexamic acid forms a complex with plasminogen that inactivates it. Once it is inactivated, it can no longer lyse the fibrin cross-links, and the fibrin mesh that is supporting the clot remains intact. It is important to note that TXA does not promote clot formation. TXA inhibits an important step in clot breakdown. If a patient does not have the necessary clotting factors for clot formation (disseminated intravascular coagulation or other coagulopathic disorders) then TXA will not help them build stable clots. The clots must be present for TXA to be effective. Thus, any patient who has active clotting which may be pathologic, such as in the brain or coronary arteries, should not be given TXA, as it will result in these clots persisting and possibly cause detrimental effects. The risks of TXA administration must be balanced with the perceived benefits.

There is limited data available on the ideal dosing and therapeutic regimen for TXA administration in pediatric patients. Although it has been determined to be safe, there may be variability in the dosage or administration criteria between programs. For adolescent patients, the dosing regimen is similar to that for adults, and there is less variability in therapeutic regimen (Table 3-2).

## Ongoing Management

As you continue to treat this patient, careful and continual reassessment of respiratory and circulatory status is necessary. Superficial cuts and lacerations can be dressed as time allows and splinting of the fractured extremity can be performed as appropriate.

| Table 3-2  TXA in Pediatric Patients | | |
|---|---|---|
| **Criteria for the Use of Tranexamic Acid in Pediatric Trauma** | | |
| Systolic blood pressure low (<80 mm Hg <5 years and <90 mm Hg ≥5 years) | | |
| Poor blood pressure response to crystalloid 20–40 mL/kg | | |
| Obvious significant bleeding | | |
| **Age** | **Loading Dose (administer within 3 hours)** | **Subsequent Dose** |
| 12 and over | 1 g intravenously over 10 minutes | 1 g intravenous infusion over 8 hours |
| Less than 12 | 15 mg/kg intravenously over 10 minutes (maximum dose 1 g) | 2 mg/kg/hr intravenous infusion over 8 hours or until bleeding stops |

Adapted with permission from Beno, S., Ackery, A.D., Callum, J. et al. Tranexamic acid in pediatric trauma: why not?. *Crit Care* 18, 313 (2014). https://doi.org/10.1186/cc13965

## Case Questions

- What is the most appropriate treatment destination and why?
  - After bleeding control and airway management, rapid initiation of transport to a trauma facility specialized in pediatric care is one of the most important steps that can be taken to save this patient's life. Data indicates that morbidity and mortality are decreased when pediatric trauma patients are cared for at pediatric trauma centers. Prehospital practitioners should know all available pediatric resources within their jurisdiction and be familiar with their capabilities. If there is going to be an extended extrication or prolonged transport time, air medical transport should be strongly considered.
- Will you allow the father to ride in the ambulance?
  - A caregiver should be allowed to ride with this patient if at all possible. The presence of caregivers can be a calming influence for children. The medical practitioners at the receiving facility may have important health questions that only the caregiver can answer. If you are unable to allow the father to ride, obtain a reliable contact phone number, and inform him that he should answer any calls coming to that number until they arrive at the hospital, as it could be medical practitioners attempting to reach him. In this case, the father was allowed by EMS personnel to ride with his child to the hospital.

- Can you safely transport this patient in your ambulance?
  - The child was large enough to be safely transported on the stretcher with appropriate safety belts attached.

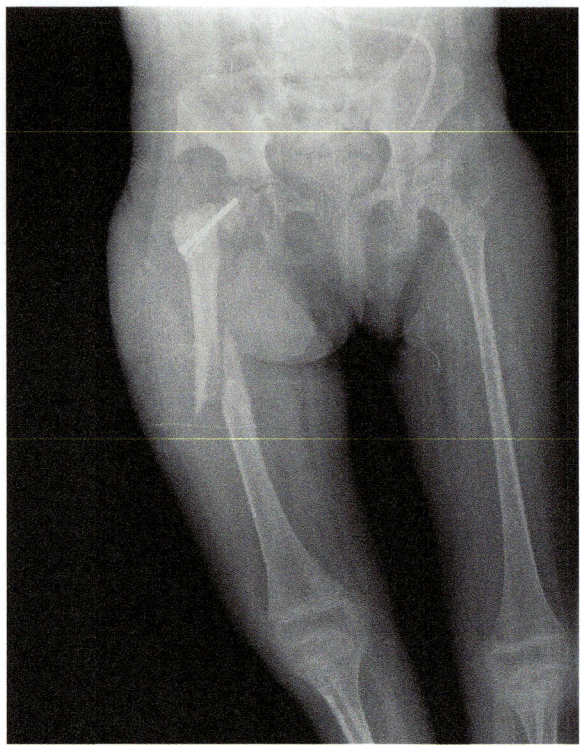

**Figure 3-20** A femur fracture may sever the femoral artery, leading to significant blood loss.
© martin81/Shutterstock.

## CASE WRAP-UP

Diagnosis: Significant blood less secondary to damaged femoral artery (**Figure 3-20**) and a minor liver laceration

On arrival to the pediatric level 1 trauma center, the patient was immediately assessed by the trauma team. The decision was made to begin administering blood products due to the suspicion of intra-abdominal injury and the large volume of blood loss reported on scene.

The patient was sent for emergent imaging of the head, neck, chest, abdomen, and pelvis, which revealed a minor liver laceration in addition to the obvious fracture of the femur. The femur fracture severed the femoral artery, which led to significant blood loss. No other fractures or organ injuries were found.

The fracture required extensive orthopedic surgery and will likely require further surgical intervention and intensive rehabilitation. The liver laceration was managed conservatively and is expected to heal without surgical intervention. The patient is expected to make a full recovery.

## CASE TAKEAWAY POINTS

Signs of poor tissue perfusion despite what appears to be an adequate blood pressure should be considered an ominous sign that the patient is at risk for rapid deterioration. In pediatric trauma, and trauma in general, it can be easy to be distracted by bleeding that is visible and obvious. In this particular case the bleeding from the leg was life threatening and required immediate control. Practitioners may assume that bleeding has been controlled when obvious bleeding has stopped; however, a thorough physical exam is necessary to identify any other potential bleeding sites. In this case, there was clear evidence of intra-abdominal bleeding noted on physical exam, and appropriate measures to maintain perfusion were taken, including fluid resuscitation.

Unrecognized internal bleeding is present in approximately 10% of pediatric major trauma patients. The most likely internal organs to be involved are the spleen and liver.

Transport planning and decision making should be a top priority in pediatric trauma management.

## CASE STUDY

### Case 2

#### Dispatch

You and your partner respond to a local farm for a 4-year-old female who has been thrown from a horse. The outside temperature is 77°F (25°C).

#### Case Questions

- What are your initial concerns?
  - The initial concerns for this patient include that she has likely fallen from a height greater than her own. This could result in multisystem trauma. Additionally, there was a large animal involved, and she could have been trampled or stomped on. It is also important to consider whether she was thrown from the horse or if she experienced a medical emergency such as a seizure that caused her to become incapacitated and fall.
  - You will need to gain access to the patient. This could be difficult based on the design of the facility and how close you can approach in the ambulance. Scene safety may also be a factor with roaming livestock that may be agitated due to the commotion.

### Initial Observations

As you arrive at the front entrance, you are guided to the horse-riding grounds. There is paved access all the way up to where the patient is waiting. You exit the ambulance to see a 4-year-old female sitting in a woman's lap. The woman identifies herself as the girl's equestrian coach. She informs you that the patient is complaining of chest pain and difficulty breathing (**Figure 3-21**).

- Pediatric Assessment Triangle
  - Appearance
    - Alert and anxious
  - Work of breathing
    - **P**atient has rapid, shallow respirations. Chest movement appears symmetric
    - **F**laring not present
    - **R**etractions not present
    - **A**udible airway sounds—no abnormal airway sounds heard
    - **P**ositioning—the patient does not appear to be tripoding or otherwise positioning her airway
  - Circulation
    - Skin appears warm and dry

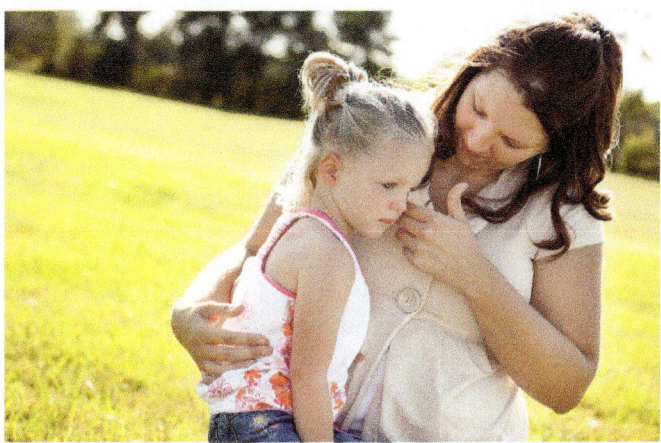

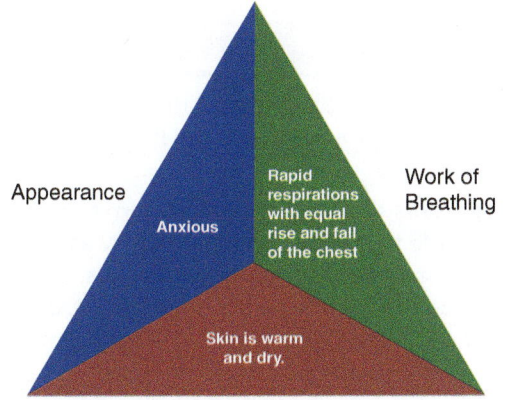

**Figure 3-21** Your patient is a 4-year-old girl who fell from a horse.

## Case Questions

- Based on your initial impression, is this patient "Quick" or "Not Quick"?

  - This patient is "Not Quick" currently. No immediate life threats were identified on the initial observations. Although further history and examination may change this patient's priority, there is currently time to continue the evaluation on scene.

- Have you identified possible red flags?

  - The patient was noted to have rapid respirations. Careful attention must be given during the rest of the physical exam to determine if this is simply due to anxiety, or if there is an underlying illness or injury that is causing this patient's respiratory distress.

  - In this particular case, the rapid respiratory rate combined with the chest pain is concerning for more than just anxiety and warrants careful examination.

## Primary Survey

The primary survey for this patient reveals the following:

**X**—No bleeding found

**A**—Open and patent

**B**—Respirations rapid with equal rise and fall of the chest

**C**—Radial pulses rapid, strong, and regular. Capillary refill time brisk. Skin warm and dry.

**D**—GCS score 15 (E4, V5, M6)

**E**—Sitting in coach's lap

## Case Questions

- Based on the findings noted in the primary survey, what would your initial interventions and treatment include?

  - Measures should be taken to calm the child if possible to facilitate the secondary assessment. This may involve breathing exercises, distraction techniques (phone, tablet, or other device) and pain control if warranted.

  - Supplemental oxygen may help the patient's respiratory distress.

## Detailed Assessment

### History Taking

As you take measures to calm the patient and apply a nasal cannula, you begin to take additional history which reveals the following:

**OPQRST:**

- **O**nset—Sudden chest pain and difficulty breathing after falling from a horse. The estimated height of the fall was approximately 10 feet. The patient remembers the fall and did not lose consciousness.

- **P**rovocation/palliation—Nothing makes it better or worse.

- **Q**uality—The patient is unable to articulate the quality, she only says, "it hurts to breathe."

- **R**adiation—None

- **S**everity—Patient states, "it hurts bad!" and is tearful. The coach says she has fallen from a horse before and her reaction this time is very different. The coach is concerned.

- **T**iming—Started approximately 10 minutes ago immediately after the fall

**SAMPLER:**

- **S**igns/symptoms—Increasing difficulty breathing. The patient is now exhibiting accessory muscle use that was not present on the initial impression. She is unable to speak in full sentences. You quickly listen again and note decreased lung sounds on the left side. There is asymmetric chest wall motion.

- **A**llergies—No known allergies to medications, foods, or the environment

- **M**edications—None

- **P**ast medical history—None

- **L**ast oral intake—Breakfast 2 hours ago

- **E**vents leading up to the emergency—Thrown from a horse after it was spooked

- **R**isk factors—None

It is clear that during the detailed assessment and history taking, this patient is actively decompensating. She is transitioning from "Not Quick" to "Quick."

As you update your partner, you say that you have changed your mind and want to load up and go. You should also go through a list of possible differential diagnoses and consider what immediate actions may need to be taken if this patient continues to decompensate.

## Vital Signs

You and your partner have moved the patient to the ambulance and the monitor is attached. The following vital signs are obtained (**Figure 3-22**):

**Heart rate:**

- 141 beats/min
- This patient is tachycardic and trying to increase cardiac output in response to some underlying process.

**SpO₂:**

- 89% RA
- There is no improvement noted after applying a nonrebreather.

**ETCO₂:**

- 38 mm Hg
- A tall shark fin waveform is developing.

**Respiratory rate:**

- 30 breaths/min
- The patient has shallow, rapid respirations. You notice increasing asymmetry in the chest wall motion.

**Blood pressure:**

- 74/30 mm Hg
- You note that the patient's pulse is now weaker than before.

**Temperature:**

- 98.6°F (37°C)

**Blood glucose:**

- Not obtained

This is a previously healthy 4-year-old female with chest pain, difficulty breathing, unequal breath sounds and evolving signs of obstructive shock. Based on the mechanism of injury and the patient's clinical presentation, a left-sided tension pneumothorax is the most likely cause.

The patient is actively decompensating and immediate intervention is necessary. The proper intervention for this life-threatening condition is needle decompression. Definitive treatment is insertion of a chest tube.

## Detailed Exam

**HEENT:**

- **H**ead: Unremarkable
- **E**yes: PERRL
- **E**ars: Unremarkable
- **N**ose: Unremarkable
- **T**hroat: Jugular vein distention (JVD) present along with mild right tracheal deviation. Both resolved after needle decompression.

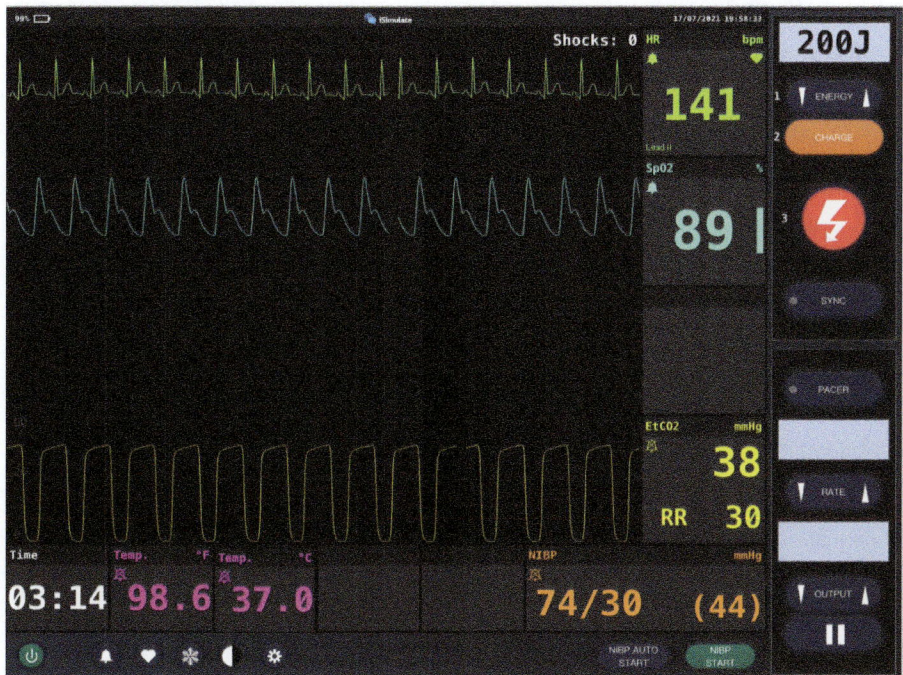

**Figure 3-22** The monitor displays your patient's vital signs.
Courtesy of iSimulate.

**Chest, heart, and lungs:**

- Pulses: Distal pulses in the upper and lower extremities present but weak
- Cardiac auscultation: Regular rate and rhythm with no rub, gallop, or murmur noted
- Lung auscultation: Clear on the right with good aeration. Diminished on the left.
- Chest exam: Asymmetric chest wall movement noted. No tenderness to palpation or apparent fractures noted.

**Neu rologic:**

- Neurovascular status intact

**Abdomen and pelvis:**

- Soft and nontender. Bowel sounds normal

**Extremities:**

- Upper extremities: No apparent injuries. Skin is pale and diaphoretic. Weak distal pulses palpated (**Figure 3-23**).
- Lower extremities: No apparent injuries. Skin is pale and diaphoretic. Weak distal pulses palpated.

**Back:**

- Unremarkable

## Chest Decompression

As described earlier in this lesson, a tension pneumothorax occurs when air escapes from the parenchyma of the lungs and begins to build pressure in the pleural space. This pressure leads to compression of the mediastinal structures and diminishes the heart's pumping capacity. Obstructive shock develops rapidly and these patients go from fairly well appearing to cardiac arrest within a matter of moments.

The recommended site for needle thoracostomy is the 4th or 5th intercostal space along the midaxillary line, or the 2nd intercostal space along the midclavicular line (**Figure 3-24**).

Using a 14- or 16-gauge needle with overlying catheter, the needle should be inserted until a pop is felt and a rush or hiss of air is heard. There is no need to advance any farther with the needle after this result is obtained. For patients younger than 13 years, a 1.5- to 2-inch needle should be sufficient. For patients older than 13 years, needles up to 3.5 inches in length may be necessary.

Once the needle and catheter are in the right position, remove the needle and leave the catheter secured in place with tape or sutures. A three-way stopcock or other one-way–type valve should be used to intermittently vent the pleural space if there is evidence of the pneumothorax reaccumulating. Additional needle

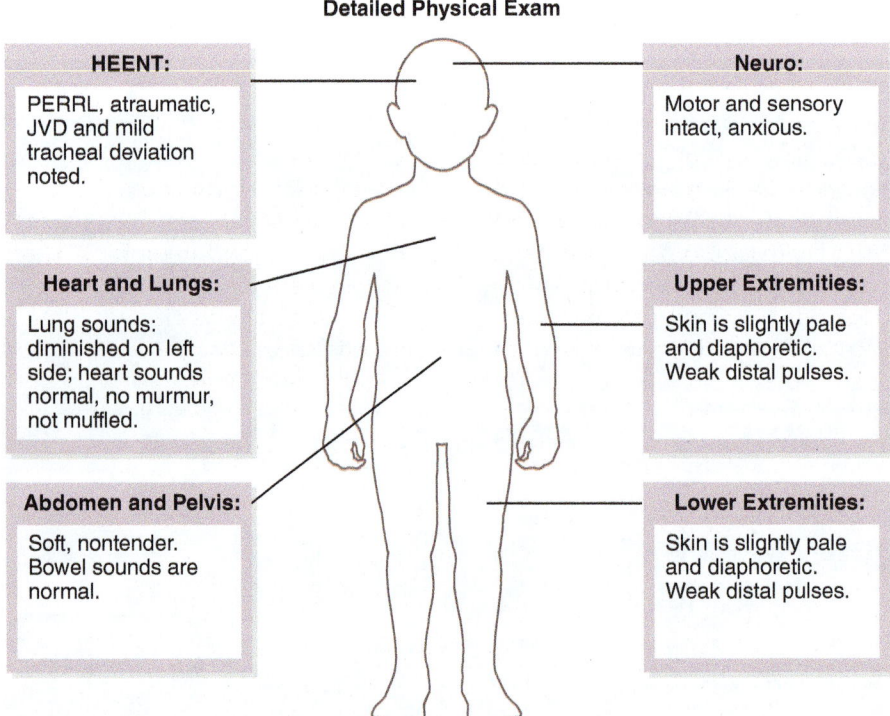

**Detailed Physical Exam**

**HEENT:**
PERRL, atraumatic, JVD and mild tracheal deviation noted.

**Neuro:**
Motor and sensory intact, anxious.

**Heart and Lungs:**
Lung sounds: diminished on left side; heart sounds normal, no murmur, not muffled.

**Upper Extremities:**
Skin is slightly pale and diaphoretic. Weak distal pulses.

**Abdomen and Pelvis:**
Soft, nontender. Bowel sounds are normal.

**Lower Extremities:**
Skin is slightly pale and diaphoretic. Weak distal pulses.

**Figure 3-23** Detailed patient exam.

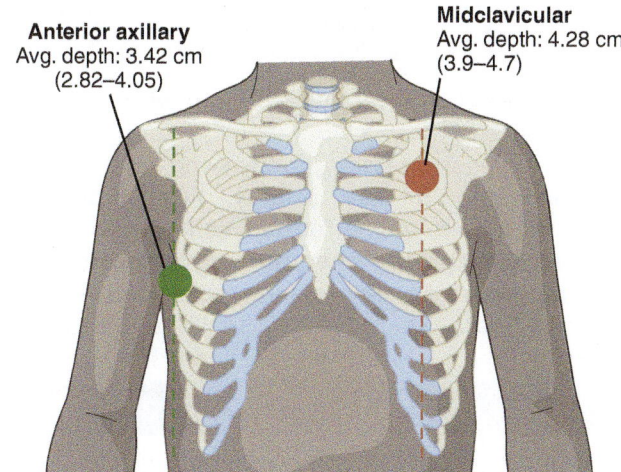

**Anterior axillary**
Avg. depth: 3.42 cm
(2.82–4.05)

**Midclavicular**
Avg. depth: 4.28 cm
(3.9–4.7)

**Figure 3-24** The recommended site for needle thoracostomy in pediatric patients is the 4th or 5th intercostal midaxillary line.

© Jones & Bartlett Learning.

decompression attempts may be necessary in cases where a large pneumothorax is present.

In cases of obstructive shock, rapid improvement is usually seen when the procedure is performed appropriately. Circulation can be rapidly restored once the compression on the heart and great vessels is relieved.

## Treatment

Initial treatment for this patient involved supportive care and respiratory support with oxygen. As she began to decompensate, it became clear she needed chest decompression. For basic life support practitioners, getting advanced life support (ALS) intercept or rapid transport to a facility capable of stabilizing the patient and then transferring from there would be appropriate. ALS practitioners can perform needle decompression in most jurisdictions as long as they have proper equipment and training. Critical care practitioners may have the ability to insert a chest tube.

In addition to chest decompression, fluid administration may be necessary to add preload to the right side of the heart and improve circulation once compression of the mediastinum has been relieved.

Rapid transport and continued reevaluation for reaccumulating pneumothorax is important for this patient.

## Ongoing Management

Continue to reassess this patient's respiratory and circulatory status throughout transport. It is possible for a pneumothorax to reaccumulate, and venting of the stopcock or valve may be necessary if the patient shows signs of obstructive shock again.

### Case Questions

- Can you safely transport this patient in your ambulance?

  - This child can be safely transported restrained in a pediatric-specific restraint system or a car seat in an ambulance in a position of comfort. While air medical transport may be a consideration for long distances or critical patients, flight physiology should be considered in a patient with a pneumothorax prior to initiating air transport. Make sure to inform the air medical service of the patient's injuries prior to them launching.

## Transport Destinations

Prehospital practitioners should be familiar with the resources available to pediatric patients in their region. For practitioners who work in the hospital environment, an established process for expediting transfer of care for critically ill and injured children to a pediatric tertiary care center should be in place.

Evidence shows that children who are treated at pediatric specialty centers have better outcomes overall. This is especially true with trauma. Morbidity and mortality are decreased when pediatric patients are treated initially at a specialized pediatric trauma center.

### CASE WRAP-UP

Diagnosis: Closed pneumothorax that progressed to a tension pneumothorax

The patient was transported safely to a level 1 pediatric trauma center. At the trauma center she was assessed by the trauma team and a chest tube was placed. She did not require surgical correction of the pneumothorax, and it was managed conservatively. She had no additional injuries and was discharged home after approximately 5 days in the hospital.

## CASE TAKEAWAY POINTS

Patients with rapidly evolving shock with preceding chest pain and dyspnea in the setting of trauma should be evaluated for possible tension pneumothorax. The signs include rapidly evolving obstructive shock, decreased breath sounds on one or both sides (in the case of bilateral pneumothoraces), JVD, tracheal deviation, chest pain, and trouble breathing with decreasing oxygen saturation. The pliable chest wall of the pediatric patient can lead to severe chest injury with little outward evidence of trauma.

Needle decompression is lifesaving in these patients and should take priority. Positive-pressure ventilation should be performed carefully as it can exacerbate the tension pneumothorax and attention should be given to peak pressures, tidal volumes, and ventilation rates.

## LESSON WRAP-UP

Trauma is the leading cause of pediatric death and disability. Many unintentional injuries can be prevented, and programs that focus on prevention have been shown to decrease the incidence of traumatic death when embraced and supported by the community and local public safety organizations.

Treatment for critically ill and injured children should focus on identification of life-threatening conditions and initiation of rapid transport to the closest appropriate facility. In some cases, this may mean bypassing local hospitals for transport directly to a pediatric-capable facility, as outcomes for pediatric patients are improved when they are treated at tertiary care centers specializing in pediatric trauma.

Continual reassessment is critical to avoid missing the evolution of life-threatening conditions while caring for the pediatric trauma patient.

## REFERENCES

Bobko J, Lai T, Smith E, et al. Tactical emergency casualty care–pediatric appendix: novel guidelines for the care of the pediatric casualty in the high-threat prehospital environment. *J Spec Oper Med*. 2013;13(4):94-107.

Callway DW, Puciaty A, Robertson J, Hannon T, Fabiano SE. Case report: life saving application of commercial tourniquet in pediatric extremity hemorrhage. *Prehosp Emerg Care*. 2017;21(6):786-788. doi:10.1080/10903127.2017.1332126

Centers for Disease Control and Prevention. 10 leading causes of injury deaths by age group highlighting unintentional injury deaths, United States—2018. Accessed October 28, 2021. https://www.cdc.gov/injury/images/lc-charts/leading_causes_of_death_by_age_group_unintentional_2018_1100w850h.jpg

Centers for Disease Control and Prevention. Leading causes of death and injury. Table: 10 Leading Causes of Death by Age Group, United States—2018. Accessed December 11, 2020. https://www.cdc.gov/injury/wisqars/pdf/leading_causes_of_death_by_age_group_2018-508.pdf

Choi PM, Hong C, Woods S, Warner BW, Keller MS. Early impact of American College of Surgeons verification at a level-1 pediatric trauma center. *J Pediatr Surg*. 2016;51(6):1026-1029.

Cornelius B, Cummings Q, Assercq M, et al. Current practices in tranexamic acid administration for pediatric trauma patients in the United States. *J Trauma Nursing*. 2021 Jan-Mar 1;28(1):21-25. doi:10.1097/JTN.0000000000000553

Cunningham A, Auerback M, Cicero M, Jafri M. Tourniquet usage in prehospital care and resuscitation of pediatric trauma patients: Pediatric Trauma Society position statement. *J Trauma Acute Care Surg*. 2018;85(4):665-667.

Goobie SM, Faraoni D. Tranexamic acid and perioperative bleeding in children: what do we still need to know? *Review Curr Opin Anaesthesiol*. 2019;32(3):343-352. doi:10.1097/ACO.0000000000000728

Halstead ME, Walter KD, Moffatt K, Council on Sports Medicine and Fitness. Sport-related concussion in children and adolescents. *Pediatrics*. 2018;142(6):e20183074. doi:10.1542/peds.2018-3074

Harcke HT, Lawrence LL, Gripp EW, et al. Adult tourniquet use in school-age emergencies. *Pediatrics*. 2019;143(6):e20183447. doi:10.1542/peds.2018-3447

Hoffman BD, Gallardo AR, Carlson KF. Unsafe from the start: serious misuse of car safety seats at newborn discharge. *Pediatrics*. 2016;171:48-54.

Kermode JC, Zheng Q, Milner EP. Marked temperature dependence of the platelet calcium signal induced by human von Willebrand factor. *Blood*. 1999;94(1):199-207.

Lier H, Krep H, Schroeder S, Stuber F. Preconditions of hemostasis in trauma: a review. The influence of acidosis, hypocalcemia, anemia, and hypothermia on functional hemostasis in trauma. *J Trauma*. 2008;65(4):951-960. doi:10.1097/TA.0b013e318187e15b

Locke T, Rekman J, Brennan M, Nasr A. The impact of transfer on pediatric trauma outcomes. *J Pediatr Sur*. 2016;51(5):843-847.

Safe Kids Worldwide. More than half of car seats are not installed correctly. September 1, 2017. https://www.safekids.org/post/more-half-car-seats-are-not-installed-correctly

Science Daily. Nearly 1 in 5 parents say their child never wears a helmet while riding a bike: national poll focuses on children's street smarts, including bike, skateboard, scooter and road safety. May 20, 2019. http://www.sciencedaily.com/releases/2019/05/190520103414.htm

Sokol K, Black G, Azarow K, et al. Prehospital interventions in severely injured pediatric patients: rethinking ABCs. *J Trauma Acute Care Surg.* 2015;79(6):983-989.

Walther AE, Falcone RA, Pritts TA, Hanseman DJ, Robinson BRH. Pediatric and adult trauma centers differ in evaluation, treatment, and outcomes for severely injured adolescents. *J Pediatr Surg.* 2016;51(8):1346-1350.

Webman RB, Carter EA, Mittal S, et al. Association between trauma center type and mortality among injured adolescent patients. *JAMA Pediatr.* 2016;170(8):780-786. doi:10.1001/jamapediatrics.2016.0805

Wolbert AS, Meng ZH, Monrose DM III, Hoffman M. A systematic evaluation of the effect of temperature on coagulation enzyme activity and platelet function. *J Trauma.* 2004;56(6):1221-1228. doi:10.1097/01.ta.0000064328.97941.fc

Wolf LL, Chowdhury R, Tweed J, et al. Factors associated with pediatric mortality from motor vehicle crashes in the United States: A state-based analysis. *J Pediatr.* 2017;187:295-302.e3

# CHAPTER 4

# Pediatric Shock

## LESSON OBJECTIVES

- Review the pathophysiology of each category of shock.
- Differentiate between compensated and uncompensated states of shock.
- Discuss management of pediatric patients in shock using the Pediatric Assessment Triangle (PAT) and XABCDE.
- Use the most appropriate pediatric shock management intervention based on the patient's assessment findings.

## Shock

Shock can be defined as a lack of tissue perfusion at the cellular level that leads to anaerobic metabolism and an inability to produce enough energy needed to support life. Shock is most often regarded as a state of generalized cellular function change from aerobic metabolism to anaerobic metabolism secondary to hypoperfusion of the tissue cells, in which the delivery of oxygen at the cellular level is inadequate to meet metabolic needs. Left untreated, shock leads to cell and organ death. Most simply put, shock is one of the ways a child's body may die.

Energy produced within the cell sustains all cellular and organ functions in the body. This energy is normally produced in a complex process that metabolizes oxygen and glucose. This process is referred to as aerobic metabolism because oxygen is required for it to occur. Energy produced is stored in the form of adenosine triphosphate (ATP) molecules. ATP molecules are broken down to release the stored energy when the energy is needed. Aerobic metabolism can produce 36 ATP from one glucose molecule (**Figure 4-1**). By-products of aerobic metabolism include carbon dioxide and water.

When oxygen is not available for aerobic metabolism, anaerobic metabolism occurs. This process uses stored body fat as its energy source, but it is not as efficient as aerobic metabolism. It produces much less energy, and harmful by-products result, such as lactic acid. Anaerobic metabolism can provide a brief period of cell survival without oxygen, but it is not sustainable. Without energy, cellular functions cease. ATP energy is required for the sodium-potassium pump, and without this part of the cell performing correctly it can lead to shock.

> **Shock is a lack of tissue perfusion that results in inefficient anaerobic cellular metabolism.**

Shock is progressive and not sudden. The body will attempt to maintain homeostasis through compensatory mechanisms. The goal is to help ensure that the patient's body maintains adequate energy production for cell survival and proper function.

## Causes of Shock

Worldwide, pediatric shock is one of the most diagnosed conditions and is one of the leading causes of pediatric morbidity and mortality, yet it is still poorly understood. It can be the result of traumatic events or from a medical cause (**Table 4-1**).

Possible traumatic causes of shock include loss of circulating blood volume such as through internal or external bleeding or though loss of body fluid volume due to plasma loss from burns. Another cause of traumatic shock is the loss of effective cardiac function to circulate oxygenated blood. Loss of cardiac function can result from tension pneumothorax, cardiac tamponade, or blunt trauma. A third cause of traumatic shock can be the loss of vascular tone which causes the loss of effective blood flow. This can occur because of spinal cord injury.

Possible medical causes of shock can be categorized in the same way as traumatic causes of shock. Loss of circulating blood volume can occur from blood loss due to internal bleeding; body fluid loss from lack of intake, vomiting, diarrhea, or osmotic diuresis from diabetes; or plasma loss due to increased permeability, as occurs with sepsis and anaphylaxis. Abnormal cardiac function can result from dysrhythmia or heart failure due to congenital heart disease, myocarditis, cardiomyopathy, poisoning, or sepsis. Loss of vascular tone that causes vasodilation and loss of effective blood flow can occur due to drug toxicity, stroke, anaphylaxis, and sepsis.

Even if treated, shock can lead to renal failure, brain damage, liver failure, metabolic derangements,

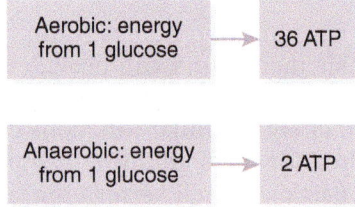

**Figure 4-1** Aerobic metabolism can produce 36 ATP from one glucose molecule, whereas anaerobic metabolism produces only 2 ATP.

© Jones & Bartlett Learning.

| Table 4-1 Causes of Shock | |
|---|---|
| **Trauma** | **Medical** |
| ▪ Blood loss | ▪ Hypovolemia |
| ▪ Tension pneumothorax |   ▪ Internal bleeding |
| |   ▪ Emesis/diarrhea |
| ▪ Cardiac tamponade | ▪ Sepsis |
| ▪ Spinal cord injury | ▪ Anaphylaxis |
| | ▪ Drug ingestion |
| | ▪ Heart failure |
| | ▪ Dysrhythmia |

© Jones & Bartlett Learning.

disseminated intravascular coagulation (DIC), multiple organ dysfunction syndrome (MODS), acute respiratory distress syndrome (ARDS), and cardiac failure.

## Shock Is Progressive

At all ages, the body attempts to preserve circulation of oxygenated blood to its vital organs. However, children will compensate differently than adults to maintain perfusion (**Figure 4-2**). Children first become tachycardic, and then their blood vessels vasoconstrict. Selective vasoconstriction shunts blood from nonvital tissues such as the skin, gastrointestinal tract, and muscles to more vital organs such as the brain, heart, and kidneys. Massive vasoconstriction is the predominant compensatory mechanism for children.

Cardiac output is determined by heart rate and stroke volume. Because children have smaller stroke volumes than adults, children primarily increase cardiac output by increasing their heart rate instead of their stroke volume. They can tolerate prolonged high heart rates for hours to days due to strong heart muscle and good coronary circulation.

Due to intact compensatory mechanisms, children will compensate longer than adults, but their decompensation will be more rapid. In other words, the progression from compensated shock to death is an accelerating process.

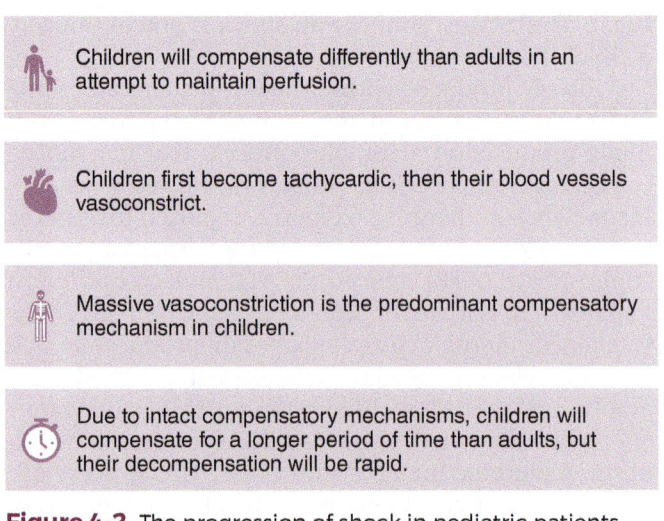

**Figure 4-2** The progression of shock in pediatric patients.

© Jones & Bartlett Learning.

**Adults typically compensate for a time and then gradually deteriorate. Children, however, will compensate for a relatively long period and then suddenly deteriorate in an accelerating process toward death (Figure 4-3).**

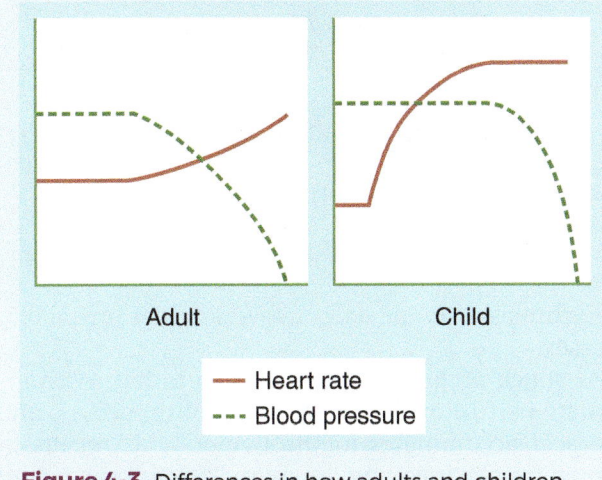

**Figure 4-3** Differences in how adults and children compensate when in shock.

© Jones & Bartlett Learning.

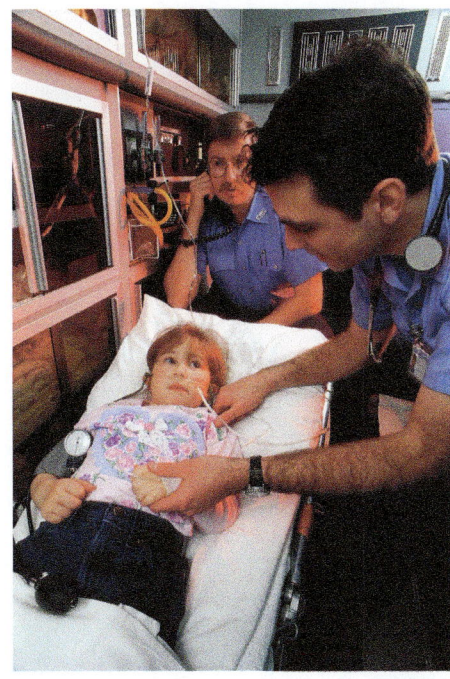

**Figure 4-4** A child whose body is compensating may be in shock but not present with altered mental status or hypotension.

© CORBIS/age fotostock.

*Do not* wait for shock symptoms to become obvious before treating for it.

## Compensated Shock

Compensated shock, also called early shock, involves inadequate tissue perfusion without evidence of end-organ dysfunction such as hypotension or altered mental status. During compensated shock, the body is experiencing a state of low volume but is still able to maintain blood pressure and vital organ perfusion by increasing the heart rate and constricting blood vessels to shunt blood toward the vital organs. In other words, the body's defense mechanisms attempt to preserve perfusion of the brain, heart, kidneys, and liver at the expense of nonvital organs such as skin, muscles, and gastrointestinal tract (**Figure 4-4**). Because of selective vasoconstriction, the last organs to become dysfunctional are the lungs and heart. Due to the preservation of the organs involved with oxygenation and circulation, compensated shock is reversible. If the cause of shock is not corrected and reversed, compensated shock will progress to decompensated shock.

There may be a progressive shift toward decompensated shock, which can evolve differently in each patient. There may also be some overlap of symptoms of compensated and decompensated shock.

### FINDINGS OF COMPENSATED SHOCK

**Neurologic/mental status changes, such as restlessness, irritability, anxiety, or confusion (Figure 4-5)**

**Mild increase in ventilatory rate**

**Normal systolic blood pressure**

**Mild to severe tachycardia (unless patient is in cardiogenic shock due to a bradyarrhythmia or in neurogenic shock)**

**Strong central pulses; weak or bounding peripheral pulses**

**Pale or normal color mucous membranes**

**Delayed or brisk capillary refill**

**Nausea, thirst**

**Mild decrease in urine output**

(*continued*)

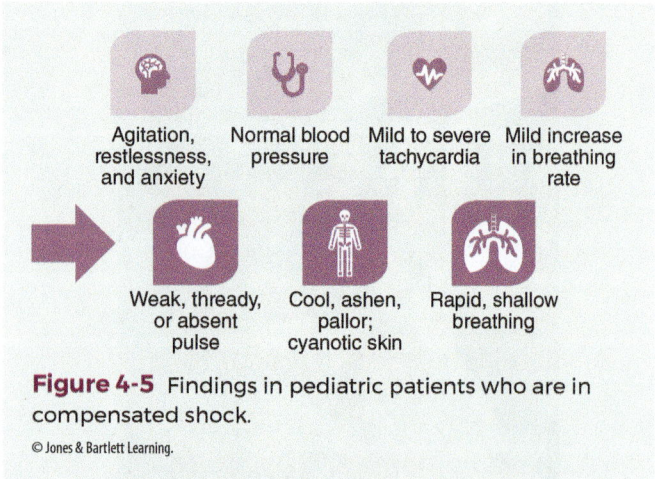

**Figure 4-5** Findings in pediatric patients who are in compensated shock.

© Jones & Bartlett Learning.

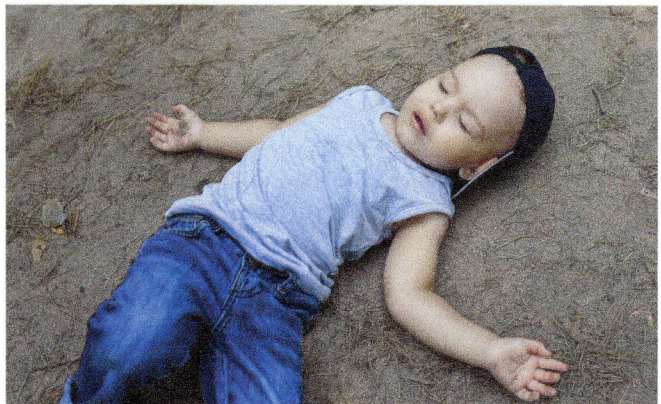

**Figure 4-6** In decompensated shock, the child's compensatory mechanisms will begin to fail.

© cash14/iStock/Getty Images Plus/Getty Image.

Peripheral vasoconstriction, a compensatory mechanism that is seen with hypovolemic, cardiogenic, and obstructive shock, is evidenced by cool, pale extremities and decreased capillary refill. In contrast, peripheral vasodilation is usually present with early distributive shock, resulting in warm, pink extremities with bounding peripheral pulses and brisk capillary refill.

## Decompensated Shock

Decompensated shock begins when compensatory mechanisms begin to fail (**Figure 4-6**). Classic signs and symptoms of shock are evident because mechanisms previously used to maintain perfusion have become ineffective. Signs of impaired perfusion due to shock include altered level of consciousness, cool extremities, mottled skin, absent distal pulses, and weak central pulses. Except for septic shock, hypotension is a late finding and indicates that cardiac arrest is imminent. Hypotension worsens cardiac perfusion, and cardiac

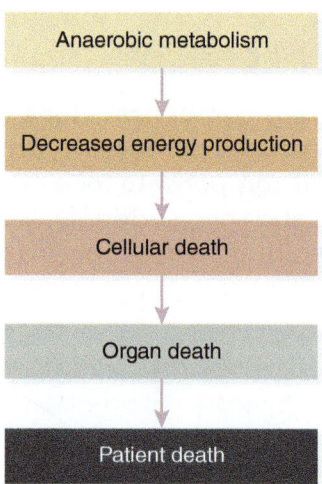

**Figure 4-7** The cascade of death.

© Jones & Bartlett Learning.

dysrhythmias may develop as ventricular irritability increases.

As shock progresses, organs begin to fail. With inadequate perfusion, anaerobic metabolism occurs, and lactic acid accumulates in the tissues. This results in cell membranes breaking down and releasing harmful enzymes. The longer organs remain poorly perfused, the less likely the patient is to respond to treatments. Decompensated shock is difficult to treat but may be reversible if appropriate aggressive treatment is begun early.

Without aggressive treatment to reestablish effective perfusion, irreversible damage to vital organs will occur due to sustained altered perfusion and metabolism. This stage of shock is referred to as irreversible shock. This stage can progress quickly and will result in multisystem organ failure, cardiopulmonary arrest, and death (**Figure 4-7**). Thus, it is critical to recognize and treat shock early.

## Types of Shock

Shock can be categorized in several ways. A common way to categorize shock is by its pathophysiology. These four classifications are hypovolemic, distributive, cardiogenic, or obstructive shock. The most common cause of shock is loss of circulating blood volume due to blood or fluid loss, called hypovolemic shock. Loss of integrity of the blood vessel walls as well as inability to control blood vessel dilation is called distributive shock. Examples of distributive shock include septic, anaphylactic, and neurogenic shock. When caused by dysfunction or failure of the heart or presence of a dysrhythmia, it is referred to as cardiogenic shock. Finally, obstruction of blood flow through the great vessels or heart is referred to as obstructive shock. Obstructions

## FINDINGS OFTEN ASSOCIATED WITH DECOMPENSATED SHOCK

**Altered mental status such as agitation or lethargy, unresponsiveness**

**Loss of muscle tone**

**Fall in systolic and diastolic blood pressures (late findings; Figure 4-8)**

**Moderate increase in ventilatory rate; possible respiratory muscle fatigue or failure**

**Moderate to severe tachycardia; possible dysrhythmias**

**Weak central pulses; thready or absent peripheral pulses**

**Delayed capillary refill**

**Pale, ashy, or cyanotic mucous membranes**

**Altered body temperature, cool extremities**

**Marked decrease in urine output**

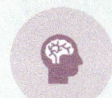  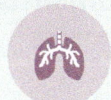

Altered mental status    Failing blood pressure    Moderate increase in respiratory rate

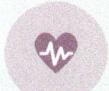  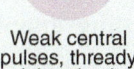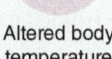 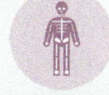

Moderate to severe tachycardia    Weak central pulses, thready peripheral pulses    Altered body temperature    Ashen, pallor, cyanotic

**Figure 4-8** Findings in pediatric patients who are in decompensated shock.

© Jones & Bartlett Learning.

**Types of shock:**

- **Hypovolemic**
- **Distributive**
- **Cardiogenic**
- **Obstructive**

of another and then another until there is complete failure and eventually death. Hypovolemic shock is the most common type of shock in the pediatric population and is the leading cause of death from shock within the pediatric population worldwide.

## General Assessment Approach

As with all pediatric patients, obtain an initial observation using the Pediatric Assessment Triangle (PAT) assessment. This will allow you to form an initial impression. As you approach the patient, parents or caregivers often volunteer a focused history, which assists in identifying the type of shock. This information can be helpful, but the purpose of the PAT and primary assessment is to identify any immediate life threats. With a pediatric patient, life-threatening conditions may not be obvious.

**Interrupt your assessment only to address a life threat.**

Perform a primary assessment using the XABCDE approach (primary survey) to identify life threats. Control any severe external bleeding, and ensure the upper airway is not obstructed. If ventilation is adequate, give supplemental oxygen in a manner that does not agitate the child. Supplemental oxygen is important to maximize oxygen-carrying capacity in the setting of decreased hemoglobin (red blood cells). If signs of respiratory failure or respiratory arrest are present, assist ventilation using a bag-valve mask (BVM) with supplemental oxygen and basic airway adjuncts. Pediatric patients can show rapid improvement when hypoxia is reversed. Intubation may *not* be required, because a pediatric patient may regain airway control and responsiveness after a period of effective ventilations with supplemental oxygen.

During the secondary assessment, initiate pulse oximetry, cardiac, and blood pressure monitoring as well as end-tidal carbon dioxide ($ETCO_2$) monitoring.

to blood flow can be due to conditions such as cardiac tamponade, tension pneumothorax, massive pulmonary embolus, or ductal-dependent heart lesions. Obstructive shock is caused by obstruction of the great vessels or heart; however, it is not discussed in this lesson.

Adequate perfusion depends on a working pump (heart), adequate fluid (blood), and an adequately sized and intact container (blood vessels). These three components have a mutual relationship with each other, and each one must be functioning adequately for the other two to work to produce adequate cardiac output. Of course, failure of one will eventually lead to failure

Checking the patient's glucose level is also necessary, because some children in shock will be hypoglycemic because of rapidly depleted carbohydrate stores. If the serum glucose is below 60 mg/dL (3.3 mmol/L), administer intravenous (IV) or intraosseous (IO) dextrose.

> **REMEMBER: Even though a pulse oximetry device on a finger may indicate adequate oxygenation, the provider still needs to evaluate whether another area of the body may not be getting the same oxygenation.**

## Hypovolemic Shock

Hypovolemic shock is the most common cause of shock in infants and children worldwide. This condition involves inadequate circulating blood volume in the vascular space (**Figure 4-9**). Possible causes include hemorrhage, plasma loss, fluid and electrolyte loss, and endocrine disease.

### Hypovolemic Shock Treatment

After assuring airway patency and effective ventilations, obtain vascular access (**Figure 4-10**). When shock is present, the most readily available vascular access site is preferred. If immediate vascular access is needed and reliable IV access cannot be rapidly achieved, early IO access is appropriate.

After vascular access has been obtained, begin fluid resuscitation when indicated. When there are signs of poor perfusion or hypotension, administration of an initial 20 mL/kg fluid bolus of an isotonic crystalloid solution, such as normal saline (NS) or lactated Ringer's (LR), is reasonable. For smaller patients, an IV tubing system that incorporates an in-line three-way stopcock (push-pull method) is often useful for rapid and precise fluid administration. After *each* fluid bolus, reassess the child's mental status, heart rate, blood pressure, and capillary refill. Monitor closely for increased work of breathing and signs and symptoms of volume overload such as pulmonary edema. Maintain normal body temperature, and keep the patient supine.

In the setting of hypovolemic shock in children due to hemorrhage, alternative management is preferred over fluid hydration when possible, including tourniquets, tranexamic acid (TXA), and in some systems, blood products. However, in the setting of hypotension, fluids should not be withheld if no other treatment proves effective or is available.

> **Hypovolemic shock = Keep calm and warm, provide oxygen, correct hypoglycemia, administer fluid resuscitation: 20 mL/kg over 5 to 10 minutes**
>
> **Hemorrhagic shock = Manage blood loss, administer fluid resuscitation if hypotensive**

## Distributive Shock

Distributive shock results from an abnormality in vascular tone (**Figure 4-11**). There are various types of distributive shock, including anaphylactic shock, neurogenic shock, and septic shock. With each type of distributive shock, a relative hypovolemia occurs when vasodilation increases the size of the vascular space. This means that the available blood volume must fill a greater space for effective flow to occur. Because the blood cannot immediately expand to fill the larger space, blood circulation is impaired. This altered distribution of the blood volume is due to relative hypovolemia rather than actual volume loss causing absolute hypovolemia, but the effect is similar.

Cases of septic shock in pediatric patients are on the rise, with an estimated annual incidence of 1.2 million cases of pediatric sepsis globally. Septic shock ranges from 1% to 26% of hospitalized pediatric patients worldwide. Mortality in pediatric patients from septic shock ranges from 5% in developed countries to 35% in developing countries. Studies attribute this high mortality rate to delayed treatment, diagnosis, and not following treatment guidelines.

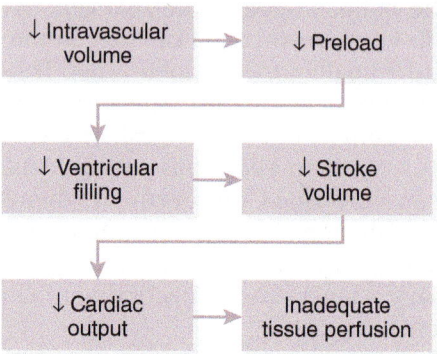

**Figure 4-9** The physiology of hypovolemic shock.
© Jones & Bartlett Learning.

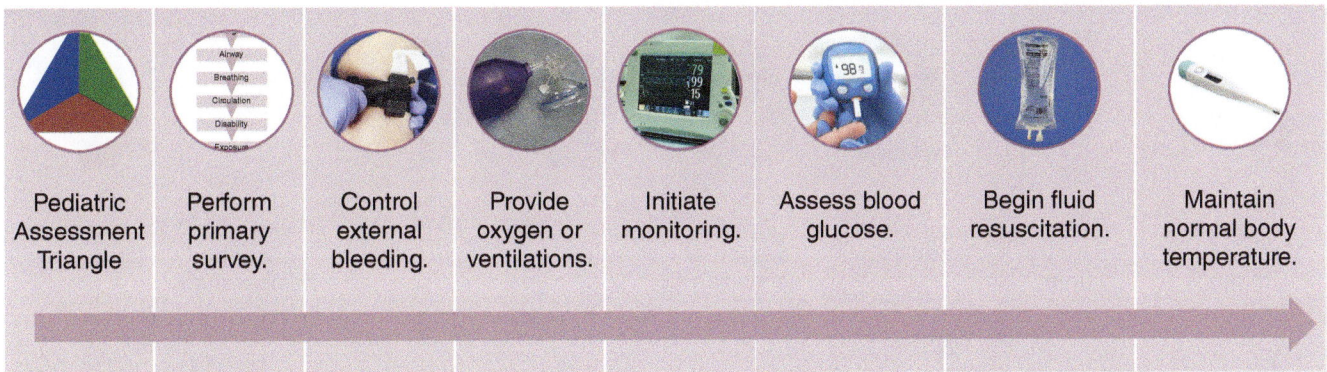

**Figure 4-10** Steps to the management of hypovolemic shock in pediatric patients.

**A.** Used with permission of the American Academy of Pediatrics, Pediatric Education for Prehospital Professionals, © American Academy of Pediatrics, 2000; **B, C & G.** Jones & Bartlett Learning.; **D.** © Jones and Bartlett Publishers. Courtesy of MIEMSS.;
**E.** © bymuratdeniz/E+/Getty Images; **F.** © simpson33/iStock/Getty Images Plus/Getty Images; **H.** © Creativeye99/iStock/Getty Images Plus/Getty Images.

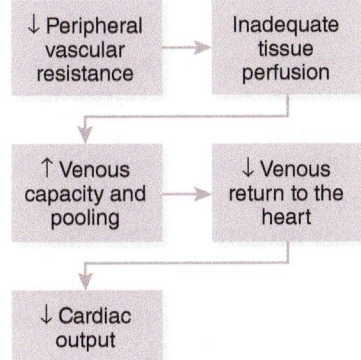

**Figure 4-11** Physiology of distributive shock.

© Jones & Bartlett Learning.

The clinical presentation of septic shock is different in infants and young children compared to most adults and some adolescents. The older group typically presents with vasodilation and normal cardiac output, so skin and extremities are warm, producing "warm shock." Neonates to young children are unable to increase cardiac output to the same degree as adults so they vasoconstrict early on, resulting in cold and poorly perfused distal extremities, referred to as "cold shock." The concern in pediatric patients is third spacing of fluids, in which blood vessels become leaky due to increased inflammation and fluid is lost to the interstitial space. The severe inflammatory response to infection leads to impaired cellular dysfunction, followed by multiple organ failure.

Severe allergic reaction, or anaphylactic shock, can occur seconds to minutes after exposure to an antigen such as a drug, vaccine, food, toxin, plant, or venom. The body's responses include venodilation, arterial vasodilation, increased capillary permeability, and pulmonary vasoconstriction. Anaphylaxis is defined as impacting two or more body systems (e.g., skin and gastrointestinal tract), but as many as 10% of cases present with hypotension only. Hypotension results from pulmonary vasoconstriction decreasing pulmonary blood flow, which decreases left ventricular filling and therefore decreases cardiac output.

Neurogenic shock occurs when spinal cord injury occurs above T6 that prevents messaging from the brain (in the form of epinephrine) from reaching other organs in the body, including the heart and blood vessels. The loss of sympathetic nervous system stimulation of the muscles in the blood vessel walls results in vasodilation. The sympathetic tachycardic response to compensate for the vasodilation is also interrupted and does not occur.

## Distributive Shock Treatment

After assuring airway patency and effective ventilations, obtain vascular access (**Figure 4-12**). When shock is present, the most readily available vascular access site is preferred. If immediate vascular access is needed and reliable IV access cannot be rapidly achieved, early IO access is appropriate.

Initiate pulse oximetry, cardiac, and blood pressure monitoring, including ETCO$_2$. Low ETCO$_2$ in septic shock is indicative of increased lactate levels and greater severity of infection. D$_{10}$W is preferred over D$_{25}$W to raise blood glucose levels should hypoglycemia be present.

If the patient is breathing adequately, give supplemental oxygen in a manner that does not agitate the child. If there are signs of respiratory failure or respiratory arrest, assist ventilation using a BVM with supplemental oxygen and basic airway adjuncts. Do not delay transport in order to intubate. Intubation

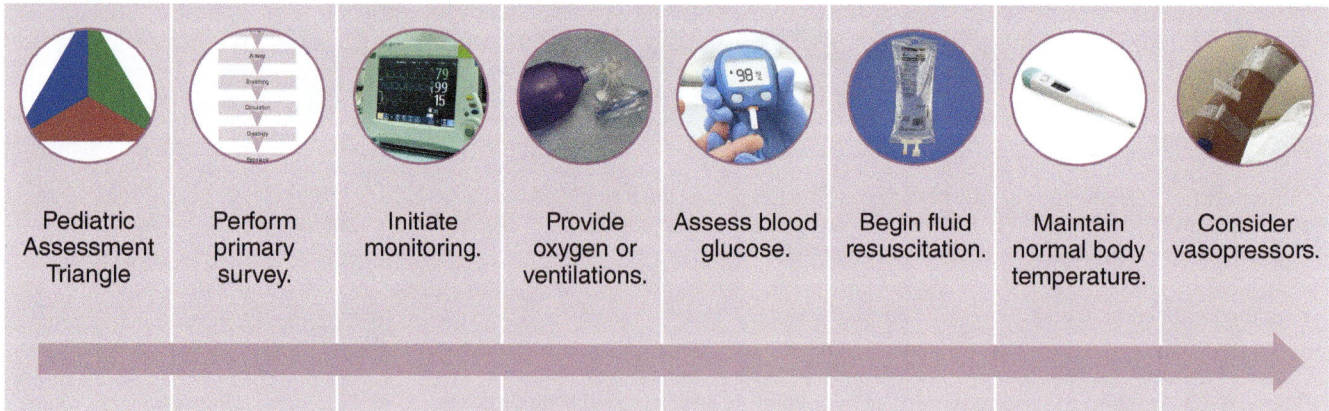

| Pediatric Assessment Triangle | Perform primary survey. | Initiate monitoring. | Provide oxygen or ventilations. | Assess blood glucose. | Begin fluid resuscitation. | Maintain normal body temperature. | Consider vasopressors. |

**Figure 4-12** Prehospital management of distributive shock.

A. Used with permission of the American Academy of Pediatrics, Pediatric Education for Prehospital Professionals, © American Academy of Pediatrics, 2000; **B & F.** Jones & Bartlett Learning.; **C.** © bymuratdeniz/E+/Getty Images; **D.** © Jones and Bartlett Publishers. Courtesy of MIEMSS.; **E.** © simpson33/iStock/Getty Images Plus/Getty Images.; **G.** © Creativeye99/iStock/Getty Images Plus/Getty Images.; **H.** © natnaree sangkaew/Shutterstock.

and mechanical ventilation may be required in *rare* cases. Consult with medical direction and follow local protocols.

Consider intubation in cases of prolonged transport times, and consult with your medical director. Rapid sequence intubation (RSI) or medication-facilitated intubation should be used with caution as induction agents, especially etomidate, may precipitate cardiac arrest in pediatric patients in septic shock. Etomidate is contraindicated in septic shock as it may suppress the stress response, making the body less capable of developing an appropriate inflammatory response. However, it does not directly cause cardiac arrest.

After vascular access has been obtained, begin fluid resuscitation. Administration of an initial 20 mL/kg fluid bolus of an isotonic crystalloid solution, such as NS or LR, is reasonable. An IV tubing system that incorporates an in-line three-way stopcock (push-pull method) is often useful for rapid and precise fluid administration.

After each fluid bolus, reassess the child's mental status, heart rate, blood pressure, and capillary refill for response. Monitor closely for increased work of breathing and signs and symptoms of volume overload, such as pulmonary edema. Maintain normal body temperature and keep the patient supine. In some agencies, vasopressors (e.g., dopamine, norepinephrine, epinephrine) may be considered if shock remains refractory after 60 mL/kg of volume resuscitation. Note guidance from the Pediatric Life Support: 2020 International Consensus on Cardiopulmonary Resuscitation and Emergency Cardiovascular Care Science with Treatment Recommendations regarding recommendations for fluid administration based on intensive care availability, and follow local protocols.

> **Distributive shock = Keep calm and warm, provide oxygen, correct hypoglycemia, administer fluid resuscitation: 20 mL/kg over 5 to 10 minutes up to 60 mL/kg, if no response to fluid, then consider vasopressor infusion**
>
> **Septic shock = Passive cooling, administer antipyretic, administer fluid resuscitation**

## Cardiogenic Shock

Cardiogenic shock is heart failure due to poor contraction or inadequate rate or rhythm, which leads to decreased cardiac output and inadequate tissue perfusion (**Figure 4-13**). Because both involve decreased cardiac output and peripheral vasoconstriction, cardiogenic shock may resemble hypovolemic shock. Usually, intravascular volume is not decreased unless the patient has also suffered vomiting and fever, such as with a viral cardiac inflammation.

Cardiogenic shock may result from redirected blood flow caused by dysrhythmias, such as supraventricular tachycardia (SVT), that cause insufficient cardiac output. Corrected congenital heart diseases may cause arrhythmias due to the surgery disrupting conduction. Decreased myocardial contractility might be caused by anomalous or abnormal coronary arteries, leading to areas of inadequate perfusion and myocardial infarction. Furthermore, genetic syndromes such as Duchenne muscular dystrophy could cause poor myocardial contractility.

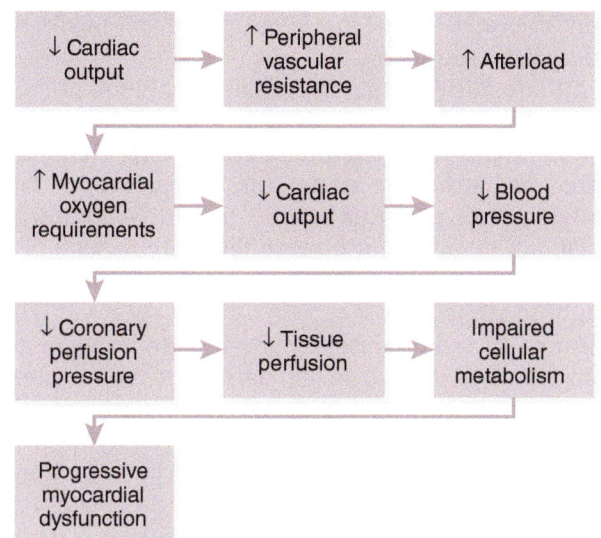

**Figure 4-13** Physiology of cardiogenic shock.
© Jones & Bartlett Learning.

Cardiogenic shock can result from inflammatory disorders such as viral myocarditis or structural disorders such as valve obstructions due to aortic stenosis, congenital defect, or hypertrophic cardiomyopathy. Other conditions that can cause cardiogenic shock include acute and chronic drug toxicity, poisoning, acute valvular regurgitation, ischemic heart disease, traumatic myocardial injury, pheochromocytoma, or thyrotoxicosis. Consider tension pneumothorax if trauma is suspected.

Cardiogenic shock is not as rare as providers may think. Clinical signs of decompensation may be similar across all types of shock, which speaks to the emphasis on patient history to understand the type of shock the patient may be experiencing (**Table 4-2**).

When collecting a SAMPLER history from the patient's caregivers, discuss medical history, including birthing complications if dealing with a neonate or young infant. Discuss in detail any physical findings

## Table 4-2 Symptoms and Signs of Cardiogenic Shock

| Possible Historical Findings in Cardiogenic Shock | Possible Physical Findings |
|---|---|
| 1. Preceding history of chest pain | 1. Tachypnea or grunting with clear lungs on examination |
| 2. Previous history of flulike symptoms associated with weakness and fatigue | 2. Unexplained dysrhythmias in the presence of a flulike illness |
| 3. Difficulty feeding because of fatigue and sweating during feeding in the breast- or bottle-fed infant | 3. Tachycardia disproportionate to the degree of fever |
| 4. No history of fever | 4. Persistent or worsening tachycardia despite fluid administration |
| 5. No history of volume loss (e.g., diarrhea, vomiting, and blood loss) | 5. Heart murmur, friction rub, or gallop on examination |
| 6. Positive history of congenital heart disease | 6. Presence of cyanosis that does not improve with the administration of oxygen |
| 7. No history of asthma despite wheezing on examination | 7. Crackles on lung examination |
| 8. Persistent wheezing despite the administration of β-agonist (e.g., albuterol [salbutamol]) | 8. Peripheral edema or pitting edema |
| 9. History of cyanosis | 9. Hepatomegaly |
| 10. Recent history of exercise intolerance | |

Used with permission of the American Academy of Pediatrics, Pediatric Education for Prehospital Professionals, © American Academy of Pediatrics, 2000.

> Cardiogenic shock is often missed or not correctly identified. Because cardiogenic shock may present like another type of shock, always be cautious of fluid resuscitation in children. Constantly monitor for fluid overload and deterioration when administering a fluid bolus. Immediately withhold further fluid administration if complications occur.

noted by the caregivers. An older child may begin to report cardiac-specific symptoms such as chest pain. Caregivers may also report that the child ingested some medications or had a recent medication prescription adjusted. It is vitally important to determine what type of medication they ingested as well as the dose. Certain cardiac medications, like calcium channel blockers or beta blockers, could result in cardiogenic shock even in low doses.

## Cardiogenic Shock Treatment

Focus on reducing myocardial oxygen demand, improving preload, reducing afterload, improving contractility, and correcting dysrhythmias (**Figure 4-14**). Reduce oxygen demand by keeping the patient calm and correcting increased work of breathing and fevers. If ventilation is adequate, give supplemental oxygen in a manner that does not agitate the child. If breathing is inadequate, ventilate using a BVM with supplemental oxygen using basic airway devices. Consider positive end-expiratory pressure (PEEP) if or

when tolerated to decrease afterload by facilitating myocardial contraction.

Initiate pulse oximetry, cardiac, and blood pressure monitoring, including $ETCO_2$. It is important that a 12-lead ECG is obtained and sent to the receiving specialized pediatric care center for interpretation. Treat any dysrhythmias identified via 3-lead ECG monitoring.

Obtain IV access at a peripheral site if possible. If the patient is hypotensive then it is reasonable to go straight to IO access.

Rapid IV fluid boluses as provided to hypovolemic or distributive shock can be harmful if administered to a patient in cardiogenic shock. Fluid administration should be performed cautiously with this type of patient, using smaller boluses administered over longer periods of time. Constantly monitor the patient for fluid overload. If the patient is hypotensive or shows signs of decreased perfusion, preload may be optimized with cautious administration of a small fluid bolus of 5 to 10 mL/kg given over 10 to 20 minutes accompanied by careful monitoring of mental status, lung sounds, work of breathing, and signs of volume overload.

The patient who has significant hypotension and is unresponsive to fluid resuscitation or who becomes

> Cardiogenic shock = Keep the patient calm and warm, provide oxygen, administer fluid resuscitation: 5 to 10 mL/kg over 10 to 20 minutes, if no response to fluid or signs of fluid overload then consider vasopressor infusion along with medical director consultation

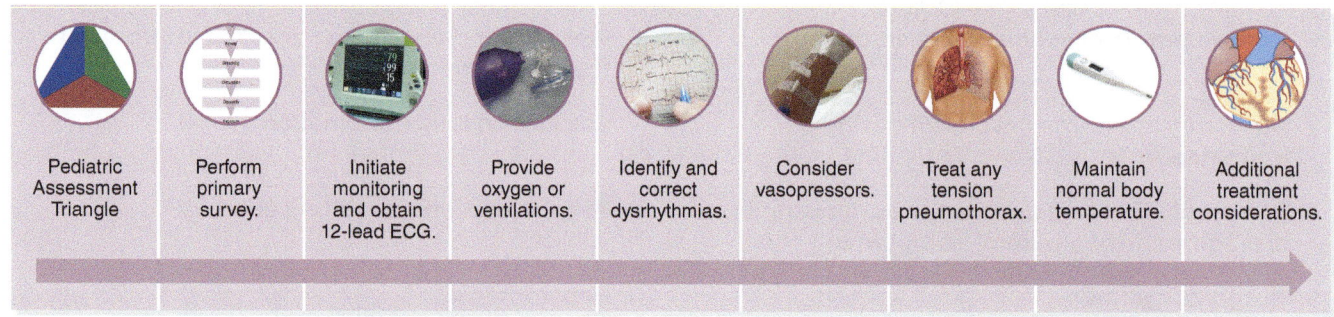

Pediatric Assessment Triangle | Perform primary survey. | Initiate monitoring and obtain 12-lead ECG. | Provide oxygen or ventilations. | Identify and correct dysrhythmias. | Consider vasopressors. | Treat any tension pneumothorax. | Maintain normal body temperature. | Additional treatment considerations.

**Figure 4-14** Prehospital management of cardiogenic shock.

volume overloaded may require vasopressors to increase blood pressure. Consider norepinephrine as a vasopressor, because it increases systemic vascular resistance and blood pressure, increases heart rate and cardiac output, and protects blood flow to organs. Refractory cardiogenic shock may require mechanical support with extracorporeal membrane oxygenation (ECMO) or a ventricular assist device (VAD).

If qualified and equipped, obtain a focused assessment with sonography for trauma (FAST) examination with point-of-care-ultrasound (POCUS), if the equipment is available and bleeding is suspected in the chest, abdomen, or pelvis. However, do not delay transport to perform POCUS.

As with any pediatric patient, maintain normal body temperature throughout transport.

## CASE STUDY

### Dispatch

It is 0900 on a fall morning. You are responding to a 5-year-old male described as a "sick child" with a fever at an apartment complex. Outside temperature is 52°F (11°C).

### Case Questions

- What are your initial concerns and possible differential diagnoses from the dispatch information?
  - "Sick child" with fever should raise considerations of viral infection, bacterial infection, dehydration, heat exposure, juvenile onset diabetes, or poisoning. Viral infection could include illness such as encephalitis, meningitis, myocarditis, influenza, or COVID-19. Bacterial infection could include meningitis, aspiration pneumonia, epiglottitis, and otitis media. Severe viral or bacterial infection can cause sepsis.
- What hazards may there be to your well-being?
  - The pediatric population often become acutely ill due to exposure to something in the environment such as a virus, bacteria, toxic fumes, or bites from an insect, reptile, or mammal. You may also be at risk of exposure and illness without proper protection.
- What clues may be found during your scene assessment?
  - You should assess the scene for evidence of toxic exposure or violence and also for evidence that the patient is in a safe environment and being provided with the necessities for healthy life. Evidence of abuse or neglect must be reported.

- What personal protective equipment (PPE) options must be considered? What PPE options are available at your agency?
  - You should consider gloves, gown, eye protection, and N95 mask for the potentially infectious patient.

### Initial Observations

You arrive on scene and find your 5-year-old patient in the arms of his mother. She is standing at the doorway of her apartment. As you approach, you notice the patient appears lethargic and has not reacted to your presence or his mother's anxiety. You also notice that he has a moderately increased work of breathing despite being at rest and his skin looks flushed (**Figure 4-15**).

His mother tells you that the patient has "not been feeling well" for the last 3 days. His illness started with diarrhea and then vomiting. She also noticed that he felt "hot." She called for help today because he would not get out of bed this morning.

- Pediatric Assessment Triangle
  - Appearance
    - Lethargic
  - Work of breathing
    - **F**laring not present
    - **R**etractions—mild retractions noted
    - **A**udible airway noises—bilateral upper airway congestion heard
    - **P**ositioning—does not appear to be tripoding or otherwise positioning his airway
  - Circulation
    - Skin hot and flushed

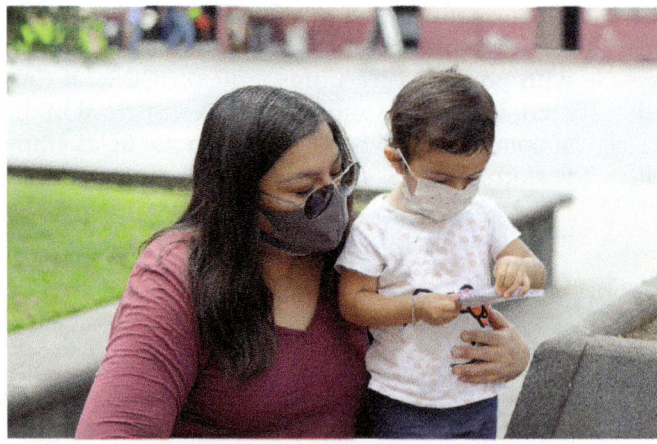

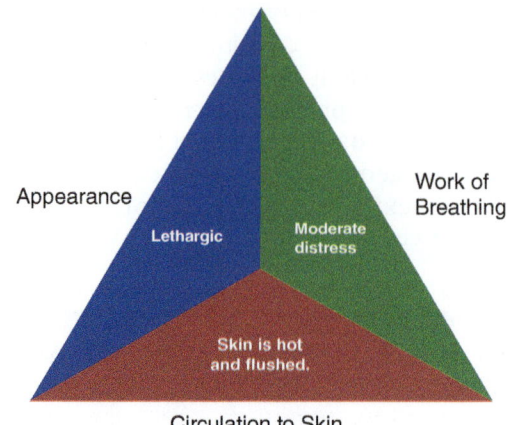

**Figure 4-15** A 5-year-old child has not been feeling well.

© Arlette Lopez/Shutterstock; Used with permission of the American Academy of Pediatrics, Pediatric Education for Prehospital Professionals, © American Academy of Pediatrics, 2000.

## Case Questions

- What is your initial impression of your patient? Is the patient "Quick" or "Not Quick"?
  - The patient is "Quick" based on the decreased level of consciousness and the increased work of breathing while at rest.
- Have you identified any possible red flags?
  - Red flags include his lethargy, his work of breathing, and his flushed skin. The history of diarrhea and vomiting raises concerns of increased fluid loss along with potentially poor fluid intake.
- Have you identified possible signs of shock?
  - Although not specific, his lethargy may be a sign of poor perfusion, suggesting shock is present. An altered level of consciousness to this degree indicates the patient is in decompensated shock. However, he has also been unwell and feverish for 3 days and so will be fatigued. In context of the case, he may be in late stage compensated shock.

## Septic Shock

Septic shock can be quite deceiving, especially in the early stages. Septic shock occurs in two clinical phases: the early warm shock phase and the subsequent cold shock phase. The early warm shock phase is characterized by peripheral vasodilation and increased cardiac output. In the cold shock phase, inflammatory response causes cardiac output to fall and peripheral vascular constriction occurs. Late septic shock is difficult to clinically

**Table 4-3** Warm Shock Versus Cold Shock

| Warm Shock | Cold Shock |
|---|---|
| Warm extremities | Cold, clammy skin |
| Bounding pulses | Rapid breathing, hypoxia |
| Tachycardia | Rapid, weak pulse |

© Jones & Bartlett Learning.

distinguish from other types of shock. Because of these two stages, providers should not use the presence or absence of fever to diagnose septic shock (Table 4-3).

Signs and symptoms of septic shock can include confusion and altered mental status, difficulty breathing, difficulty waking from sleep, fever, irritability, restlessness, lethargy, tachycardia, and change in skin color.

## Septic Shock Treatment

Treatment of the child in septic shock is more about stabilization rather than treatment. $ETCO_2$ is a reliable indicator of progression of sepsis. The lower the $ETCO_2$ level, the higher the serum lactate level. A higher serum lactate level is most often associated with cellular hypoxia but can also be due to decreased clearance of normal lactate production.

An IV or IO line should be established immediately, followed by fluid resuscitation with a 20 mL/kg fluid bolus and reassessment following the bolus administration. If there are no signs of improvement, fluid bolus administration and reassessment can be repeated two more times for a total of 60 mL/kg. Vasopressors, such as dopamine, epinephrine, or norepinephrine may be indicated for fluid-refractory shock. Fluid-refractory shock is defined as shock that persists after 60 mL/kg of fluid.

Norepinephrine is recommended for warm shock with a low blood pressure, and epinephrine is recommended for cold shock with a low blood pressure. *Dopamine is not recommended for children in septic shock*, because it has been associated with increased risk of death and infection.

If the child is hypoglycemic, then administer 10% dextrose.

## Primary Survey

Now that the PAT is completed, you direct your partner to administer high-flow supplemental oxygen by applying a nonrebreather mask to the patient. Concurrently, you begin the primary survey with the following findings:

- **X**—No bleeding found
- **A**—Open, upper congestion heard
- **B**—Moderate distress with rapid rise and fall of chest. Lung sounds reveal congestion bilaterally.
- **C**—Brachial pulses rapid, weak, and regular; capillary refill time delayed. Skin hot and flushed.
- **D**—Lethargic; Glasgow Coma Scale (GCS) score = 13 (E3, V4, M6)
- **E**—The patient's clothing is removed. No signs of trauma, rash, or urticaria.

### Case Questions

- Were any life threats identified in the primary survey?
  - Upper airway congestion could obstruct the airway; bilateral lung congestion suggests lower airway impairment of gas exchange. Delayed capillary refill and weak peripheral pulses indicate poor perfusion of the extremities; hot and flushed skin raises concern of fever creating increased oxygen demand of the cells and uncontrolled vasodilation preventing effective blood circulation.
- What further treatment is required based on the primary survey findings?
  - The patient is showing signs of late stage compensated distributive shock. This must be treated early and aggressively by initiating IV access and administering fluid resuscitation of up to 3 boluses of 20 mL/kg over 5 to 10 minutes each. Supplemental oxygen is continued, and fever is reduced following local protocol.

- Why is oxygen needed?
  - Oxygen is needed to maximize delivery to tissues at the cellular level to encourage aerobic metabolism and minimize anaerobic metabolism for energy production.

## Detailed Assessment

### History Taking

After suctioning the upper airway, an IO is established, and a resuscitation tape estimates your patient's weight as 18 kg. The first bolus of normal saline solution is administered as you collect the patient's history from the mother:

**OPQRST:**

- **O**nset—Gradual, according to mother
- **P**rovocation/palliation—Nothing apparent
- **Q**uality—Unable to assess
- **R**adiation—Unable to assess
- **S**everity—Unable to assess
- **T**iming—3 days, according to mother

**SAMPLER:**

- **S**igns/symptoms—Loss of appetite, diarrhea, vomiting, subjective fever, congestion
- **A**llergies—No known allergies
- **M**edications—Acetaminophen last night
- **P**ast medical history—Respiratory syncytial virus (RSV), strep throat
- **L**ast oral intake—Has not had anything to eat or drink today, had a popsicle last night
- **E**vents leading up to the emergency—Has gotten worse over the last 3 days. Physician advised to call EMS if breathing got worse.
- **R**isk factors—History of RSV/strep throat, age, delayed capillary refill

### Case Questions

- Why is it important to continuously reevaluate the patient's mental status?
  - The patient's mental status provides important feedback on the effectiveness of your therapies, as does heart rate and breathing rate. Deterioration of mental status may indicate the need for advanced airway management, whereas improvement may

indicate the need to remove airway adjuncts and advanced airways or provide sedation.

- What is the significance of previous RSV infection?
  - RSV infection at an early age is associated with recurrent bronchospasm and asthma in later life. This can complicate any current respiratory illness.
- What is the significance of the patient's age with respect to risk factors?
  - At 5 years of age, the patient's upper airway is not fully developed and can complicate airway management with adjuncts and advanced airways as well as with positive-pressure ventilation. He will also have a smaller tidal volume, a reduced oxygen reserve, and higher metabolism, which will require more oxygen than an adult patient.
- What is the significance of delayed capillary refill as a risk factor?
  - Delayed capillary refill on a pediatric patient is a sign of decreased peripheral circulation. This indicates the patient is beginning to transition from compensated shock to decompensated shock.

## Vital Signs

While collecting the patient history from the mother, you and your partner have assessed vital signs with the following findings (**Figure 4-16**):

**Heart rate:**

- 165 beats/min
- The patient is tachycardic and is attempting to increase cardiac output in response to early sepsis.

**SpO$_2$:**

- 92% on room air and 99% with supplemental oxygen
- Oxygen saturation improves with supplemental oxygen delivery.

**ETCO$_2$:**

- 28 mm Hg
- The waveform is boxed.
- The patient is presenting with a low ETCO$_2$. There is an inverse relationship between ETCO$_2$ levels and serum lactate levels. Therefore, carbon dioxide levels fall as lactate levels rise.

**Respiratory rate:**

- 32 breaths/min
- The patient is tachypneic and is in moderate distress with rapid rise and fall of the chest.

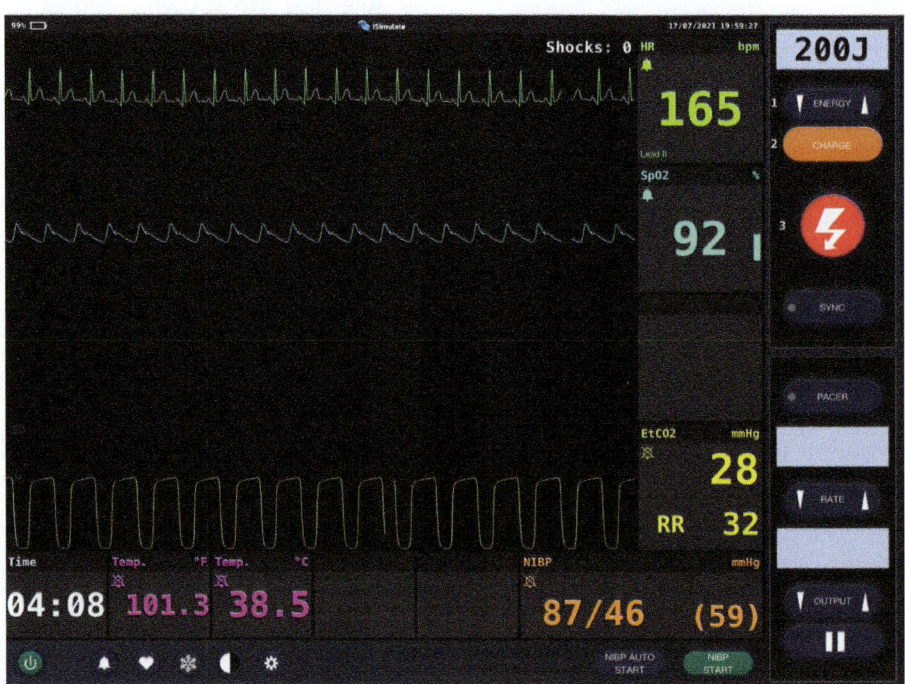

**Figure 4-16** Patient's vital signs. What do these vital signs tell you about this patient?

Courtesy of iSimulate.

**Blood pressure:**

- 87/46 mm Hg
- The patient has a normal blood pressure for his age.

**Temperature:**

- 101.3°F (38.5°C)
- The temperature is elevated, which likely indicates an infection.

**Blood glucose:**

- 167 mg/dL (9.3 mmol/L)
- The patient's blood glucose is elevated, likely due to the stress and inflammatory response of sepsis.

**ECG:**

- Shows sinus tachycardia.

## Case Questions

- Is oxygen needed?

  - Yes, oxygen should be administered as soon as altered level of consciousness, increased work of breathing, cyanosis, or signs of decreased perfusion are noted.

- Why is the $ETCO_2$ reading low?

  - Lowered $ETCO_2$ levels can occur when the patient is tachypneic with adequate gas exchange. Hyperventilating lowers $CO_2$ levels in the blood as increased amounts of $CO_2$ are exhaled. The respiratory system acts as a buffer to acidosis, the accumulation of acid in the bloodstream. Acidosis develops when lactic acid is produced due to impaired circulation and anaerobic cellular metabolism.

- What basic measures may be used to cool this patient?

  - In addition to the administration of antipyretic medication, the patient should be undressed and skin-to-skin contact should be avoided. Do not provide active cooling such as application of cold packs.

- What can be done to improve cardiac output?

  - Cardiac output can be improved with the administration of IV fluid and vasopressors if needed.

## Detailed Exam

Your final assessment is to perform a thorough physical assessment of the patient. You assess the following (**Figure 4-17**):

**HEENT:**

- **H**ead: Dry mucous membranes
- **E**yes: PERRL, sunken eyes
- **E**ars: Unremarkable
- **N**ose: Dried mucus
- **T**hroat: Unremarkable

**Chest, heart, and lungs:**

- Pulses: Brachial pulses are rapid, weak, and regular
- Lung auscultation: Congested bilaterally
- Cardiac auscultation: Heart sounds are normal, no murmur
- Chest exam: Respirations rapid with good rise and fall

**Neurologic:**

- Circulation, motor, and sensory intact
- Decreased mental status

**Abdomen and pelvis:**

- Soft, nontender
- Bowel sounds normal

**Extremities:**

- Upper extremities: Delayed capillary refill, flushed skin
- Lower extremities: Flushed skin

**Back:**

- Unremarkable

## Case Questions

- Given the age of this child, would you perform a head-to-toe assessment or toe-to-head assessment?

  - A head-to-toe assessment is appropriate for any age of patient that has a decreased level of consciousness as this patient does. Performing a toe-to-head assessment is appropriate for the alert young pediatric patient as it is less threatening and therefore, less stressful for the patient.

## Treatment

Different levels of providers are guided by their respective scopes of practice. Typically, a basic-level provider is expected to continue to closely monitor the airway and

**Detailed Physical Exam**

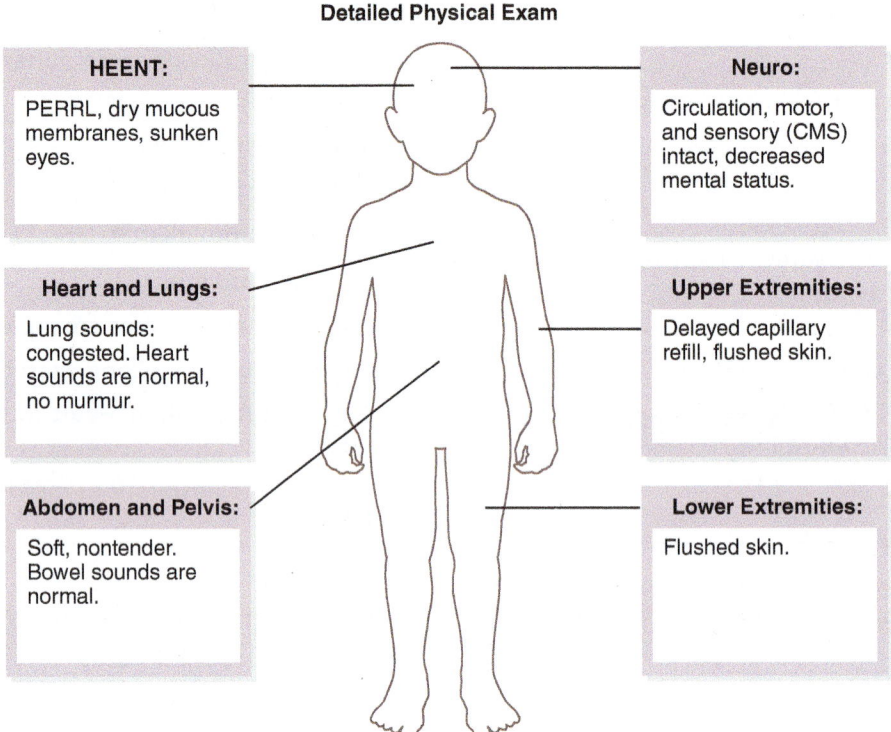

**HEENT:**

PERRL, dry mucous membranes, sunken eyes.

**Neuro:**

Circulation, motor, and sensory (CMS) intact, decreased mental status.

**Heart and Lungs:**

Lung sounds: congested. Heart sounds are normal, no murmur.

**Upper Extremities:**

Delayed capillary refill, flushed skin.

**Abdomen and Pelvis:**

Soft, nontender. Bowel sounds are normal.

**Lower Extremities:**

Flushed skin.

**Figure 4-17** Detailed patient exam.
© Jones & Bartlett Learning.

ventilations. Consider assisting ventilations if you notice the patient's ventilations becoming less effective as he fatigues from the increased work of breathing. Administer antipyretic medication and continue passive cooling. Keep the patient as calm as possible to further decrease oxygen demand.

In addition to these treatments, providers at an advanced level should provide fluid resuscitation. If the patient's cardiac output does not respond to fluid or if signs of fluid overload become apparent, administer vasopressors if within local scope of practice. Critical care providers can also obtain blood cultures and administer empiric broad-spectrum antibiotic therapy if permitted by their local medical direction.

All levels of providers must closely monitor the patient and frequently reassess for rapid deterioration.

## Case Questions

- What are your goals for this patient?
  - The foundation of treatment is supportive care and rapid transport. Be prepared for rapid deterioration requiring more advanced airway management and positive-pressure ventilations. Promptly recognize early

decompensated shock and escalate therapy appropriately.

- What are your differential diagnoses for this patient now?
  - Differential diagnoses should include juvenile onset diabetes, influenza, strep throat, COVID-19, toxic aspiration, sepsis, and status asthmaticus.
- For the advanced and critical care providers: what is the amount of fluid required for each bolus? What is the total amount of fluid without signs of fluid overload before considering vasopressors?
  - Each bolus is 20 mL/kg. The weight of the patient is estimated to be 18 kg so the calculation is 20 mL/kg × 18 kg = 360 mL for each bolus. The total amount of fluid is 60 mL/kg so the calculation is 60 mL/kg × 18 kg = 1,080 mL.

## Ongoing Management

During transport, the first fluid bolus is administered over 5 minutes. The patient is reassessed after the first bolus and the blood pressure has increased to 96/67 mm Hg and the heart rate decreased to 134 beats/min. The respiratory rate decreases to 28 breaths/min with no changes to lung sounds or accessory muscle use noted. The $ETCO_2$ increases to 30 mm Hg. There are no further changes during transport.

> **Not all emergency departments maintain a foundational infrastructure to meet the needs of children (i.e., "pediatric readiness"), but all can and should. Efforts should be taken to understand the pediatric capabilities of possible destination facilities to ensure the ED is ready to meet the needs of this child. This may not be the closest appropriate facility. Follow local protocol when considering bypassing a hospital in favor of a designated children's hospital. As with all critical patients, notify the ED of your patient's age and status prior to arrival.**

## Case Questions

- Where is the most appropriate treatment destination and why?
  - The most appropriate destination is a hospital that specializes in pediatric care. This patient is quite sick and requires prompt empirical administration of a broad-spectrum antibiotic for best outcome. This can be accomplished at any ED and an emergency transfer to a specialized pediatric unit can be arranged for resuscitation therapies based on more invasive hemodynamic monitoring and lab data. Follow local protocols directing transport destination.
- How would you safely transport this child in your ambulance?
  - Policies, equipment, and procedures for pediatric transport may vary from jurisdiction to jurisdiction but all are subject to legal requirements. Specialized pediatric restraints attached to the stretcher or built into the ambulance seating are common options.
- Will you allow a parent to ride in the ambulance?
  - Although EMS services vary in their regulations, the safest option for transport of the patient's parent is with a seat belt in a forward-facing position in the front seat beside the driver. However, family-centered care is a priority, so allowing one parent to ride with the EMS crew, if possible, is recommended. The parent should be encouraged to assist in the care of their child as safety allows. The operator of the ambulance is ultimately legally responsible for ensuring all passengers are properly restrained; always follow your local protocols.

## CASE WRAP-UP

Diagnosis: Influenza B with associated compensated shock and early sepsis

At the hospital, swab indicated influenza B with strep throat. Fluid boluses were continued to correct the patient's hypovolemia resulting from fever, fluid loss through vomiting and diarrhea, and decreased fluid intake. The child had not received his flu vaccine this season. The patient was discharged with full recovery after spending a week in the hospital.

## CASE TAKEAWAY POINTS

An estimated 10% to 20% of the population in the United States contracts influenza each year. Influenza is a viral infection of the upper respiratory system. Influenza types A and B are responsible for epidemics of respiratory illness that occur almost every winter and are often associated with increased rates of hospitalization and death.

Efforts to control the impact of influenza are focused on types A and B. One of the reasons the flu remains a problem is because the viruses alter their structure, exposing adults and children to new types of the virus each time. The Centers for Disease Control and Prevention (CDC) estimates that since 2010, flu-related hospitalizations among children younger than 5 years have ranged from 7,000 to 26,000 in the United States. The CDC reported 170 pediatric deaths during the 2019–2020 flu season.

## LESSON WRAP-UP

Prehospital providers need to have a high index of suspicion for shock due to history and mechanism of injury. Early recognition and rapid interventions are the key in treating shock and preventing the patient from decompensating.

Assessment of pulse quality and perfusion status are key indicators of shock. Compensated shock is characterized by poor perfusion with a normal blood pressure while decompensated shock is characterized by poor perfusion and low blood pressure. Compensatory mechanisms involve respiratory rate and heart rate, so be particularly concerned when the patient is tachypneic and tachycardic while at rest and without fever.

Address any airway and breathing issues immediately. Obtain vascular access quickly if shock treatment

**A healthy-looking child at rest with tachycardia and delayed capillary refill is in shock until proven otherwise.**

is needed. The antecubital fossa is the preferred site for older children, but this vein may not be accessible in younger patients. When IV access is not readily accessible, opt for an IO route. Deliver crystalloid fluids for fluid resuscitation at a rate of 20 mL/kg over 5 to 10 minutes unless cardiogenic shock is suspected. When managing cardiogenic shock, administer 5 to 10 mL/kg over 10 to 20 minutes. Sometimes fluid is all they need.

## REFERENCES

Bakker J. Increased blood lactate levels: a marker of...? Acute care testing.org. June 2003. https://acutecaretesting.org/en/articles/increased-blood-lactate-levels-a-marker-of

Dellinger RP, Levy MM, Rhodes A, et al. Surviving Sepsis Campaign: international guidelines for management of severe sepsis and septic shock, 2012. *Intensive Care Med.* 2013;39:165-228. doi:10.1007/s00134-012-2769-8

Fleischmann-Struzek C, Goldfarb DM, Schlattmann P, Schlapbach LJ, Reinhart K, Kissoon N. The global burden of paediatric and neonatal sepsis: a systematic review. *Lancet Respir Med.* 2018;6(03):223-230.

Frazier A, Hunt EA, Holmes K. Pediatric cardiac emergencies: children are not small adults. *J Emerg Trauma Shock.* 2011;4(1):89-96. doi:10.4103/0974-2700.76842

Hartman ME, Linde-Zwirble WT, Angus DC, Watson RS. Trends in the epidemiology of pediatric severe sepsis. *Pediatr Crit Care Med.* 2013 Sep;14(7):686-693. doi:10.1097/PCC.0b013e3182917fad

Maconochie IK, Aickin R, Hazinski MF, et al.; Pediatric Life Support Collaborators. Pediatric life support: 2020 international consensus on cardiopulmonary resuscitation and emergency

cardiovascular care science with treatment recommendations. *Circulation.* 2020 Oct 20;142(16 Suppl 1):S140-S184. doi:10.1161/CIR.0000000000000894

Martin K, Weiss SL. Initial resuscitation and management of pediatric septic shock. *Minerva Pediatr.* 2015;67(2):141-158.

Pasman EA. Shock in pediatrics. *Medscape.* July 12, 2019. https://emedicine.medscape.com/article/1833578-overview

Rodriguez-Gonzalez M, Sanchez-Codez MI, Lubian-Gutierrez M, Castellano-Martinez A. Clinical presentation and early predictors for poor outcomes in pediatric myocarditis: a retrospective study. *World J Clin Cases.* 2019;7(5):548-561. doi:10.12998/wjcc.v7.i5.548

Ventura AMC, Shieh HH, Bousso A, et al. Double-blind prospective randomized controlled trial of dopamine versus epinephrine as first-line vasoactive drugs in pediatric septic shock. *Crit Care Med.* 2015;43(11):2292-2302.

Walkzman M. Initial management of shock in children. *UpToDate.* June 7, 2011. https://somepomed.org/articulos/contents/mobipreview.htm?3/20/3393

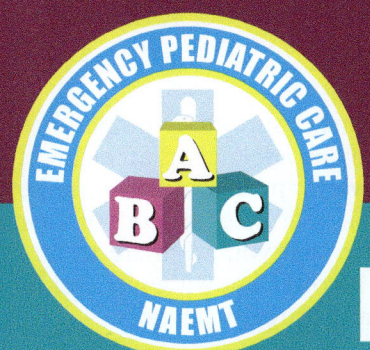

# CHAPTER 5

# Pediatric Medical Emergencies

## LESSON OBJECTIVES

- Discuss management of pediatric medical emergencies.
- Differentiate between medical emergencies in pediatrics.
- Discuss management of pediatric patients with medical emergencies using the Pediatric Assessment Triangle and XABCDE.
- Discuss the assessment and management of pain in the pediatric patient, along with the impact of untreated pain.

## Introduction

According to recent data, nearly 1 in 5 children accessed emergency care in 2015. The vast majority of these patients were treated and discharged from the emergency department without requiring inpatient admission or hospitalization. In that same year, the most common presenting conditions were as follows:

- Respiratory illness
- Injury (accidental or intentional, including toxicologic ingestions)
- Neurologic conditions

For patients presenting with an isolated medical emergency, respiratory illness and seizure disorder made up the majority of the chief complaints seen.

Fever is also a commonly reported chief complaint. While it is rarely an emergency, it is a nonspecific sign that there may be a more severe underlying illness such as infection or sepsis.

Infants and children younger than 5 years account for 2 out of 5 patients seen for treatment in the emergency department.

## Altered Mental Status

Pediatric patients presenting with altered mental status should be assumed to have a life-threatening illness or injury until proven otherwise. The differential diagnosis

for the causes of altered mental status is broad, and a detailed history and physical exam is often necessary to identify the specific cause. Table 5-1 describes the AEIOU-TIPS mnemonic, which may be helpful to work through possible differential diagnoses when treating a pediatric patient with altered mental status.

## Assessing Mental Status

Mental status assessment in infants and children can be difficult. The tools we commonly use, such as asking about person, place, time, and event, may not be developmentally appropriate for younger children.

The Glasgow Coma Scale (GCS) score is commonly utilized in the assessment of mental status, but it is important to remember that it is not intended for use in the medical emergency population. Despite this limitation, acute decompensation or decline in the GCS score is ominous and generally indicates patient deterioration.

The AVPU scale can be used to quickly assess mental status in the field and may be modified to be developmentally appropriate for the patient. AVPU describes the patient's level of responsiveness to one of four categories:

- Awake
  - The patient is awake and alert without any stimuli needed.
- Verbal
  - The patient responds to verbal stimuli or commands.

**Table 5-1** Altered Mental Status

| A | Alcohol |
|---|---|
| E | Epilepsy |
|   | Endocrine |
| I | Insulin |
|   | Intussusception |
|   | Intoxication |
| O | Oxygen |
| U | Uremia |
| T | Trauma |
|   | Temperature |
|   | Tumors |
| I | Infection |
| P | Psychiatric |
| S | Stroke |

© Jones & Bartlett Learning.

- Pain
  - The patient responds to painful stimuli, such as pressure to the nail bed or a sternal rub.
- Unresponsive
  - The patient does not arouse to any stimuli and is completely unresponsive.

Family members and caregivers can be helpful in assessing the mental status of children, especially when the patient may be acting shy or is intimidated by strangers. It is completely appropriate to ask caregivers, "Do you feel like your child is acting normally?" If they answer "no," ask what specifically is concerning about their behavior. Parental or caregiver concern about behavior is an important warning sign that the patient may have altered mental status.

# AEIOU-TIPS

## Alcohol

Accidental or intentional consumption of alcohol may lead to intoxication or coma. Prehospital practitioners should carefully assess the scene for clues of alcohol consumption when responding to pediatric altered mental status calls. In some cases, toddlers may have accidently consumed a parent or caregiver's drink. In other cases, it may be a teen who was intentionally ingesting the alcohol. It is important to make sure that you perform a thorough history and provide adolescents an element of privacy during the interview and exam. They may be reluctant to admit to alcohol or drug use in front of their parents. Emphasize to them that you are there to care for them, and part of that involves knowing whether or not they have consumed any drugs or alcohol.

## Epilepsy

Seizures are a common chief complaint in children suffering from a medical emergency. In many cases, the patient's first seizure activity prompts the call to emergency medical services (EMS). Therefore, many patients who go on to be diagnosed with epilepsy may initially present via EMS to the emergency department with an unprovoked seizure.

Some seizures may be related to ingestion of alcohol or drugs, while for others, hypo- or hyperglycemia may be the etiology. It is important to take a thorough history and perform a complete exam.

The seizure activity may have terminated spontaneously prior to the arrival of EMS. In these cases, clues that a seizure has occurred include the following:

- Injuries to the inner mouth, such as tongue or lip lacerations from biting
- Loss of bowel or bladder control
- Description of visual disturbance, hallucination, or other aura-type phenomenon immediately prior to the episode
- Stereotypical postictal phase

Patients who have already been diagnosed with epilepsy may experience seizures due to a number of factors. Illness is known to lower a patient's seizure threshold. Gastrointestinal (GI) illness resulting in vomiting may reduce the absorption of the patient's seizure medications. Missed doses of medication can prompt breakthrough seizures. In some cases, patients who have experienced a growth spurt may have outgrown their current seizure medication dose, making it subtherapeutic and less effective.

## Endocrine

Endocrine disorders are a common cause of altered mental status. Blood glucose abnormalities, including both hyper- and hypoglycemia, can lead to altered mental status, coma, and death.

Children with a known history of diabetes may have over- or underdosed their insulin, leading to dramatic swings in blood glucose levels. Some patients may have had insulin administered and then forgotten to eat or eaten less than anticipated. This is particularly true in toddlers who may refuse to eat a meal.

Diabetic children who are ill, particularly with GI pathogens, are susceptible to dramatic swings in glucose levels when diarrhea and/or vomiting are present.

Children with new-onset diabetes commonly present in diabetic ketoacidosis. When taking a history, look for the pathognomonic triad of polydipsia, polyphagia, and polyuria to aid in diagnosing this condition. There may also be a recent history of weight loss, and cachectic appearance may be present on physical exam.

Thyroid disorders may be present in infants and children. The physical exam may reveal signs of thyrotoxicosis, such as hyperthermia, agitation, tachycardia, weight loss, and sweating. Alternatively, if hypothermia, fatigue, bradycardia, and decreased alertness are present, severe hypothyroidism should be considered.

## HYPOTHYROIDISM IN INFANTS

**Mothers with a history of autoimmune thyroiditis, sometimes called Hashimoto's thyroiditis, may pass thyroid-stimulating hormone (TSH) receptor–blocking antibodies on to their newborn. These antibodies prevent TSH from binding to the appropriate receptor and lead to hypothyroidism in the child. The antibodies typically subside by about age 3 months and the child typically recovers without long-term issues.**

**Infants younger than 3 months with altered mental status and a maternal history of autoimmune thyroiditis should be screened for hypothyroidism.**

## Insulin

As discussed previously, improper administration of insulin can lead to dramatic swings in glucose levels. Diabetics who were previously well-controlled can easily go into hypo- or hyperglycemic crisis when insulin is not administered properly.

Adolescents and teens are prone to noncompliance with their insulin regimen. This is sometimes because they do not want to be perceived as different from their peers. They may skip insulin administration in order to hide their illness from their friends.

Some patients may have their insulin delivered via an automatic pump device. These devices sometimes malfunction or fail. Pump problems should be considered when evaluating a diabetic patient using this type of device for insulin delivery.

Oral diabetic medications may be unintentionally ingested by toddlers. Obtain a thorough history, including asking about medications in the home that the patient may have inadvertently ingested.

In some cases of medical child abuse (factitious disorder by proxy, Munchhausen by proxy) exogenous insulin may be administered to the child to induce hypoglycemia and prompt medical evaluation and treatment. Careful documentation of the history that a caregiver gives can aid in revealing medical child abuse if it is present.

## Intussusception

Intussusception is a GI disturbance caused by the telescoping of one segment of bowel into an adjoining segment. Incidence of intussusception peaks at age 18 months and is rarely seen in patients older than 2 years. Males are more commonly affected than females.

In most cases there is no identifiable cause for why the bowel telescoped into itself (idiopathic). In some cases, a pathologic lead point is identified. These lead points are inflamed or malformed areas of the bowel that serve as an area for adjoining segments to "bite" onto and begin the telescoping process.

Patients with intussusception will generally have episodic abdominal pain accompanied by significant inconsolability, with intervening periods of relative comfort. These episodes may be separated by a few minutes (usually less than 15) and represent the natural peristalsis of the GI tract, repeatedly running through the intussuscepted segment with peristaltic waves leading to the severe bouts of pain. Ambulatory children may squat during these episodes. Nonambulatory children may draw their legs up to their chest. A late finding of intussusception is bloody, so-called currant jelly stools.

## Intoxication

Intoxication with any number of substances can lead to altered mental status. In some cases, the patient may have intentionally ingested the substance in an attempt to become intoxicated or cause self-harm. In other cases, the patient may have ingested the substance(s) unknowingly.

Intoxication should be high on the differential diagnosis for all cases of altered mental status. While certain substances have a known toxidrome that may aid in identification, it is reasonable to empirically obtain a urine toxin screen in the emergency department setting as part of the altered mental status work-up.

EMS practitioners should pay close attention to clues at the scene that may aid in identifying whether substances have been ingested and what those substances may have been.

With the widespread decriminalization of marijuana, there has been a rise in children gaining access to legally obtained marijuana edible products. This has led to an increase in children presenting with acute marijuana intoxication. These patients may present with a wide variety of symptoms. Most commonly, children are described as having decreased responsiveness, slurred speech, and sluggish or slow behaviors. Some case reports describe symptoms of agitation, euphoria, or excitability. It is always reasonable to suspect coingestion of other substances or ingestion of marijuana that has been laced with additional substances.

## Oxygen

Hypoxia is a well-known cause for altered mental status in pediatric patients. Refer to the notes for Lesson 2, *Respiratory Emergencies,* for more information on hypoxia, its causes, and treatment.

## Uremia

Children with chronic kidney disease are susceptible to increased urea levels in the blood as kidney function declines. This leads to numerous symptoms, including altered mental status, seizures, coma, bleeding, and pericarditis. Some patients may have a known kidney disease, whereas others may have underlying chronic kidney disease that has yet to be diagnosed.

One cause of uremia is chronic or recurrent kidney infection that leads to scarring and dysfunction of the renal system. In some cases, the pathogens causing the urinary tract infections produce an enzyme called urease. The presence of excessive urea (such as when chronic kidney disease and infection are present) combined with urease can lead to high levels of ammonia as a result of urea breakdown by urease. These high levels of ammonia lead to encephalopathy, which may be accompanied by confusion and altered mental status.

## Trauma

Traumatic experiences can lead to altered mental status even in the absence of visible injury or bleeding. Children often do not know how to process traumatic events and may be confused, agitated, catatonic, or otherwise altered.

In situations where significant blood loss may be present, altered mental status is an ominous sign

and indicates poor cerebral perfusion. This should be treated as symptomatic shock until proven otherwise.

## Temperature

Environmental exposure leading to hypo- and hyperthermia can cause altered mental status. Children are unable to regulate their body temperature as well as adults and can suffer from environmental emergencies even in temperatures that are relatively comfortable to adults. When concern exists that a patient may be having a temperature-related emergency, a core temperature should be taken (rectal).

### MALIGNANT HYPERTHERMIA

Malignant hyperthermia is a condition in which there is activation of a skeletal muscle receptor with a genetic defect that causes excessive release of calcium. The downstream effects of this excessive activation include pathologic and uncontrolled increase in core body temperature. Common triggers include inhaled volatile anesthetics and succinylcholine. Prehospital practitioners should be aware of this and monitor for malignant hyperthermia in any patient receiving medications known to trigger the condition.

In addition to dramatic rise in temperature, precipitous rise in end-tidal $CO_2$ ($ETCO_2$) despite appropriate ventilation can be another sign of evolving malignant hyperthermia.

Treatment for malignant hyperthermia involves active cooling and temperature control, along with the administration of dantrolene. If there is suspicion for malignant hyperthermia in the field after administration of succinylcholine, the receiving facility should be notified so they can have dantrolene on standby when the patient arrives.

## Tumors

Acute onset of altered mental status combined with other focal neurologic findings such as ataxia, dysarthria, paralysis, visual disturbance, or other deficits may be the initial findings when an intracranial tumor has grown to the point where it is causing mass effect on adjacent structures. In some cases, the symptoms may be nonspecific and difficult to differentiate from other causes of altered mental status. In other cases, a thorough neurologic exam reveals specific deficits that can isolate the location of the neoplasm with a high degree of accuracy. Differentiating between mass effect from a tumor and cerebrovascular accident or stroke can be difficult in the field. Identifying that a neurologic deficit is present and transporting to the appropriate facility are the most important prehospital steps. Imaging and specific diagnosis will take place at the receiving hospital.

## Infection

Infection of the blood (bacteremia) and infection of the central nervous system (CNS; meningitis, encephalitis) will often have associated altered mental status. The mental status changes may be due to sepsis and shock, as is the case with bacteremia, or from direct invasion of the CNS by pathogens, as is seen in meningitis.

Patients with decreased immunity, such as neonates and patients undergoing chemotherapy, are particularly susceptible to overwhelming infection. Signs may include fever, confusion, and agitation. Neonates may have poor oral intake, lethargy, increased irritability, and a bulging fontanelle.

## Psychiatric

Psychiatric emergencies occur in patients of nearly all ages. A history of mental health issues may aid in diagnosing a psychiatric emergency. Underlying acute illness such as infection, endocrine imbalance, or CNS neoplasm can also be triggers for psychiatric or behavioral emergencies. The potential for an organic cause of psychiatric emergency should always be considered. More information on pediatric behavioral health emergencies is presented in Lesson 11, *Pediatric Behavioral Health*.

## Stroke

As discussed, cerebral hypoperfusion can lead to acute altered mental status. Although children are not classically thought to be at high risk for stroke or cerebrovascular incident (CVA), there are certain underlying illnesses that increase the risk of these conditions. Some children may have a condition called an arteriovenous malformation (AVM). An AVM is an overgrowth of tangled arterial and venous vasculature. These form in utero early during fetal development. The true incidence of AVM is unknown as many patients never experience clinical symptoms. When the

AVM is large or placed under stress, it can rupture, leading to significant intracranial bleeding. The most common symptom of this is acute-onset severe headache. In some cases, it may wake the patient from sleep. Infants who are not able to describe their pain may present with inconsolability and focal neurologic deficit.

Other patients at risk for stroke include individuals with sickle cell disease and blood clotting disorders. It is important to take not only a good patient history, but also ask if any family members had a stroke at an early age.

# Hypoglycemia

Hypoglycemia is a common cause of altered mental status in pediatric patients. All pediatric patients with altered mental status should have a blood glucose level checked early on in their work-up, as this is inexpensive to check, relatively noninvasive, high yield, and easily corrected.

## Signs of Hypoglycemia

When the serum blood glucose begins to decline, glucose stores (in the form of glycogen) are mobilized from the liver. This process is regulated by the hormone glucagon. In addition to glucagon, epinephrine also raises blood glucose levels. Part of the fight-or-flight response stimulated by the sympathetic nervous system is to mobilize glucose stores to fuel the brain and muscles to enable the body's ability to flee or defend against a threat. This same response can be seen when glucose levels become dangerously low. Adrenergic, cognitive, and behavioral symptoms of hypoglycemia can be seen in **Table 5-2**.

| Table 5-2 Symptoms of Hypoglycemia | | |
|---|---|---|
| **Adrenergic** | **Cognitive** | **Behavioral** |
| ■ Pallor | ■ Fatigue | ■ Irritability |
| ■ Sweating | ■ Lethargy | ■ Agitation |
| ■ Tachycardia | ■ Headaches | ■ Erratic behavior |
| ■ Tremor | ■ Seizure | ■ Quietness in an otherwise gregarious child |
| ■ Palpitations | ■ Coma | |
| | | ■ Tantrums |

© Jones & Bartlett Learning.

Not all patients have the same response to hypoglycemia. Some patients will be symptomatic at a much lower or higher blood glucose level than expected, and the symptoms may not reflect the severity of their hypoglycemia. Some patients may be awake and alert with a mild headache and a blood glucose level of 38 mg/dL, whereas others may be acutely altered and confused with a blood glucose level of 58 mg/dL.

# Pathophysiology of Hypoglycemia

The most common cause of hypoglycemia in children outside of infancy is mismanagement of type 1 diabetes. Infants 12 months or younger more commonly experience hypoglycemia due to poor feeding and intercurrent GI illness. This is due to low glucose reserves (inadequate glycogen stores) and the inability to mobilize glucose from glycogen when oral intake is low.

Outside of the traditional causes of hypoglycemia, the following causes are rare, but should be considered:

- Hyperinsulinemia
  - Hyperinsulinemia is a condition in which too much insulin is produced by the body. This can be the result of hyperactive beta islet cells or an insulin-producing tumor.
- Exogenous insulin administration
  - Some patients may have been given exogenous insulin leading to acute hypoglycemia. In some cases, this may be an accidental miscalculation of a routine dose. In other cases, it may be a form of medical child abuse in which a parent or caregiver gives the patient exogenous insulin to cause clinical symptoms and prompt medical evaluation or treatment of the child.
- Inborn errors of metabolism
  - Neonates and infants may experience glucose homeostasis issues due to deficiencies in enzymes and proteins necessary for glucose metabolism. These are generally tested for on state newborn screening, however in some cases there is a false negative on this screening and patients present later in infancy.
- Gluconeogenesis disorders
  - Patients who lack the proper enzymes or hormones necessary to build, store, break down, or mobilize glycogen stores will have glycemic control issues. These disorders are unique because patients will be stable when they ingest glucose and have the functional necessity to use glucose. When such patients fast and must rely on glycogen, they become hypoglycemic as they are unable to mobilize glycogen stores.
- Toxins
  - Certain ingestions will have a toxidrome that includes hypoglycemia. Oral diabetic medications such as sulfonylureas increase insulin production, which can lead to acute hypoglycemia. Parents and caregivers should always be questioned about what medications the child may have accessed. Beta blockers, salicylates, and ethanol ingestion can also cause acute hypoglycemia. A thorough history is necessary to identify possible ingestion in these cases.
- Illness
  - GI illness and poor oral intake is a well-known cause of hypoglycemia. Other illnesses such as malaria and any overwhelming infection causing sepsis can also have concomitant hypoglycemia as metabolic demand is significantly elevated.

## Hypoglycemia Severity

Treatment for hypoglycemia depends on the severity and the patient's level of consciousness. In general, the severity of hypoglycemia is based on the following ranges:

- Mild
  - 55–70 mg/dL
- Moderate
  - 40–55 mg/dL
- Severe
  - Less than 40 mg/dL

These ranges represent a guideline for hypoglycemia severity. The actual patient presentation will vary between individuals. Some individuals tolerate hypoglycemia much better than others. For this reason, the actual clinical value must be considered within the context of the symptoms the patient is experiencing to make an overall assessment of the severity.

## Mild to Moderate Hypoglycemia Management

There are three options to treat hypoglycemia based on the severity of the patient's condition and their level of consciousness.

Oral glucose, sometimes referred to as enteral glucose, is the least invasive method for treating hypoglycemia. It typically can be administered in mild or moderate hypoglycemia if the patient is alert enough to swallow without the risk of aspiration.

Oral glucose can be safely administered through an enteral feeding tube or gastrostomy tube (G-tube). Practitioners should flush the tubing with 30 mL or more of water to prevent clogging and ensure that the entire dose is given.

After administration of enteral glucose, the blood glucose level should be rechecked in 10 to 15 minutes, or sooner if the patient's condition deteriorates. If the blood glucose level remains low and the patient is alert enough to swallow without the risk for aspiration, an additional dose may be administered.

## Severe Hypoglycemia Management

In patients with glucose levels below 40 mg/dL or any level of hypoglycemia accompanied by altered level of consciousness, enteral administration of glucose may not be safe or achieve the intended effects within a reasonable amount of time.

There are two options for treatment of severe hypoglycemia. The first is intravascular dextrose (D-Glucose). This can be given via intravenous (IV) or intraosseous (IO) line. In general, the concentration of glucose administered through a peripheral line should not exceed 25%.

### CONVERTING D50 FOR PEDIATRIC USE

While 50% dextrose (D50) is commonly given in adults, it is not recommended in children younger than 8 years. D50 can be diluted into either D25 or D10 by doing the following:

- To dilute D50 to D25:
  - Expel 25 mL of volume from the 50 mL ampule.
  - Replace the expelled volume with 25 mL of normal saline.
  - This will result in a dextrose concentration of 25% (D25).
- To dilute D50 to D10:
  - Expel 40 mL of volume from the 50 mL ampule.
  - Replace the expelled volume with 40 mL of normal saline.
  - This will result in a dextrose concentration of 10% (D10).

D10 is generally preferred in pediatric patients as it has less potential to cause sclerosis to the vasculature as it is infused. High dextrose concentrations tend to have higher potential for vascular sclerosis.

### DEXTROSE DOSING

A quick method for determining the proper volume of IV dextrose to administer to a patient for hypoglycemia is to divide 50 by the dextrose concentration, and then multiply that answer by the patient's weight in kilograms to determine to total volume to be administered. An example with D10 would look like the following:

You have a 13-kg patient and you want to administer a D10 bolus.

50 (constant)/ 10 (dextrose concentration) = 5 mL/kg (volume to be administered)

5 mL/kg × 13 kg = 65 mL (total volume to be administered)

A similar example with D25 would appear as follows:

You have a 17-kg patient and you want to administer a D25 bolus.

50 (constant)/ 25 (dextrose concentration) = 2 mL/kg (volume to be administered)

2 mL/kg × 17 kg = 34 mL (total volume to be administered)

As you become more comfortable with dextrose administration in pediatric patients, you may be able to skip the first step by simply remembering that a D10 bolus is 5 mL/kg, and a D25 bolus is 2 mL/kg.

The second option for severe hypoglycemia treatment is glucagon. Glucagon is a naturally occurring hormone that breaks down stored glycogen into glucose that can be used by the body. Glucagon is available as an intramuscular (IM) injection, and in some areas may be available for intranasal (IN) administration. IN administration is an excellent option for practitioners who are not authorized to provide IM injections. The dosing for glucagon is as follows:

- Patients weighing 20 kg or more, or older than 5 years:
  - 1 mg IM or IN
- Patients weighing less than 20 kg, or younger than 5 years:
  - 0.5 mg IM or IN

> Since glucagon relies on the body's glycogen stores in order to increase blood glucose levels, patients with poor nutrition or depleted glucose stores are less likely to respond. These patients will likely receive greater clinical benefit from dextrose administration. This should be considered when the patient's response to glucagon administration is not as favorable as desired.

# Hyperglycemia

Hyperglycemia is defined as a blood glucose level greater than 200 mg/dL. Blood glucose can be elevated for several reasons. In some cases it may be a normal physiologic response to stress. In these cases, the patient does not generally suffer ill effects and the body is able to restore glucose homeostasis without direct intervention.

In other cases, the patient may have an underlying pathology that is causing hyperglycemia.

## Diabetes Mellitus

There are two types of diabetes: type 1 and type 2. Type 1 was previously referred to as juvenile-onset diabetes, as this was the most common form seen in children and adolescents. With the increase in childhood obesity, type 2 diabetes, previously referred to as adult-onset diabetes, is being increasingly seen in patients younger than 18 years.

### Type 1 Diabetes Pathology

Type 1 diabetes is an autoimmune disorder in which antibodies destroy the beta islet cells in the pancreas and the body is no longer able to produce endogenous insulin. Most of these patients will have some degree of endogenous insulin production for many years and reach a tipping point where a terminal number of beta islet cells have been destroyed and endogenous insulin is no longer sufficient to maintain metabolic homeostasis. Most type 1 diabetics do not present in infancy, rather they present in childhood and adolescence. These patients will often be cachectic, and when the serum insulin level is checked, it will be dramatically low. These patients are completely dependent on exogenous insulin to manage their glucose homeostasis. Measured serum insulin levels in these patients will be very low, as the beta islet cells have been destroyed and are no longer producing insulin.

The prototypical type 1 diabetic patient is a child or adolescent who is underweight, dehydrated, and has a prodrome of polyuria, polydipsia, and polyphagia. These patients will be cachectic, in a starvation state, with muscle and fat breakdown taking place. Despite the hyperglycemia, the body is unable to use the glucose due to lack of endogenous insulin.

Many type 1 diabetics will have a recent history of febrile illness. The increased metabolic state that children enter when experiencing a febrile illness may precipitate diabetic ketoacidosis in a type 1 diabetic.

## Type 2 Diabetes Pathology

Type 2 diabetes is a process in which the body has been subjected to excessively high levels of insulin due to dietary and genetic factors. This prolonged exposure to high insulin levels causes a downregulation in cellular insulin receptors, leading to insulin resistance. In this case, the patient's serum insulin level is high, however the cellular response to insulin will be inadequate due to receptor downregulation and resistance. Treatment for these patients includes medications to enhance cellular response to endogenous insulin, along with medications to enhance endogenous release of insulin. Type 2 diabetics who are poorly controlled for extended durations may reach a point at which their beta islet cells stop functioning, leading to insulin deficiency and a dependence on exogenous insulin to maintain glucose homeostasis, similar to type 1 diabetes.

The prototypical patient with type 2 diabetes is obese and generally an adolescent or adult. Physical exam may reveal acanthosis nigricans—a dermatologic finding that results from insulin resistance and high circulating insulin levels (**Figure 5-1**). This is most often seen on the back of the neck and in the axillary folds.

## Hyperglycemic Emergencies

There are two main types of hyperglycemic emergencies: diabetic ketoacidosis (DKA) and hyperglycemic hyperosmolar state (HHS).

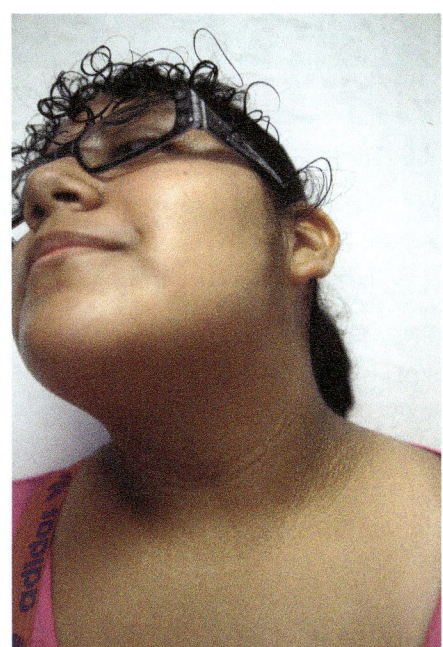

**Figure 5-1** Classic acanthosis nigricans on the neck of a patient with insulin resistance. It is a thick, velvety buildup of darkened skin. It can also be seen in the axillary folds of the arms and legs.

© Benedicte Desrus/Alamy Stock Photo.

## Diabetic Ketoacidosis

DKA is a hyperglycemic, dehydrated state in which the body must use alternative fuel sources to support metabolism. Although glucose is elevated, insulin is deficient or absent and glucose cannot be used. The serum concentration of catecholamines, glucagon, and cortisol increase the lipolysis and ketogenesis in an effort to meet the cellular energy needs. This leads to a metabolic cascade resulting in ketosis and acidosis.

The most common cause of DKA is undiagnosed type 1 diabetes. This will be the presenting illness in 25% of new type 1 diabetics. Established type 1 diabetics are also at risk of developing DKA when their illness is poorly managed, they are ill, or they miss doses of insulin. DKA in established diabetics is usually easier to diagnose as it is known that the patient has diabetes and the suspicion for DKA is higher. Drug and alcohol use in diabetic adolescents, combined with poor glucose control and missed doses of insulin, can also lead to DKA.

The classic presentation of DKA in the undiagnosed diabetic includes the triad of polyuria, polydipsia, and polyphagia. The serum glucose is high, and glucose has the osmotic effect of pulling free water into the intravascular space. The excess glucose is excreted by the kidneys along with free water, leading to polyuria. The excessive urination and shift of fluids leads to severe dehydration. This dehydration stimulates a significant thirst response, and parents may report an increase in oral fluid intake. Inability to use glucose leads to a starvation state, and patients may have a history of increased appetite. However, the nausea that accompanies the acidosis and dehydration may curtail eating.

The profound metabolic acidosis seen in DKA leads to respiratory compensation in the form of a deep, rapid respiratory rate called Kussmaul breathing. Some new-onset DKA patients will present with a chief complaint of respiratory distress due to this breathing pattern, only to find out it has been precipitated by DKA. The excessive ketones may be detected on the breath of patients in the form of a fruity or chemical odor, however this is not always the case.

> DKA is often an insidious process, developing over weeks to even months. A thorough and detailed history is necessary to make the diagnosis. Often when the diagnosis is made based on lab values at the hospital, and the family is asked more specific questions about the history, they begin to recall that the patient was indeed eating, drinking, and urinating more over the weeks leading up to the presentation. This history is often unclear to the parents until they are asked about it directly. The challenge in eliciting this history is ensuring the right questions are asked.

## Hyperglycemic Hyperosmolar State

HHS is most associated with poorly controlled type 2 diabetes. Profound insulin resistance combined with illness, injury, or other physiologic stress leads to a precipitous rise in the serum glucose. Serum glucose in this condition is generally much higher than DKA. This process evolves more quickly than DKA and ketosis is most often absent or very mild. The acidosis present is usually mild. Altered consciousness and seizures can be present in up to 50% of cases.

> DKA and HHS are distinct clinical entities with specific diagnostic criteria. There is a small subset of patients that will present with crossover features of both disease processes. The management of these complex cases requires a multidisciplinary team at a pediatric tertiary care center.

| Table 5-3 DKA Versus HHS | |
| --- | --- |
| **DKA** | **HHS** |
| <ul><li>Usually younger children, no diabetic history</li><li>Hyperglycemia<ul><li>Generally less than 600 mg/dL</li></ul></li><li>Profound metabolic acidosis<ul><li>Venous pH <7.3</li><li>pH may be less than 7.1 in severe cases</li><li>bicarb <15 mEq/L</li><li>Serum bicarbonate deficit alone can be used for diagnosis in some settings</li></ul></li><li>Ketosis<ul><li>Blood and urine ketones required for diagnosis of DKA</li></ul></li><li>Altered consciousness may be present in severe cases, but generally mental status is preserved</li></ul> | <ul><li>Usually older adolescents, history of type 2 diabetes</li><li>Severe hyperglycemia<ul><li>Generally >600 mg/dL</li></ul></li><li>Mild to moderate metabolic acidosis<ul><li>Venous pH is generally >7.25</li><li>Arterial pH is generally greater than 7.3 and can even be normal in some cases</li></ul></li><li>Small to no ketones present in blood or urine</li><li>Altered consciousness, including seizures present in approximately 50% of cases</li></ul> |

© Jones & Bartlett Learning.

Table 5-3 presents a comparative summary of characteristics of DKA and HHS.

# Hyperglycemia Management

Whether the patient is in DKA or HHS, the mainstay of treatment is evaluating and treating dehydration. In most cases, blood gas analysis and serum chemistry will not be available in the prehospital setting and differentiating between the two conditions may not be possible.

The first step is to assess the degree of dehydration. Clinical exam features such as poor skin turgor, dry mucous membranes, and prolonged capillary refill suggest a moderate to severe degree of dehydration. If the patient's weight is known and it is clear they have lost a significant amount of weight in a short period of time, it can be assumed that a large amount of that weight is free water. This can also serve as a starting point for rehydration.

Rehydration therapy should be performed slowly. It is reasonable to accomplish this goal with 10 mL/kg boluses of isotonic crystalloid. Repeat boluses may be given to support hemodynamic parameters such as level of consciousness, blood pressure, pulse, and capillary refill.

Serum potassium may appear normal or elevated at the time of presentation, however the overall body content of potassium is low. This is due to intracellular potassium shifting to the extracellular space in exchange for hydrogen in an effort to increase the pH and mitigate the metabolic acidosis. The potassium deficit puts the patient at risk of arrhythmias. The most high-risk period is during rehydration and at the initiation of the insulin infusion. Once the patient begins to get insulin, the serum potassium drops precipitously as the insulin drives potassium ions back into the cell. DKA patients often require electrolyte repletion as part of their long-term metabolic correction strategy. Due to the potential for electrolyte abnormalities, all patients with hyperglycemia should have an electrocardiogram (ECG) performed and should be placed on a cardiac monitor.

The primary therapy for HHS is rehydration, circulatory support, and slow glucose correction. HHS patients will be profoundly dehydrated.

Both DKA and HHS patients are at risk for cerebral edema. When large volumes of fluid are given, followed by insulin infusions, there is a dramatic shift of fluid into the cells. Tissues in the body that are particularly glucose dependent are susceptible to swelling and edema. This is especially true for the cerebral tissues. When administering fluid to a patient with a level of consciousness that is already altered, it can be difficult to note signs of increasing intracranial pressure. Vital signs should be monitored closely and any clinical findings that are consistent with elevated intracranial pressure (hypertension, bradycardia, irregular breathing) should be aggressively treated.

# Fever

A fever is defined as a temperature of 100.4°F (38°C) or higher in children. Fever is a natural response to infection. When the body encounters an infection, pyrogenic cytokines are produced, including interleukins 1 and 6. These cytokines are transported via the bloodstream to the hypothalamus, the region in the brain responsible for temperature homeostasis. In response to these cytokines, a new "set point" is established, metabolic rate increases, muscles activate (in the form of shivering or rigors), and perfusion to the skin is diminished as the body produces and retains heat. All of these processes act together to increase body temperature and generate a fever. Due to the increased blood flow and metabolism required to generate a fever, tachycardia and tachypnea are often present when patients are febrile.

The body increases temperature in the face of infection for several reasons. Elevated temperatures create a suboptimal environment for the reproduction of many bacteria and viruses, slowing their spread. Elevated temperature also enhances endogenous neutrophil production and T-lymphocyte proliferation. Both of these processes aid in fighting infection.

## Fever Myths

As fever is the body's natural response to infection, in most cases fevers are not dangerous and require no treatment unless the patient is uncomfortable. Fever alone is not necessarily an emergency. Parents will often focus on things they can see and treat, such as the child's temperature. In addition to this, many parents do not understand the definition of a fever and will often treat nonfebrile temperatures of 99°F to 100°F (37.2°C to 38°C), unnecessarily giving medications. Nearly half of parents do not correctly dose antipyretic medications, with 15% giving too much medication. This overdose of fever medication can endanger the kidneys and liver.

Another misconception is that the severity of the fever alone is an indicator of the severity of infection. Some patients who are in fulminant septic shock may only have low-grade temperatures, whereas other patients with temperatures above 102°F (38.9°C) may appear clinically well. Temperature should not be used as the sole determinant of illness severity.

## Fever Emergencies

In general, fever is not a medical emergency unless it is associated with signs and symptoms of respiratory distress, poor perfusion, or altered mental status. Fevers reaching 104°F (40°C) or higher are more likely to be associated with severe infection when any of the previously mentioned findings are present.

There are two specific patient populations in which fever of any level is a medical emergency requiring further work-up in the emergency room:

- Febrile neonates
  - Infants younger than 3 months with fever should be evaluated by a physician.
    - Less than 28 days old with a fever requires a full septic workup including:
      - Complete blood count (CBC)
      - Inflammatory markers
      - Blood culture
      - Urine culture
      - Lumbar puncture for cerebrospinal fluid studies
    - Infants 28 days to 2 months of age can get limited work-up in a stepwise fashion.
  - Infants have immature immune systems and are susceptible to overwhelming infection that can lead to rapid decompensation.
- Immunocompromised individuals
  - Any patient with compromised immune system function should have an evaluation for fever.
  - The most common pediatric patients with immunocompromise are those undergoing chemotherapy.
  - Any febrile patient actively being treated with chemotherapy should have an evaluation by a physician.

> **Parents of children with febrile seizure history may be more aggressive in attempting to control fevers in an effort to prevent recurrence of seizure activity. This is appropriate and should be documented in the past medical history.**

## Fever Management

Fever is managed with antipyretic medications and, in some cases, passive and active cooling measures. The decision to give antipyretics is made based on local protocols. The dosing information for the most used pediatric antipyretic medications is as follows:

Acetaminophen

- 10–15 mg/kg by mouth every 4 hours
- Do not exceed 75 mg/kg total dosage in 24 hours

Ibuprofen

- 10 mg/kg by mouth every 6 hours
- Use caution in patients with renal impairment
- Do not use in infants younger than age 6 months

# Seizures

Seizures can be defined as a sudden occurrence of abnormal or hyperexcitable electrical activity in the brain. There is a variety of seizure presentations depending on what part of the brain is suffering from the aberrant electrical activity (**Figure 5-2**).

Not all seizures are associated with generalized tonic-clinic (GTC) activity or altered mental status. Seizures in neonates and infants can be very subtle and difficult to recognize. Lip smacking, twitching of the face or extremities, eye deviation, jaw clenching, and cyanosis are all possible signs that a seizure is occurring. Neonates do not have the neurologic maturity to present with GTC activity. Often spasms, tongue thrusting, and lip smacking may be the only signs present. It may be necessary to ask specific questions about the activity that occurred, as the event being described by parents may be very subtle.

A comparative summary of the features of focal and generalized seizures is shown in **Table 5-4**.

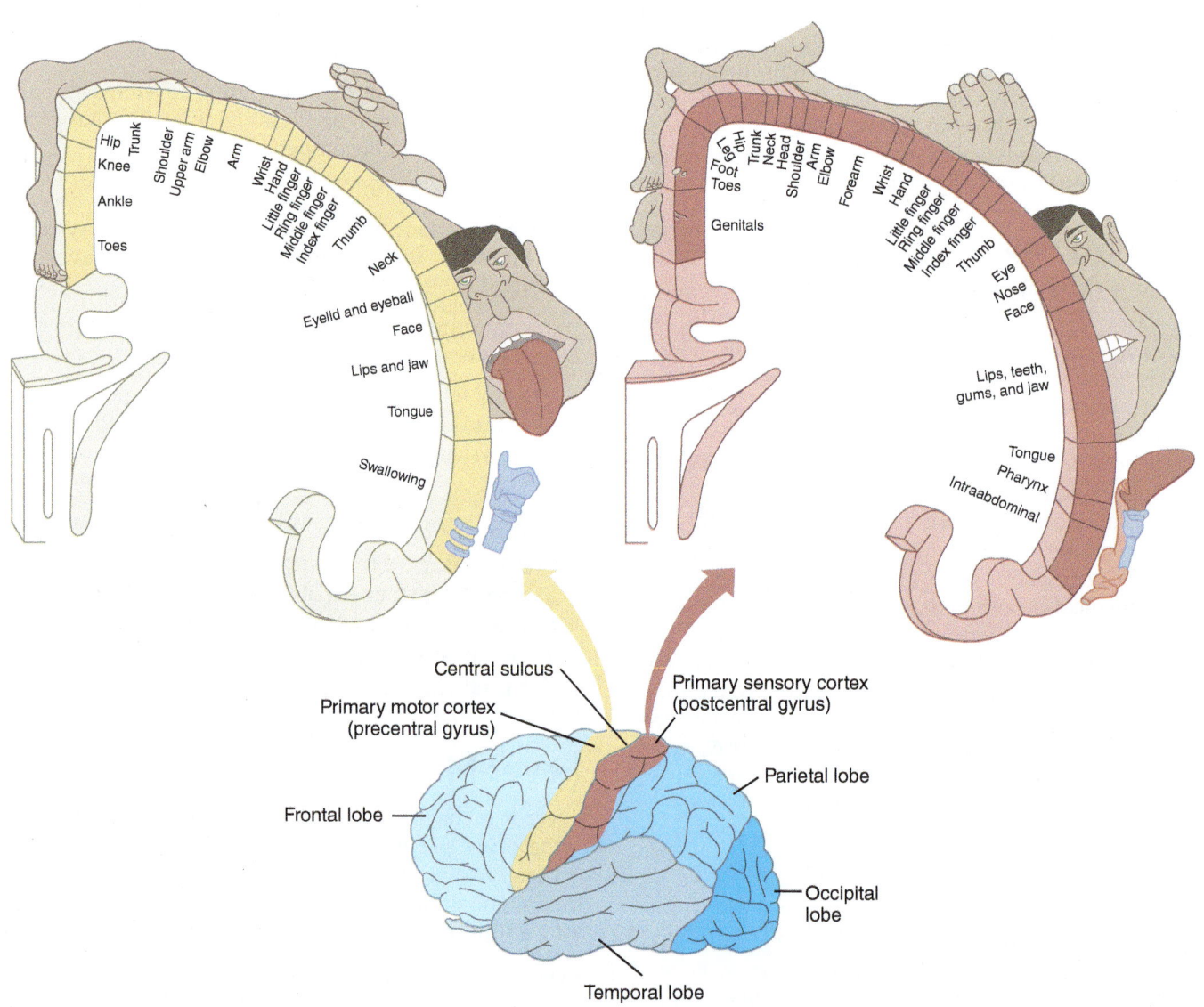

**Figure 5-2** The phenotypic presentation of a seizure depends on what part of the brain is impacted.

© Jones & Bartlett Learning.

**Table 5-4** Seizure Classification

| Focal (Partial) | Generalized |
|---|---|
| ■ Seizure activity originates within networks limited to a single hemisphere. | ■ Seizure activity engages bilateral networks. |
| ■ Patients may be completely alert and aware. | ■ Motor activity can be present or absent. |
| ■ Focal motor activity starts in one region and spreads to adjacent anatomic regions as the aberrant electrical activity propagates through the brain. | ■ Absence seizures (a generalized subtype) are staring spells without motor activity. The patients are not aware of these spells and have no recall of the event. There is usually no respiratory depression. |
| ■ May begin with eye or head deviation, or with vocalization or arrest in speech. | |
| ■ Sensory seizures (a subset of focal seizures) may originate with paresthesia, disorientation, vertigo, or other sensory phenomena (sight, sound, smell, taste, etc.). | |

© Jones & Bartlett Learning.

**With smartphones being nearly universal, some parents may have video of the seizure-like activity for you to review. This can be very important for the pediatric neurologist to evaluate in determining what kind of seizure activity, if any, occurred.**

**Depending on the policies in your jurisdiction, it may be appropriate to have parents record the seizure activity if it occurs during transport, so that it may be reviewed later. Never delay caring for a seizure to capture video evidence.**

# Commonly Encountered Seizure Emergencies

The two most common pediatric seizure emergencies requiring EMS response are febrile seizures and status epilepticus.

## Febrile Seizures

A febrile seizure is seizure activity occurring in a child aged 6 months to 5 years in the presence of a fever (temperature greater than 100.4°F [38°C]) without CNS infection. Febrile seizures can be simple or complex based on the length of activity and the number of episodes in 24 hours.

A simple febrile seizure is 15 minutes or less with only a single episode in 24 hours. There should be no lingering neurologic deficit or focal neurologic findings after the seizure has stopped and the postictal state is complete. Simple febrile seizures generally do not require any additional work-up, and parents are given anticipatory guidance for seizure precautions with future infections. Any evaluation for a simple febrile seizure is usually directed at finding and treating infectious sources of fever if possible.

Complex febrile seizures last longer than 15 minutes or have more than one occurrence in 24 hours. In addition to identifying any treatable infectious cause of fever, patients with complex febrile seizure activity will generally require an electroencephalogram (EEG) and possibly head imaging. All patients with febrile seizures should be transported to the hospital for evaluation and observation, as it is not possible to know if seizure activity will recur or become prolonged.

Any patient who fails to return to their neurologic baseline after the seizure activity has terminated requires evaluation at a hospital. In these cases, there may be a serious underlying etiology such as infection, bleeding, or intracranial mass.

### Febrile Seizure Management and Prognosis

Febrile seizures that spontaneously resolve in less than 5 minutes should receive supportive care. In most cases the activity will have terminated prior to the arrival of EMS. When seizure activity persists longer than 5 minutes, treatment is the same as would be given to nonfebrile seizures, with the exception of antipyretic administration after the activity is terminated if allowed by protocol. Full seizure treatment is discussed in the next section.

The likelihood of additional febrile seizures with subsequent fever episodes is fairly high at 30% to 35%. Despite the high recurrence rate, the overall prognosis is very good. Approximately 1% to 2% will go on to be diagnosed with epilepsy. Very few children have long-lasting neurologic deficit due to febrile seizures. Those who do have long-term deficits likely suffered from prolonged hypoxia and may have benefitted from aggressive pharmacologic seizure control.

## Status Epilepticus

Status epilepticus is seizure activity that persists longer than 5 minutes. Status epilepticus is a medical emergency. Even if you can terminate the seizure activity, be aware that the patient's seizure threshold has likely been lowered, and recurrence is likely unless additional therapy is initiated.

### CAREGIVER ADMINISTRATION OF MEDICATIONS

Rectal diazepam is a form of diazepam packaged in a syringe that can be administered to seizing patients rectally. This medication is provided to parents and caregivers of children with a known seizure disorder so that they can treat prolonged seizure activity while awaiting EMS arrival.

IN midazolam is a newer option to achieve the same goal. You may encounter parents who have been prescribed IN midazolam kits for their children.

It is important to ask if any medications were given to stop the seizure when obtaining a history.

## Seizure Management

Most seizures will terminate or resolve spontaneously prior to EMS arrival on scene and usually only require supportive care during transport. In status epilepticus, the priorities are airway and breathing support, while taking measures to terminate the seizure activity.

Positioning patients on their sides so that they do not choke on vomit and secretions can aid in maintaining a patent airway. Supplemental oxygen and assisted ventilations should be provided to hypoxic patients with poor respiratory drive.

A blood glucose level can be obtained rapidly and is an easily corrected source of seizure activity. This measurement can be performed while obtaining vascular access.

Benzodiazepines are the first-line medication therapy for seizures. Midazolam is used most commonly due to its rapid onset and flexible routes of administration. Delays in treatment with antiseizure medications result in increased seizure refractoriness. The longer it takes to treat the seizure, the harder it is to terminate. Multiple doses may be needed. EMS practitioners should be aware that respiratory depression becomes more likely with subsequent benzodiazepine doses.

If seizure activity continues despite maximized use of a benzodiazepine, you should proceed to a second-line drug. The selection of a second-line agent is dependent on local protocols and guidelines.

Table 5-5 lists medications that can be used to terminate seizure activity.

| Table 5-5 Antiseizure Medications | | | | |
|---|---|---|---|---|
| **First-Line Medications** | | | | |
| **Medication** | **Dose** | **Route** | **Pros** | **Cons** |
| Midazolam | 0.1 mg/kg | IV, IM, IO, IN | Rapid onset | Medium duration of action (30 min) |
| Diazepam | 0.1 mg/kg | IV, IO | Rapid onset<br>Inexpensive<br>No refrigeration | Sedating<br>Respiratory depression<br>Short duration of action for seizure control (15 min) |
| | 0.5 mg/kg | PR | Rapid onset<br>No IV required | Sedating<br>Respiratory depression |
| Lorazepam | 0.05–0.1 mg/kg | IV, IO | Rapid onset<br>Long duration of action (24 hours) | Must be stored away from heat and extreme temperatures |

| Second-Line Medications | | | | |
|---|---|---|---|---|
| **Medication** | **Dose** | **Route** | **Pros** | **Cons** |
| Valproic acid | 40 mg/kg | IV, IO | Rapid onset<br><br>Lower risk of respiratory depression | Hepatoxicity |
| Fosphenytoin | 20 mg/kg (phenytoin equivalents or PE) | IV, IO | Inexpensive<br><br>Long duration of action (12–28 hours) | Hypotension and respiratory depression |
| Keppra | 60 mg/kg | IV, IO | Rapid onset | Somnolence, dizziness, and hostility |

© Jones & Bartlett Learning.

## CASE STUDY

## Case 1

### Dispatch

You and your partner respond to a residence for a 2-year-old male with fever and altered mental status. It is a summer afternoon with an outside temperature of 90°F (32.2°C).

### Case Questions

- What are your initial concerns?
  - Altered mental status is an ominous sign in pediatric patients.
- Based on the dispatch information, what are the possible differential diagnoses for this patient?
  - Altered mental status in pediatric patients has a broad differential diagnosis. This could include the following:
    - Trauma (accidental or nonaccidental)
    - Intracranial bleed
    - Concussion
    - Respiratory distress with hypoxia
    - Infection
      - CNS (meningitis)
      - Pneumonia
      - Urinary tract infection (UTI)
    - Seizure
    - Ingestion or poisoning
      - Carbon monoxide
      - Alcohol
      - Fertilizer
      - Pesticide
    - Metabolic disorder
      - DKA
      - Hypoglycemia
  - The scene size-up, history, and clinical exam will be critical in determining what is going on with this patient. Careful assessment of the patient and identification of any possibly ingested chemicals, medications, or other materials may be helpful. History taking with attention to the onset of the altered mental status and fever (acute versus chronic) and the behavior of the parents may aid in narrowing the differential diagnosis. Identifying medical conditions in the history that could cause altered mental status is also important.

## Initial Observations

As you arrive at the front entrance of the home you are met by the father who appears extremely anxious and distressed. He informs you that they recently traveled out of the country to see family.

- Pediatric Assessment Triangle (**Figure 5-3**)
  - Appearance
    - Lethargic
  - Work of breathing
    - **F**laring not present
    - **R**etractions not present but effort labored and respirations shallow and rapid
    - **A**udible airway sounds not present

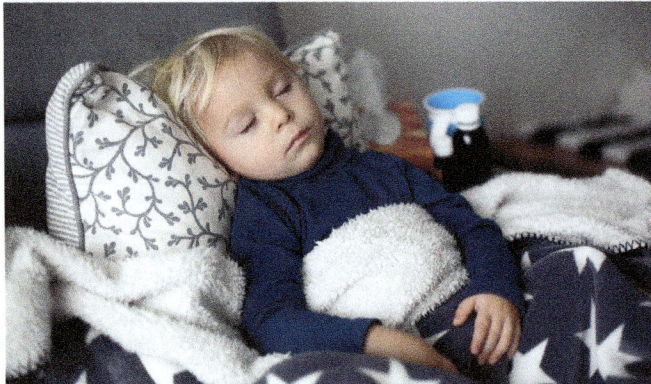

**A**

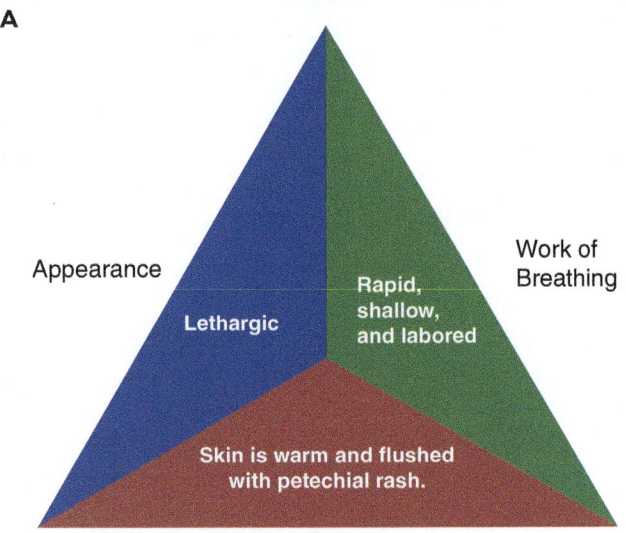

**B**

**Figure 5-3** The patient appears lethargic with rapid, shallow, and labored breathing.

- **P**ositioning—the patient not actively positioning themselves
- Circulation
  - Skin warm and flushed with petechial rash noted on legs

### Case Questions

- What additional precautions might be necessary based on these findings?
  - The petechial rash and fever are concerning for infectious disease, especially considering the patient has recently traveled internationally.
  - Appropriate personal protective equipment should be worn to reduce the risk of disease transmission.
- Based on your initial impression, is this patient "Quick" or "Not Quick"?
  - This patient is "Quick."
  - Any pediatric patient with altered level of consciousness requires rapid stabilization, treatment, and transport. The lethargy, respiratory distress, and petechial rash all indicate that the patient is very ill.
  - The altered mental status is the major red flag in this case. The flushed skin may be evidence of flash capillary refill, which should be evaluated on physical exam. If flash capillary refill is present, the concern for distributive (in this case septic) shock increases.

## Standard Precautions

There are various forms and styles of personal protective equipment (PPE) available to healthcare practitioners. The type you wear will depend on the guidelines and protocols of your agency and which vendors they use to procure equipment (**Figure 5-4**).

Gloves should be worn during all patient contact to mitigate the potential for exposure to any infectious agent or body fluid. If aerosol generating procedures (AGPs) are being performed (nebulizers, high-flow nasal cannula, intubation, deep suctioning), then goggles, face shields, and surgical masks should also be used.

Impermeable gowns should be worn in addition to the PPE listed earlier when splash or liquid exposures are possible. A gown should also be worn with patients

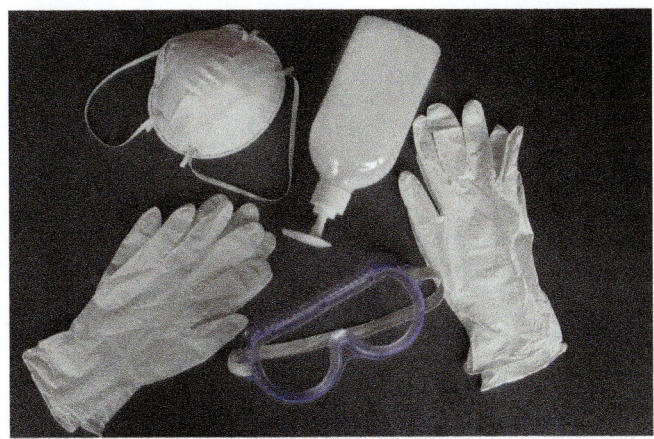

**Figure 5-4** Proper PPE lessens the safety risk to EMS practitioners.
© Isabel Pavia/Moment/Getty Images.

who are producing aerosols or receiving AGPs to prevent aerosol and droplet deposition onto your uniform. Patients who are persistently coughing or breathing heavily can also generate aerosols. Consider an N95 mask when appropriate. When in doubt, level up your PPE. If you are unsure whether a mask or N95 is appropriate, go with the higher level—the N95.

PPE should be donned in a systematic fashion, and partners should always cross-check one another to ensure that everything is being worn properly. When doffing PPE, take care to avoid self-contamination. Potential or known exposures should be reported and handled per local policy and guidelines.

When EMS practitioners arrive, maintain 6 feet of distance whenever possible. As the situation evolves, you may need to adjust or add PPE. Wash your hands with soap and water or alcohol-based rub before and after patient care. Remember that certain pathogens, such as *Clostridioides difficile* (C diff), are not killed by alcohol hand rubs, and soap and water must be used in certain circumstances.

Patients with an active cough or those who may be immunocompromised should be given a mask to wear. This limits their personal exposure and decreases the exposure they impart on others.

In addition to PPE, time and distance are also important components of exposure reduction. Interactions longer than 15 minutes at distances closer than 6 feet pose the most significant risk for exposure and contraction of airborne- and droplet-transmitted pathogens. Interactions longer than 15 minutes inside an enclosed space with poor ventilation, regardless of distance from other individuals, also poses increased risk. When distance cannot be increased, and time is likely to exceed 15 minutes, standard precautions, including eye protection, mask, and gown, should be taken when there is the potential for exposure to an airborne or droplet-borne pathogen. This is especially applicable when riding in the cab or passenger compartment of the ambulance.

Part of determining whether it is safe for family to accompany the patient is evaluating whether they cause a potential exposure risk to healthcare practitioners. At a minimum, parents and caregivers should wear a surgical face mask when riding in the ambulance with EMS personnel. Depending on the situation, they may be required to wear additional PPE to limit exposure potential. Parents and caregivers who are unable to don and tolerate appropriate PPE present a safety risk to healthcare personnel and should follow in their personal vehicle.

It is not rude or inappropriate to provide a gentle reminder if any person, caregiver, or fellow crewmember is presenting a potential exposure risk by not wearing their PPE properly.

**An unfortunate side effect of the COVID-19 pandemic has been increased "PPE fatigue" and burnout. It is important to remain vigilant and always wear PPE properly when applicable.**

## Primary Survey

The primary survey for this patient reveals the following:

**X**—No bleeding

**A**—Open and patent

**B**—Rapid, labored, and shallow respirations

**C**—Brachial pulses are weak. Capillary refill is slow. The skin is warm and flushed.

**D**—GCS is 11 (E2, V4, M5).

**E**—Lying on couch. There is a diffuse petechial rash noted on the legs, chest, and back.

## Case Questions

- Based on the findings noted in the primary survey, what would your initial interventions and treatment include?

  - The initial treatment for this patient should include aggressive resuscitation focused on airway, breathing, and circulation. Supplemental oxygen should be applied. The respiratory effort should be assisted if necessary to provide adequate tidal volumes for ventilation. Vascular access should be obtained with the intention of providing volume resuscitation.

- Are there any indications of trauma?

  - There is no apparent trauma based on the initial impression and primary survey; however, the patient appears septic.

## Detailed Assessment

### History Taking

**OPQRST:**

- **O**nset—Sudden
- **P**rovocation/palliation—None
- **Q**uality—None
- **R**adiation—None
- **S**everity—Unknown
- **T**iming—24 hours

**SAMPLER:**

- **S**igns/symptoms—Altered mental status, weak brachial pulse, tachypnea
- **A**llergies—No known allergies to medications, foods, or the environment
- **M**edications—None
- **P**ast medical history—Recent upper respiratory infection that was self-limited

- **L**ast oral intake—Not eating or drinking much in the last 24 hours
- **E**vents leading up to the emergency—Significantly worse in the last 24 hours
- **R**isk factors—Recent travel, incompletely vaccinated

In a physiologically unstable child such as this one, the on-scene assessment and treatment should be limited to critical information and lifesaving interventions. In this case, refining the history of recent international travel is important information to gather and pass on to the receiving facility.

Additional questions to consider asking for this patient include the following:

Known potential exposures to infection:

- Patient just returned from a 2-week trip to Guinea 48 hours prior to calling EMS.
- Asking parents where they traveled, how long they were there, and if anyone else in their party is sick can be helpful in isolating where and when the exposure occurred.

Fever curve:

- This patient has had a fever for the past 24 hours.
- Understanding the curve and trajectory of the fever can help determine infection timing and severity. A persistent fever that has been the same each day might be less concerning than a fever that started out mild and has increased in duration and severity each day.
- Clarifying the timing of the fever and response to antipyretic medications is important.
- Determine how and what medicines have been given and at what times and doses.

Associated signs and symptoms:

- This patient has a petechial rash. The parents report that he was crying and holding his head the day prior to calling EMS at the onset of the fever. He has not been drinking.

Immunization status:

- Every pediatric patient should be asked about their immunization status.
- When infection is likely, physicians will start empiric antibiotics to cover the most likely pathogens.
- Fully immunized children are susceptible to fewer pathogens, therefore empiric antibiotic treatment is narrower than empiric treatment for a patients of the same age and exposure profile who lack immunizations.

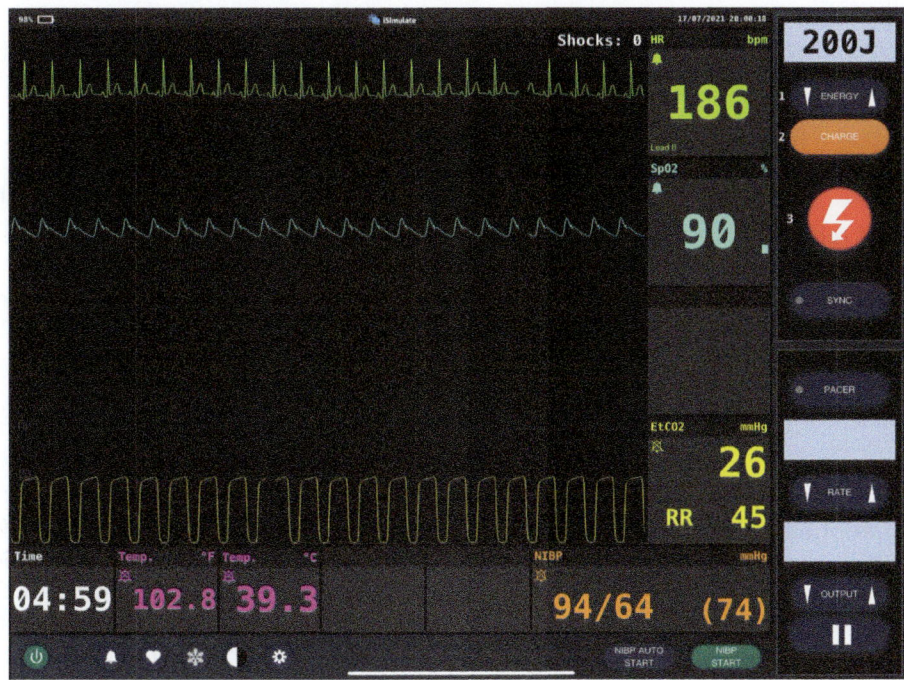

**Figure 5-5** Note the patient's SpO₂ and ETCO₂ levels.
Courtesy of iSimulate.

## Vital Signs

As you were discussing the history, the patient was attached to the monitor and the following vital signs were obtained (**Figure 5-5**):

**Heart rate:**

- 186 beats/min
- This is tachycardic for this patient.
- The tachycardia may be exacerbated by the fever.

**SpO₂:**

- 90% on room air (RA)
- Improves with supplemental oxygen

**ETCO₂:**

- 26 mm Hg
- There is an inverse relationship between ETCO₂ and serum lactate levels.
- As serum lactate rises, the patient becomes more acidotic, and the minute ventilation increases in an effort to produce respiratory compensation.
- As minute ventilation increases, carbon dioxide is off-loaded via the respiratory system, and ETCO₂ levels decline.
- In the background of respiratory compensation, systemic and pulmonary perfusion are also

reduced in distributive shock patients, decreasing the ability to deliver carbon dioxide to the lungs for off-loading via the respiratory system.

- ETCO₂ levels less than 25 mm Hg in patients with suspected sepsis are predictive of serum lactate levels >4 mmol/L.
- Serum lactate levels >4 mmol/L are associated with dramatically higher mortality and morbidity.

**Respiratory rate:**

- 45 breaths/min
- As discussed earlier, this patient is tachypneic.
- Tachypnea is likely the result of the fever and the distributive shock state.

**Blood pressure:**

- 94/64 mm Hg

**Temperature:**

- 102.8°F (39.3°C)

**Blood glucose:**

- 94 mg/dL

**Weight:**

- 23 kg

This is a previously healthy unvaccinated 2-year-old male with recent international travel to Guinea presenting with 24 hours of fever, irritability, headache, poor oral intake, and altered mental status with a diffuse petechial rash and signs of distributive shock, likely secondary to sepsis.

## Detailed Exam

### HEENT (Figure 5-6):

- **H**ead: The patient is reluctant to turn his head and resists flexion or extension of the neck.
- **E**yes: PERRL
- **E**ars: Unremarkable
- **N**ose: Unremarkable
- **T**hroat: Unremarkable

### Chest, heart, and lungs:

- Pulses: Palpable peripheral pulses, thready
- Cardiac auscultation: Tachycardic; regular rhythm; no rubs, gallops, or murmurs auscultated
- Lung auscultation: Tachypnea; lung sounds clear
- Chest exam: Intercostal retractions noted

### Neurologic:

- Lethargic with altered mental status

### Abdomen and pelvis:

- Soft, nontender
- Nonblanching rash present

### Extremities:

- Upper extremities: Nonblanching rash present
- Lower extremities: Nonblanching rash present
- Capillary refill time slow

### Back:

- Nonblanching rash present

## Treatment

Basic life support (BLS) treatment for this patient includes supportive care targeted at optimizing airway, breathing, and circulation. High-flow oxygen and assisted ventilations will help meet the increased metabolic demand. One of the most critical interventions is to take steps to prevent additional disease transmission.

Advanced life support (ALS) personnel should initiate fluid resuscitation. In fulminant distributive shock secondary to sepsis, up to three 20 mL/kg isotonic crystalloid boluses may be given to support hemodynamic

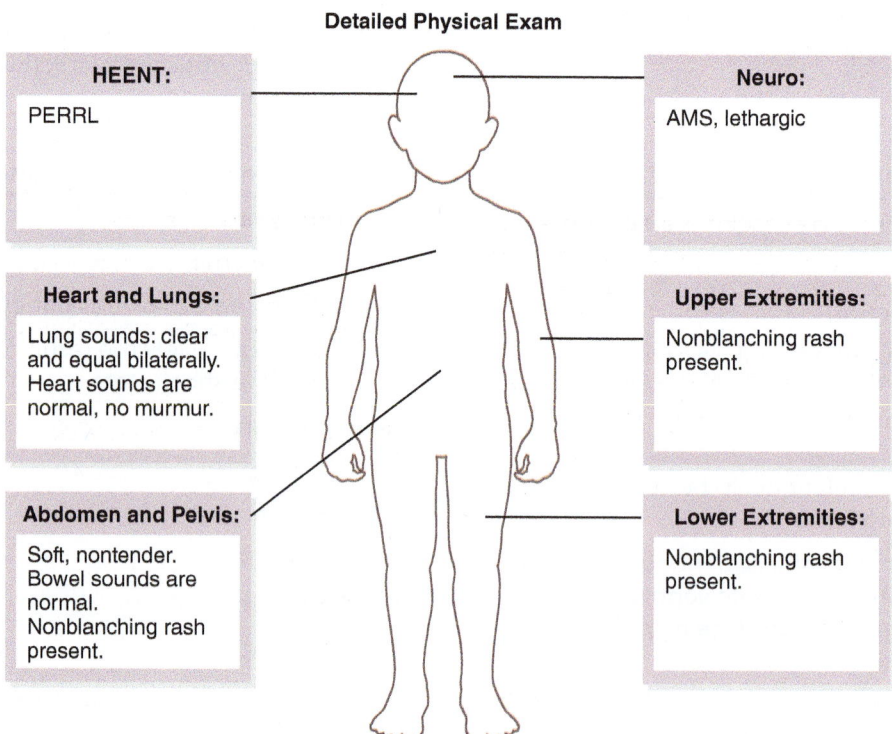

**Detailed Physical Exam**

| HEENT: | Neuro: |
|---|---|
| PERRL | AMS, lethargic |

| Heart and Lungs: | Upper Extremities: |
|---|---|
| Lung sounds: clear and equal bilaterally. Heart sounds are normal, no murmur. | Nonblanching rash present. |

| Abdomen and Pelvis: | Lower Extremities: |
|---|---|
| Soft, nontender. Bowel sounds are normal. Nonblanching rash present. | Nonblanching rash present. |

**Figure 5-6** This patient presents with a nonblanching rash and slow capillary refill time.

status. Medical personnel should constantly reassess the patient respiratory status to make sure that volume overload does not occur. If the patient begins to have crackles or rhonchi, they may be developing pulmonary edema, which could be exacerbated by additional fluid.

Critical care personnel should focus on the BLS and ALS care outlined previously. In some cases, empiric antibiotics may be started in transport by critical care personnel. When this is the case, every effort should be taken to obtain cultures prior to antibiotic administration, as culture results may be altered by the antimicrobial medications. Antibiotic therapy should not be delayed solely to obtain cultures.

> In pediatric distributive shock, norepinephrine is the vasopressor of choice due to its nearly pure alpha agonist properties. It provides the most potent vasoconstriction. Administration of this medication through a peripheral line is possible but presents risk of ischemia and necrosis to the local tissues. Ideally a central line should be used.

Be prepared for rapid deterioration of this patient. He is critically ill and may decompensate with little or no warning.

## Narrowing the Differentials

At the beginning of this case there was an extensive list of differential diagnoses provided. Whereas the case has clearly demonstrated a patient with distributive shock secondary to sepsis with likely meningitis, what clues effectively rule out the other possible differentials?

- Trauma
  - The fever heavily favors infectious etiology.
  - Although the patient could have a febrile illness and trauma, this shock presentation is not consistent with hypovolemic shock, which normally has peripheral vasoconstriction, not vasodilation as seen in this case.
  - Additionally, this patient has decreasing blood pressure. If there was a closed head injury with herniation, we would expect to see Cushing triad response with elevated blood pressure and decreasing heart rate.
- Hypoxia
  - The patient is hypoxic, which favors respiratory illness.

  - The clear lung sounds make respiratory illness less likely, but do not rule it out.
- Infection
  - CNS infection, UTI, or pneumonia could all cause the symptoms seen here if the infection were severe enough to lead to sepsis.
  - This is the most favored diagnosis currently.
- Neurogenic
  - No seizure activity was reported, so this is unlikely a postictal phase or otherwise seizure related.
  - Aneurysm could cause the headache and altered mental status; however, in the presence of fever and diffuse rash, this is the less likely explanation.
- Poisoning:
  - No known exposures were reported, and there were no clues on the scene pointing to possible accidental exposure.
- Metabolic disorders:
  - These are still possible, but again, the fever favors an infectious etiology.
  - Although illness can be a trigger for some metabolic issues, the presence of petechial rash suggests septicemia.
- Cardiac arrhythmias:
  - The ECG shows sinus tachycardia, and no abnormal rhythms have been identified.
- Intestinal obstruction:
  - Obstruction and rupture leading to severe infection is possible.
  - Clues that would favor this diagnosis would include a preceding history of abdominal pain, nausea, and/or vomiting. None of these was reported.

## Ongoing Management

The patient was continuously reassessed throughout transport. He was stable on a nonrebreather; however,

> Soft blood pressures that are fluid nonresponsive are an ominous sign that the patient may rapidly decompensate at any time. This finding indicates that without additional measures such as vasopressors, the patient may rapidly decompensate and die.

you prepared positive-pressure ventilation and intubation equipment just in case. Two 20 mL/kg boluses were administered with little change in blood pressure.

## Case Questions

- What is the most appropriate treatment destination and why?

  - The most appropriate destination for this patient is a pediatric tertiary care facility with pediatric subspecialty support, particularly intensive care and extracorporeal membrane oxygenation. In cases where bypassing less specialized facilities would only cause minimal delay, it may be appropriate to go to the pediatric facility. In cases where the delay in advanced care may be excessive, transporting to a closer facility that can obtain central access, administer vasopressors, and facilitate transfer to a pediatric subspecialty center may be appropriate.

- Can you safely transport this patient in your ambulance?

  - The patient's father hands you the car seat so that you may safely transport the patient in the ambulance.

- Will you allow the father to ride in the ambulance?

  - The father agrees to wear a mask, gown, and gloves, and you are able to transport him in the front of the ambulance.

### ECMO

**Extracorporeal membrane oxygenation (ECMO) is a form of heart lung bypass that can circulate and oxygenate a patient's blood while they recover from a reversible illness or injury. Placing the patient on heart lung bypass allows the organs time to rest while any reversible cause of illness is addressed. ECMO is reserved for patients who have reversible pathologies with no comorbidities that would prevent a favorable outcome once those reversible causes are addressed. Not every hospital has the capability to place pediatric patients on ECMO. It is important to know the capabilities of the transport destinations in your jurisdiction.**

## CASE WRAP-UP

Diagnosis: Meningococcal septicemia

On arrival to the transport destination, a third 20 mL/kg bolus was given with no response. The patient's blood pressure continued to drop and his oxygen saturation and heart rate began to trend down. During the intubation attempt he became pulseless and CPR was started. Despite high-quality CPR and aggressive resuscitation, return of spontaneous circulation was not obtained, and the patient died approximately 30 minutes after arriving to the hospital. *Neisseria meningitides* were found on autopsy, and it is presumed that patient contracted meningococcal disease while traveling with his family.

This case serves as an example of how patients with distributive shock secondary to sepsis can decompensate rapidly, even in facilities where personnel and equipment are readily available for resuscitation.

## CASE TAKEAWAY POINTS

Meningitis is the second leading cause of infection-related deaths in the world. Although developed countries tend to see meningitis-related deaths infrequently due to high immunization rates and readily available access to medical care, these deaths still occur.

Populations at risk for meningitis related deaths include:

- Neonates, due to their immature immune systems

- Immunocompromised patients (patients on chemotherapy, HIV/AIDS, immunosuppressed)

- Unvaccinated and incompletely vaccinated patients

- Patients with exposures to atypical pathogens (foreign travel, exotic pets, IV drug use)

Meningitis has several bacterial causes. The following are the most common pathogens involved:

- *Streptococcus pneumoniae* (most common in infants and young children who are unvaccinated)

- *N. meningitides* (children younger than 1 month with risk factors such as travel or known exposures)

- Group B *Streptococcus* (Generally only seen in children younger than 3 months)

Although it is rare, meningitis still occurs in children in developed countries. Signs of meningitis include the following:

- Fever

- Headache

- Photophobia

- Nausea/vomiting

- Confusion or altered mental status

- Lethargy

- Irritability

- Petechial rash (nonblanching)

  - Using a clear device to press against the rash and see if it blanches can aid in determining if the rash is petechial or not (**Figure 5-7**).

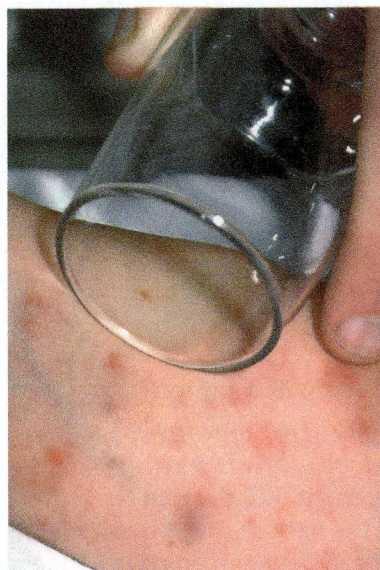

**Figure 5-7** Note how the red spots (petechiae) do not blanch when pressure is applied to them. A nonblanching rash in a febrile patient with altered mental status should be considered meningitis until proven otherwise.
© Mediscan/Alamy Stock Photo.

- Nuchal rigidity (the reluctance or inability to flex or extend the neck) associated with fever is almost pathognomonic for meningitis.

  - Flexing or extending the neck puts traction on the inflamed meninges and causes exquisite pain.

- Kernig sign

  - Inability to straighten the leg when the hip is flexed to 90 degrees in the supine position (**Figure 5-8**)

  - This is very painful in patients with meningitis.

- Brudzinski sign

  - Flexion of the hips and knees when the head of the patient is lifted from a flat surface while lying supine (**Figure 5-9**)

  - This is due to the pain caused by moving the neck.

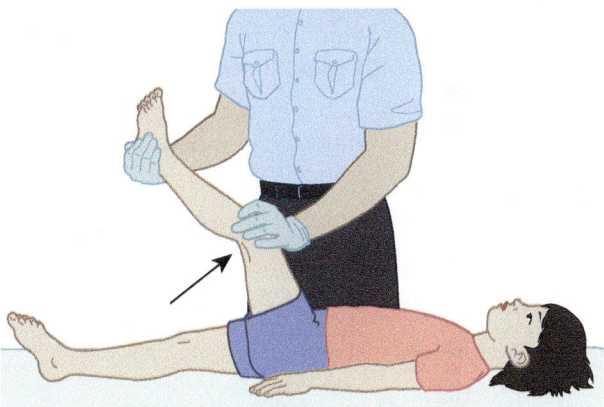

**Figure 5-8** Kernig sign—with the patient supine and the hip flexed to 90 degrees, the patient will resist extension at the knee due to discomfort as traction is applied to the meninges.
© Jones & Bartlett Learning.

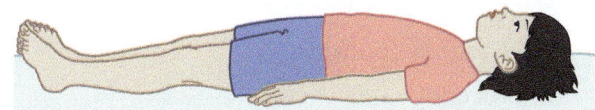

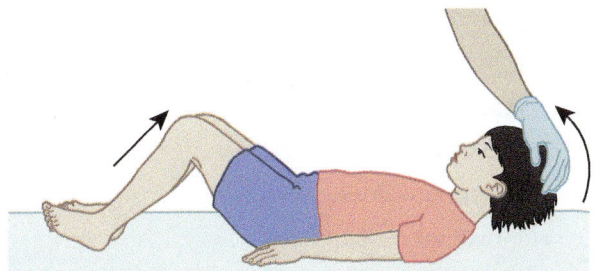

**Figure 5-9** Brudzinski sign—with the patient supine, the neck is flexed, and the hips and knees reflexively flex to reduce traction on the meninges and alleviate discomfort.
© Jones & Bartlett Learning.

## CASE STUDY

### Case 2

#### Dispatch

At 7:15 p.m. you and your partner respond to a household for an 11-month-old male experiencing lethargy (**Figure 5-10**). It is a cool, clear autumn evening and the outside temperature if 55°F (12.7°C).

#### Case Questions

- What are your initial concerns?
  - The primary concern for this patient is the altered mental status.
- Based on the dispatch information, what are the possible differential diagnoses for this patient?
  - Altered mental status in pediatric patients has a broad differential diagnosis. This could include the following:
    - Trauma (accidental or nonaccidental)
    - Intracranial bleed
    - Concussion
    - Respiratory distress with hypoxia
    - Infection
      - CNS (meningitis)
      - Pneumonia
      - UTI
    - Seizure
    - Ingestion or poisoning
      - Carbon monoxide
      - Alcohol
      - Drugs
      - Fertilizer
      - Pesticide
    - Metabolic disorder
      - DKA
      - Hypoglycemia
    - Intestinal obstructions
      - Volvulus
      - Bowel perforation
      - Intussusception

  - As with the previous case, careful assessment of the scene may reveal clues about likely diagnoses.

#### Initial Observations

You arrive at the front door where both parents meet you. The child is being held by the father.

- Pediatric Assessment Triangle
  - Appearance
    - Intermittently lethargic
  - Work of breathing
    - **F**laring not present
    - **R**etractions not present
    - **A**udible abnormal airway sounds not present
    - **P**ositioning—patient not actively positioning himself
  - Circulation
    - Skin normal in appearance

The parents tell you that the child has had several episodes of vomiting with intermittent abdominal pain. He has had decreased appetite and no bowel movements in the past 24 hours. Parents report he has had four wet diapers.

#### Case Questions

- Based on your initial impression, is this patient "Quick" or "Not Quick"?
  - This patient is "Quick." There is intermittent lethargy. Any patient with altered mental status should be designated as "Quick" and treated as critically ill.
- Have you identified any red flags?
  - Intermittent lethargy is a specific term used to describe patients with episodic periods of altered mental status that recur in minutes to hours. The patient may be completely back to baseline in between episodes. The episodes may increase in frequency over time.
  - Lethargy and/or altered mental status in any pediatric patient is a red flag that they are critically ill.

**C**—Radial pulses are strong and capillary refill time is less than 2 seconds.

**D**—GCS is 14 (E4, V4, M6).

**E**—In father's arms. Skin is normal in appearance.

- Based on the findings noted in the primary survey, what would your initial interventions and treatment include?
  - This patient has been vomiting and has reduced urine output (only four diapers in last 24 hours). Obtaining vascular access for rehydration and administering an antiemetic to relieve nausea and vomiting are both appropriate initial treatments.

**Ondansetron can prolong QT interval in patients. Patients with electrolyte disturbance, such as those who have had protracted vomiting or diarrhea, are more susceptible to QT prolongation and arrhythmia. Close monitoring in at-risk patients is advisable.**

## Detailed Assessment

### History Taking

As the monitor is applied to the patient and IV access is established, you begin to work through the patient's history.

**OPQRST:**

- **O**nset: Gradual over the last 12 hours
- **P**rovocation/palliation: Palpation of the abdomen causes pain. Bouts of pain occur spontaneously, lasting a few minutes, then resolve; the pain is relieved spontaneously without any apparent intervention.
- **Q**uality: Unable to obtain
- **R**adiation: Unable to obtain
- **S**everity: The patient is in obvious discomfort.
- **T**iming: 12 hours

**SAMPLER:**

- **S**igns/symptoms: Vomiting, lethargy, abdominal pain

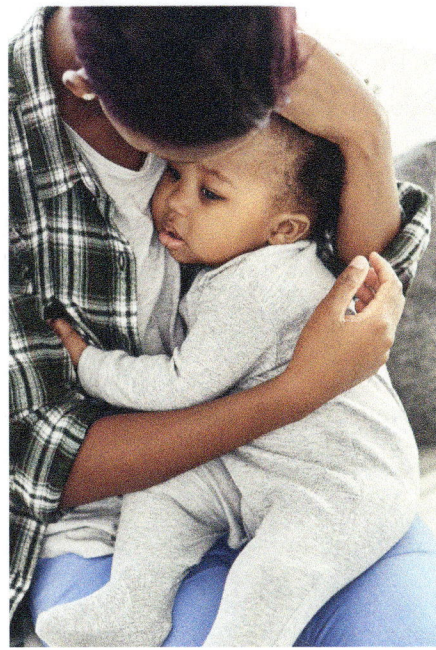

**A**

**Appearance** — Intermittent lethargy

**Work of Breathing** — Respirations appear normal.

**Circulation to Skin** — Skin is normal in appearance.

**B**

**Figure 5-10** This child is experiencing intermittent abdominal pain with vomiting.

A. © PeopleImages/iStock/Getty Images Plus/Getty Images; B. Used with permission of the American Academy of Pediatrics, Pediatric Education for Prehospital Professionals, © American Academy of Pediatrics, 2000.

## Primary Survey

The primary survey for this patient reveals the following:

**X**—No bleeding found

**A**—Patent

**B**—Respirations are regular and normal in depth. Lung sounds are clear bilaterally.

- **A**llergies: No known allergies to medications, foods, or the environment
- **M**edications: None
- **P**ast medical history: None
- **L**ast oral intake: Breakfast
- **E**vents leading up to the emergency: Worsened over the last 12 hours with no apparent cause
- **R**isk factors: Age

## Vital Signs

As you were discussing the history, the patient was attached to the monitor and the following vital signs were obtained (**Figure 5-11**):

**Heart rate:**

- 150 beats/min
- This is tachycardic—which may be a result of the pain the patient is in or anxiety about medical practitioners.

**SpO₂:**

- 97% RA
- There is no apparent respiratory distress or compromise; no oxygen or respiratory support is needed at this time.

**ETCO₂:**

- 39 mm Hg
- The patient is ventilating well.

**Respiratory rate:**

- 32 breaths/min

**Blood pressure:**

- 94/61 mm Hg

**Temperature:**

- 98.6°F (37°C)

**Blood glucose:**

- 106 mg/dL

**Weight:**

- 10 kg per the length-based tape

**ECG:**

- Sinus rhythm with no QT prolongation

This is an 11-month-old male with no previous medical history presenting with episodic abdominal pain progressing in intensity over the past 12 hours accompanied by multiple episodes of emesis and bloody stool.

The patient is currently stable, but acutely ill and requires rapid treatment, stabilization, and transport.

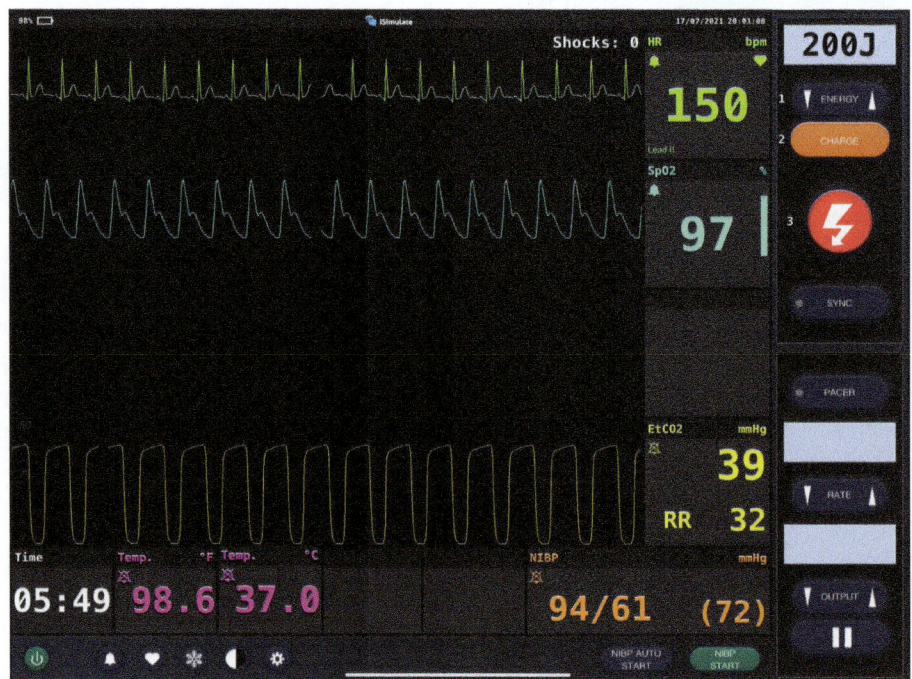

**Figure 5-11** Note the patient's vital signs and consider if they are typical for his age.
Courtesy of iSimulate.

## Detailed Exam

**HEENT (Figure 5-12):**

- **H**ead: Unremarkable
- **E**yes: PERRL
- **E**ars: Unremarkable
- **N**ose: Unremarkable
- **T**hroat: Unremarkable

**Chest, heart, and lungs:**

- Pulses: Peripheral pulses easily palpated
- Cardiac auscultation: Tachycardic; regular rhythm; no rubs, gallops, or murmurs auscultated
- Lung auscultation: Clear and equal bilaterally
- Chest exam: Unremarkable

**Neurologic:**

- Neurovascular status intact
- The patient is anxious and intermittently lethargic.

**Abdomen and pelvis:**

- A sausage-shaped mass can be palpated in the right abdomen. Bowel sounds are hypoactive.

**Extremities:**

- Upper extremities: Unremarkable, capillary refill time brisk
- Lower extremities: Unremarkable; patient draws legs toward abdomen when crying.

**Back:**

- Unremarkable

## Pediatric Pain Management

Many healthcare practitioners are reluctant to give pain medication to pediatric patients. This results in pediatric pain being undertreated or ignored.

Pain is defined as any unpleasant sensory or emotional experience associated with possible or definite tissue damage. There are three dimensions of pain, as follows:

- Biologic
  - This includes the physiologic response to pain.
  - Processes such as inflammation, mechanical or ischemic tissue damage, or damage to the neurologic system fall into the biologic pain dimension.

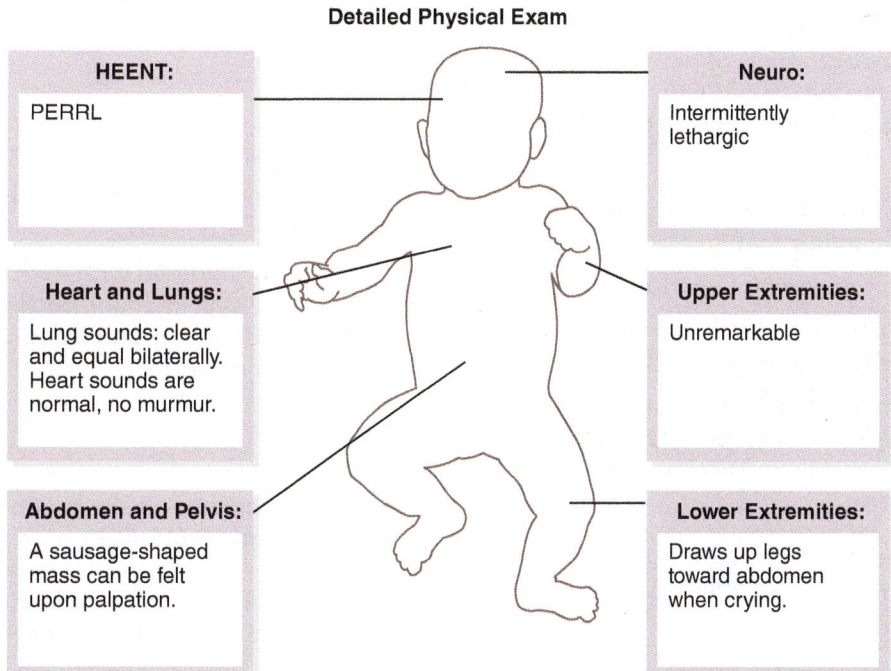

**Detailed Physical Exam**

**HEENT:**
PERRL

**Neuro:**
Intermittently lethargic

**Heart and Lungs:**
Lung sounds: clear and equal bilaterally. Heart sounds are normal, no murmur.

**Upper Extremities:**
Unremarkable

**Abdomen and Pelvis:**
A sausage-shaped mass can be felt upon palpation.

**Lower Extremities:**
Draws up legs toward abdomen when crying.

**Figure 5-12** Patient's detailed physical exam.

© Jones & Bartlett Learning.

- Psychological
  - This includes anxiety related to how pain is experienced. Previous experience with pain and anticipation of pain are also included in the psychological dimension.
- Social
  - This includes consideration of how the pain is reported.
  - Consider whether the pain is reported by the patient or the caregiver.
  - Pain reported is not necessarily pain experienced.
  - A numeric scale or visual pain scale such as the Wong-Baker Faces scale should be used to assess pain in patients who are cognitively developed enough to self-report.

Pain that goes untreated in pediatric patients has real and long-term consequences. Untreated pain in infants can lead to sensory issues, particularly with regard to pain sensation. Older children who are aware they are in pain and not receiving treatment may be reluctant to seek help from healthcare practitioners in the future. Pain can increase fear, and fear can increase pain during a medical evaluation, making it more difficult to accomplish a quality physical exam.

Pain is treated by interrupting the mechanisms that produce it or modifying how we experience it. Tissue-damage leads to activation of nerve endings in those tissues. Once activated, transduction of the pain signal occurs. Transduction is treated with the following various therapies:

- Local antiseptics to stop infection from spreading and causing further inflammation
- Splinting to prevent movement and further tissue damage
- Rest, ice, compression, and elevation (RICE)
- Ibuprofen (a nonsteroidal anti-inflammatory drug [NSAID]) is taken systemically, but acts at a local level to reduce inflammation, thereby reducing pain.

Transmission is the act of the pain signal traveling to the brain. To modify how this signal travels, pharmacologic therapies are used.

- Mild or moderate pain usually responds well to acetaminophen 15 mg/kg IV or PO every 4 hours (not to exceed 75 mg/kg in 24 hours or 4 g in 24 hours, whichever is less).

- Severe pain can be treated with opioids.
  - Fentanyl
    - 1 mcg/kg/dose IV every 30 to 60 minutes
    - 1–2 mcg/kg/dose IN every 30 to 60 minutes
    - Fentanyl can cause severe chest wall rigidity if pushed too fast. Be prepared for this possibility. The patient may require administration of a paralytic in order to support ventilation and break the rigidity.
  - Morphine
    - Neonates: 0.05 mg/kg IM, IV, IO, subcutaneous (SQ)
    - Infants and children: 0.05–0.1 mg/kg IM, IV, IO, SQ
    - Adolescents: 2–4 mg IV or IO, may be repeated as needed so long as level of consciousness and respiratory drive remain intact.
  - Ketamine
    - Ketamine is an effective analgesic in pediatric patients. It is used less frequently than other options because it impacts the ability to perform an accurate mental status exam more than other agents we have discussed.
    - Ketamine causes catecholamine release and is an excellent choice for trauma with any concern for large volume loss or hypotension.
    - Ketamine may increase intracranial pressure, so consider this when administering to a patient with trauma.

Perception relates to any unpleasant sensory or emotional experiences related to possible or actual pain.

- Perception of pain is continuously accompanied by negative emotions.
- Perception is treated with nonpharmacologic methods. Visual imagery, pacifier, bottle, music, holding, distraction, and caregiver assistance all help with perception.

## Treatment

BLS care for this patient includes maintaining airway, breathing, and circulation along with taking steps to keep the patient comfortable. ALS care should include establishing IV access and initiation of pain management if appropriate. Critical care for this patient should include these steps, along with preparation for any decompensation.

## Narrowing Differentials

As was done in the previous case, the differential should be narrowed to the most likely possible diagnoses. In this case, the constellation of symptoms combined with the focal finding in the abdomen (sausage-shaped mass) are indicative of an intussusception.

Lack of fever moves infectious causes lower on the list. The episodic nature of the pain is due to the peristaltic movement of the GI tract, and the blood is present because of ulceration caused by the telescoping of the bowel into itself. Patients will squat or draw their legs up during these episodes of pain in an attempt to alleviate the intense discomfort.

## Ongoing Management

The patient's mental status was reassessed throughout transport. No further changes were noted, and the patient remained stable.

### Case Questions

- What is the most appropriate treatment destination and why?
  - The patient is transported to the closest appropriate facility. In this case, a facility with pediatric surgical capabilities was selected in case the patient requires abdominal surgery.
- Can you safely transport this patient in your ambulance?
  - The patient was transported in his own car seat, and a parent was allowed to accompany him.

## CASE WRAP-UP

Diagnosis: Intussusception

The patient was taken to the pediatric tertiary care hospital where imaging of the abdomen was performed with ultrasound. The classic "bull's-eye" or "target" sign was seen, indicating intussusception (**Figure 5-13**). Morphine 0.05 mg/kg IV was administered to alleviate an episode of pain while the surgery team evaluated the patient.

An air contrast enema was performed. In this procedure, air and contrast are placed into the colon via an enema tube. The contrast allows the colon to be visualized, and the air inflates the colon in such a way that any telescoped segments will expand and reduce to their normal position. In some cases the intussuscepted areas will return to the telescoped position and the procedure will be repeated. If unsuccessful, surgery may be necessary, which was not the case with this patient.

The patient was observed for 24 hours and discharged home without further complication.

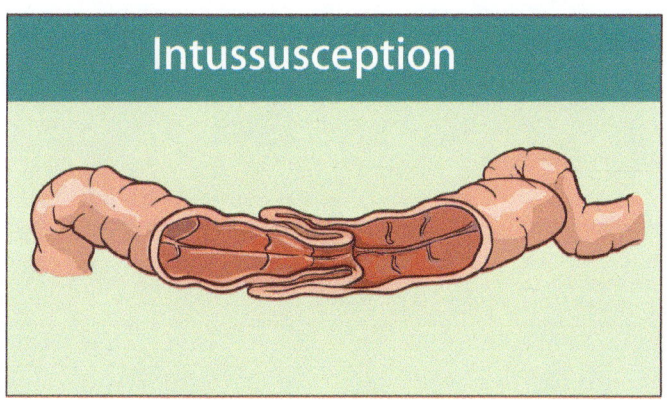

**A**

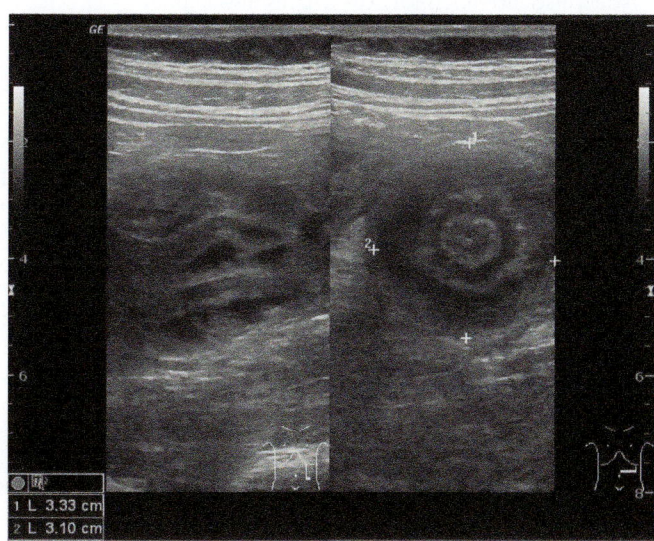

**B**

**Figure 5-13** Note the classic "target" or "bull's-eye" sign visible on the ultrasound image.

A. © corbac40/Shutterstock; **B.** Case courtesy of Dr Maulik S Patel, Radiopaedia.org, rID: 9265.

## CASE TAKEAWAY POINTS

Intussusception most commonly occurs in patients who are 6 months to 3 years old. The majority are younger than 2 years. It is the most common cause of bowel obstruction in this age group.

There is no identifiable cause in 75% of cases (idiopathic). In some cases a pathologic lead point such as a polyp or diverticulum is seen and can be surgically removed to prevent future episodes from occurring.

If left untreated, the bowel will become ischemic, which will lead to necrosis and death of that segment. Necrotic segments of bowel must be surgically resected. If the necrotic loops of bowel are not removed, the patient will perforate, become septic, and die.

## LESSON WRAP-UP

Many pediatric patients present with altered mental status. The differential diagnosis for altered mental status is broad, however history and clinical exam can easily narrow it down to just a few potential causes in most cases. In cases where no identifiable cause is apparent after history and physical exam, the information you gathered will be critical to helping physicians at the receiving hospital determine what advanced testing is necessary to treat and diagnose the patient.

Altered mental status in pediatric patients is a huge red flag and should not be treated lightly.

Pain management in the pediatric population is critical and should not be overlooked due to inexperience or practitioner discomfort with providing analgesia to pediatric patients.

## REFERENCES

Berg AT, Shinnar S, Darefsky AS, et al. Predictors of recurrent febrile seizures: a prospective cohort study. *Arch Pediatr Adolesc Med*. 1997;151(4):371-378. doi:10.1001/archpedi.1997.02170410045006

Centers for Disease Control and Prevention. Scientific brief: SARS-CoV-2 transmission. Updated May 7, 2021. Accessed October 15, 2021. https://www.cdc.gov/coronavirus/2019-ncov/science/science-briefs/sars-cov-2-transmission.html

McDermott KW, Stocks C, Freeman WJ. Overview of pediatric emergency department visits, 2015. *Healthcare Cost and Utilization Project*. Agency for Healthcare Research and Quality. August 2018. Accessed October 15, 2021. https://hcup-us.ahrq.gov/reports/statbriefs/sb242-Pediatric-ED-Visits-2015.pdf

Offringa M, Bossuyt PM, Lubsen J, et al. Risk factors for seizure recurrence in children with febrile seizures: a pooled analysis of individual patient data from five studies. *J Pediatr*. 1994;124(4):574-584. doi:10.1016/s0022-3476(05)83136-1

Safari E, Torabi M. Relationship between end-tidal $CO_2$ ($ETCO_2$) and lactate and their role in predicting hospital mortality in critically ill trauma patients: a cohort study. *Bull Emerg Trauma*. 2020;8(2):83-88.

Wang GS, Roosevelt G, Le Lai M-C, et al. Association of unintentional pediatric exposures with decriminalization of marijuana in the United States. *Ann Emerg Med*. 2014;63(6):684-689. doi:10.1016/j.annemergmed.2014.01.017

Wolfsdorf J, Glaser N, Sperling MA. Diabetic ketoacidosis in infants, children, and adolescents. *Diabetes Care*. 2006;29(5):1150-1159.

# CHAPTER 6

# Pediatric Cardiac Events

## LESSON OBJECTIVES

- Identify the major classifications of pediatric cardiac rhythms.
- Differentiate between pediatric cardiac events.
- Discuss the management of pediatric dysrhythmias.
- Explain the epidemiology of sudden cardiac arrest.
- Discuss management of postresuscitation care.

## Introduction

The majority of cardiac dysrhythmias in pediatric patients occur due to respiratory compromise causing hypoxia, which leads to dysrhythmia and arrest. There is a small subset of pediatric cardiac events that are the result of underlying cardiac anomaly, disease, or injury. It is important to be able to accurately assess the pediatric patient and determine the underlying cause of the cardiac event in order to efficiently treat it. This lesson provides the foundational information necessary to the initial emergency stabilization of pediatric patients experiencing cardiac events.

## The Normal Pediatric ECG

The human heart experiences structural remodeling as a patient progresses into adolescence and adulthood. Reflecting that remodeling, the pediatric electrocardiogram (ECG) undergoes a series of expected changes over time (**Figure 6-1**). Thus, the neonatal ECG appears quite different than that of an adolescent patient.

### Normal QRS and Expected Axis

There are variable age-related changes in the 12-lead ECG across the age continuum. Shortly after birth, expect to see right-sided axis prominence. The rightward

axis is most pronounced at age 1 to 2 months and begins to normalize to a more traditional leftward axis thereafter. A normal axis is expected by around age 6 months. Any infant who has persistent right axis deviation may have an underlying congenital heart abnormality or cardiomyopathy.

> The smaller pediatric heart has fewer myocardial cells to depolarize and repolarize compared to the adult heart. Fewer cells to depolarize results in shorter ECG intervals. As the child grows and develops, so does the myocardium. The ECG intervals will gradually lengthen to the expected adult range as the myocardium develops over time.

### Right Ventricular Dominance

As described, right ventricular dominance is physiologically normal in infancy and gradually decreases over time. This dominance causes characteristic R wave findings not typically seen in adult ECGs.

In children and young adults, $V_1$, $V_2$, and $V_3$ will generally have dominant R waves present. An

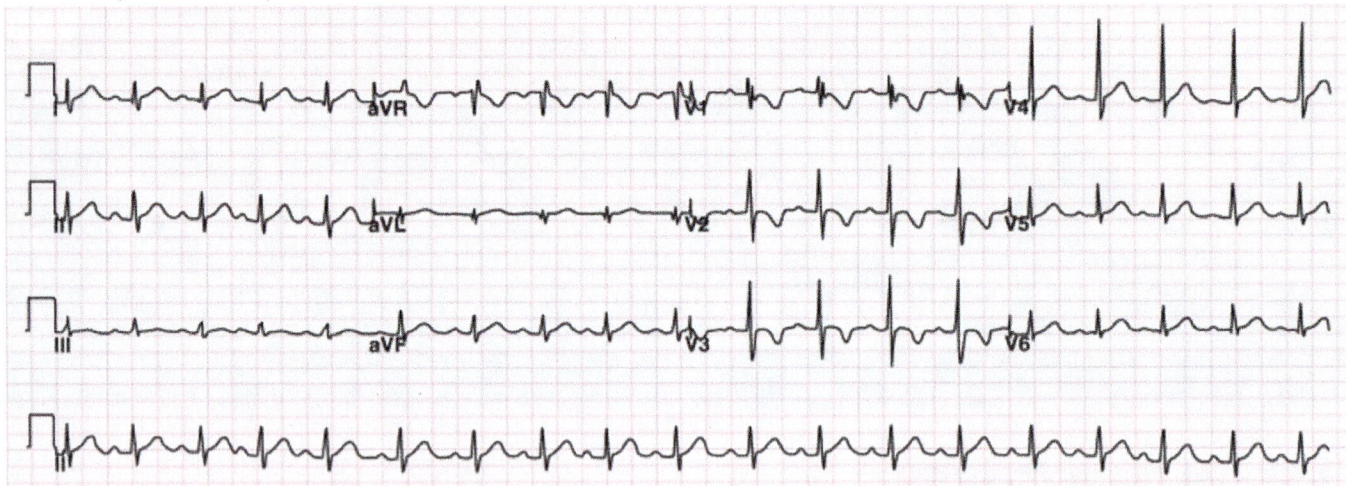

**Figure 6-1** A normal, or expected, ECG for a pediatric patient.

From Arrhythmia Recognition: The Art of Interpretation, courtesy of Tomas B. Garcia, MD.

| Table 6-1 Possible Causes of T Wave Abnormalities | |
|---|---|
| **Peaked** | **Flat or Inverted** |
| ▪ Hyperkalemia | ▪ Hypokalemia |
| ▪ Left ventricular hypertrophy | ▪ Pericarditis |
| | ▪ Myocarditis |
| | ▪ Newborns |
| | ▪ Hypothyroidism |

© Jones & Bartlett Learning.

RSR′ may be found in lead $V_1$ and is not considered pathologic outside of other findings or symptoms. The presence of RSR′ in lead $V_1$ generally resolves by age 3 years; however, it may remain a nonpathologic finding in a small number of patients up to age 12 years.

## T Waves

The conformation of the T waves changes as the pediatric patient grows. Upright T waves in the right precordial leads ($V_1$–$V_3R$) are seen in the first 2 to 3 days of life. The precordial T waves should invert by approximately 1 week of life. This is known as a *juvenile T wave pattern*. When upright T waves persist past age 1 week, it raises concern for abnormalities in cardiac conduction due to structural or intrinsic causes (**Table 6-1**).

As the patient grows older, the intermediate lead T waves will revert back to an upright position, typically following a $V_3$, $V_2$, $V_1$ progression. This reversion is generally complete by age 8 years. In some cases, the juvenile T wave pattern will persist into adolescence or adulthood for idiopathic reasons.

The lateral leads ($V_5$ and $V_6$) are expected to be upright in all ages. In a small number of cases the lateral leads may be inverted for the first 1 to 3 days of life; however, inversion that persists past this point is highly suspect for left ventricular hypertrophy.

## Q Waves

Q waves are most prominent in leads I, III, aVF, $V_5$, and $V_6$. Q wave amplitude in these leads generally doubles in the first few months of life, with maximal amplitude seen between ages 3 and 5 years. After this peak is seen, the amplitude will decrease over time back to that which was seen in the newborn period (**Table 6-2**).

> **Regarding Q waves, in general:**
>
> **Q waves should be present in leads $V_5$ and $V_6$.**
>
> **Q waves should not be present in lead $V_1$.**

## Pediatric Cardiac Rhythms

In the United States, approximately 55 per 100,000 children will be seen in the emergency department for cardiac dysrhythmias annually. Not all of these patients

**Table 6-2** Q Wave Abnormalities

| Abnormality | Potential Cause |
| --- | --- |
| High amplitude (>5 mm) | Hypertrophy secondary to volume overload |
| High amplitude with prolongation (>5 mm, >0.03 sec) | Hypertrophy secondary to infarction with remodeling and fibrosis |
| Present in $V_1$ | Right ventricular hypertrophy (beyond physiologic RVH of the neonatal period) |
| Absent in left precordial leads | Right bundle branch block |

© Jones & Bartlett Learning.

present via emergency medical services (EMS), and the conditions they present for can be as benign as a "tickling in the chest," to as serious as sudden cardiac arrest. In some cases, the patient may present with a chief complaint seemingly unrelated to the heart, only to find out during the history and exam that they have a dysrhythmia. Additional details for each rhythm, including identification and treatment, will be included in the sections that follow.

## Tachycardia

Tachycardia is the term used to describe any heart rate above the expected normal value for that patient's age range (see Lesson 1, *Pediatric Development and Assessment*, for a review of expected vital signs by age). Most cases of tachycardia in pediatric patients are the result of the body compensating for illness or injury. Tachycardia is almost universally present when patients are febrile. Hypovolemia, anxiety, pain, and any disease process causing decreased perfusion or increased metabolic demand will generally lead to

> In cases for which tachycardia is a compensatory response and not related to underlying congenital heart disease, the heart rate will typically not exceed 220 beats/min in infants and 180 beats/min in children.

tachycardia. Elevated heart rate may also be present due to underlying endocrine disorders such as hyperthyroidism. Certain pathologic tachycardias can also be the result of prolonged hypoxia, such as ventricular tachycardia (VT) seen in victims of submersion injury or suffocation.

Although most presentations of tachycardia are not related to congenital heart disease or conduction issues, there is a subset of cardiac-specific causes that can result in tachydysrhythmias. When encountering patients with a rapid heart rate, it can be helpful to first classify the rhythms as wide or narrow complex. From there, they can be further subdivided as symptomatic and nonsymptomatic. Working through the rhythms in this fashion will allow prehospital practitioners to pursue treatment using the proper tachycardia algorithm.

> In most cases, specific identification of the underlying rhythm beyond wide and narrow is not necessary for emergency treatment and stabilization. Focus on differentiating wide versus narrow, and symptomatic versus asymptomatic. This will allow you to quickly establish the correct treatment algorithm.

There is a wide variety of signs and symptoms that can be seen in patients with tachycardia. The presentation may evolve over time as the patient's perfusion decreases and they become more symptomatic. Table 6-3 provides a list of signs and symptoms that may be encountered with tachycardic patients.

> Some pediatric patients may have trouble articulating what pain or pressure in their chest feels like. In some cases, patients may describe a "tickling" in their chest or feel as if their heart is "flip flopping." Some patients may also mistake these feelings as being in their throat or neck.

### Sinus Tachycardia

When the rate is less than 220 beats/min in infants and 180 beats/min in children, there is a high probability that the rhythm is sinus tachycardia. Signs that

| Table 6-3 Physical Findings in Tachycardia | |
| --- | --- |
| **Infants (younger than 12 months)** | **Children (1 year and older)** |
| ■ Fussiness<br>■ Irritability or inconsolability<br>■ Lethargy<br>■ Poor feeding<br>■ Sweating or choking during feeding<br>■ Mottling or decreased peripheral perfusion | ■ Lightheadedness<br>■ Dyspnea<br>■ Syncope<br>■ Weakness<br>■ Nervousness or agitation<br>■ Sweating or tremors<br>■ Palpitations<br>■ Chest pain or pressure |

© Jones & Bartlett Learning.

the rhythm is most likely sinus tachycardia include the following:

■ Rate greater than 220 beats/min in infants and 180 beats/min in children

■ Identifiable P waves that have uniform and normal morphology

■ An R-R interval that is variable

When the ECG demonstrates these findings, it is likely that the patient is in sinus tachycardia. The primary treatment for sinus tachycardia is to identify and treat the underlying cause. **Table 6-4** identifies potential causes for sinus tachycardia and their associated treatments.

## Supraventricular Tachycardia

Supraventricular tachycardia (SVT) is the most likely dysrhythmia when the following conditions are met:

■ Rate greater than 220 beats/min in infants and 180 beats/min in children

■ No identifiable P waves

■ QRS duration ≤0.09 seconds

There are two possible algorithms to follow with SVT: stable and unstable. Patient stability is judged primarily on the presence or absence of cardiopulmonary compromise. Nearly all narrow complex tachycardias originate above the level of the ventricles—making them by definition *supraventricular*.

### Stable Supraventricular Tachycardia

There are two primary treatments in the emergency management of stable SVT: vagal maneuvers and

| Table 6-4 Sinus Tachycardia Causes and Treatments | |
| --- | --- |
| Hypovolemia | ■ Provide isotonic fluid boluses of 10–20 mL/kg (10 mL/kg for infants, 20 mL/kg for children)<br>■ Assess peripheral perfusion and lung sounds to ensure cardiac overload and pulmonary congestion do not develop |
| Fever | ■ Provide antipyretic medications:<br>  ▪ Acetaminophen<br>  ▪ Ibuprofen<br>■ Remove excess clothing or blankets<br>■ Apply cool washcloths to the forehead |
| Pain | ■ Provide appropriate analgesia<br>■ Depending on choice of medication, monitor blood pressure parameters closely |
| Anxiety | ■ Use age-appropriate distraction and breathing techniques<br>■ Allow appropriate time to calm down and return to baseline between procedures<br>■ Provide preprocedure anxiolytics when appropriate<br>■ In cases of severe anxiety or agitation, medications for anxiolysis may be necessary |
| Respiratory distress | ■ Provide supplemental oxygen<br>■ Assist ventilation as appropriate<br>■ Identify and resolve underlying cause |

This list is not comprehensive but does identify some of the most common causes of sinus tachycardia.

© Jones & Bartlett Learning.

medication and fluid administration—both of which may be necessary if the rhythm does not terminate with less invasive methods.

## STABLE VERSUS UNSTABLE

The presence or absence of cardiopulmonary compromise determines whether the patient is stable. When assessing for signs of cardiopulmonary compromise, look for the following signs or symptoms:

- Acutely altered mental status
- Signs of shock or decreased peripheral perfusion
- Hypotension
- Chest pain

If there is concern that any of the these signs or symptoms are present, pursue treatment utilizing the unstable algorithm.

## HOW TO INDUCE A VAGAL RESPONSE

There are three primary ways to elicit a vagal response in children:

- Coaching through a Valsalva maneuver when the patient is developmentally appropriate.
- A bag of chilled ice water applied to the face for 10 to 30 seconds.
- Rectal stimulation with a thermometer or other appropriate probing device.

The following techniques are *not* routinely recommended in infants or children:

- Ocular pressure
- Carotid sinus massage

pharmacologic cardioversion with adenosine. Long-term management of refractory SVT may involve initiation of beta blocker or calcium channel blocker medications; however, this should be done in consultation with online medical direction and a pediatric cardiologist, when possible.

### Vagal Stimulation

In patients who are developmentally appropriate to follow instructions, coaching them through a Valsalva maneuver similar to adults is usually effective. This may involve having them bear down like when they have a bowel movement or blowing through a straw that is sufficiently small to restrict airflow and cause increased intrathoracic pressure.

In patients who are too young for effective coaching in Valsalva maneuvers, such as infants, the primary method for inducing the vagal response is to apply a plastic bag filled with ice water to the face for approximately 10 to 30 seconds. This will stimulate the mammalian diving reflex.

Rectal stimulation in infants may also be effective. This can be done with a rectal thermometer in a similar fashion to taking a rectal temperature. This elicits a bearing down response in the infant.

Some infants have been observed to spontaneously terminate the SVT rhythm during attempts at intravenous (IV) access, as they bear down in response to the discomfort associated with the needle insertion. While needle insertion solely for the purposes of vagal stimulation is not routine, this can be a benefit that is seen during attempts to gain access for

### Adenosine

When noninvasive techniques have failed to convert SVT into normal sinus rhythm and the patient remains in stable condition, the next step in treatment is administration of adenosine.

As mentioned previously, the half-life of adenosine is very short. This means that administration should be done through an IV site that is as proximal as possible. In addition to choosing a proximal site, the administration of adenosine should be performed in a coordinated manner allowing for rapid administration with a rapid flush immediately following that administration. Using an IV site that is extremely peripheral, failing to push the medication rapidly, and not flushing the line are common mistakes made during adenosine administration and limit the drug's efficacy. The dosing for adenosine is as follows:

- 0.1 mg/kg rapid IV push followed by an appropriate flush
  - Maximum initial dose is 6 mg.
- A second dose of 0.2 mg/kg rapid IV push followed by an appropriate flush may be administered if the patient is refractory to the initial dose.
  - Maximum second dose is 12 mg.
- In some cases, a third dose may be administered, but only per local protocols.

## ADENOSINE ADMINISTRATION GUIDELINES

Adenosine should be pushed rapidly with a flush immediately afterward. The administration site should be as proximal as possible. Poor administration technique is a common cause for therapeutic failure when administering adenosine.

The patient should be on cardiac monitoring and rhythm changes documented before, during, and after administration. Defibrillation pads should be applied prior to administration, and the steps for synchronized and unsynchronized shocking, along with dosages, should be reviewed prior to administration.

### Unstable Supraventricular Tachycardia

When SVT is noted and the patient has signs of cardiopulmonary compromise, then synchronized cardioversion is the first-line therapy (**Figure 6-2**). Adenosine prior to synchronized cardioversion is appropriate when it does not delay cardioversion. Cardioversion should not be delayed to administer adenosine when the patient is unstable. Do not delay cardioversion for sedation or analgesia administration in the unstable patient. The appropriate energy dosage for synchronized cardioversion is as follows:

- 0.5–1 J/kg initial dosage
- Increase to 2 J/kg for subsequent attempts

The energy required for synchronized cardioversion may vary depending on the manufacturer of the defibrillator. It is important to be familiar with the devices that your service uses.

## SVT TREATMENT PEARLS

- Treatment sequence and options may vary based on current American Heart Association (AHA) guidelines or local protocols.
- If possible, do not separate the child from the caregiver.
- Monitor patients for respiratory depression and hemodynamic instability when administering sedation.
- Continuous pulse oximetry and end-tidal $CO_2$ ($ETCO_2$) should be applied.
- Capture all rhythm changes in real time with ECG printouts.

## Ventricular Tachycardia

VT is the most likely dysrhythmia when the following conditions are met:

- Rapid rate
- No identifiable P waves
- QRS duration ≥0.09 seconds

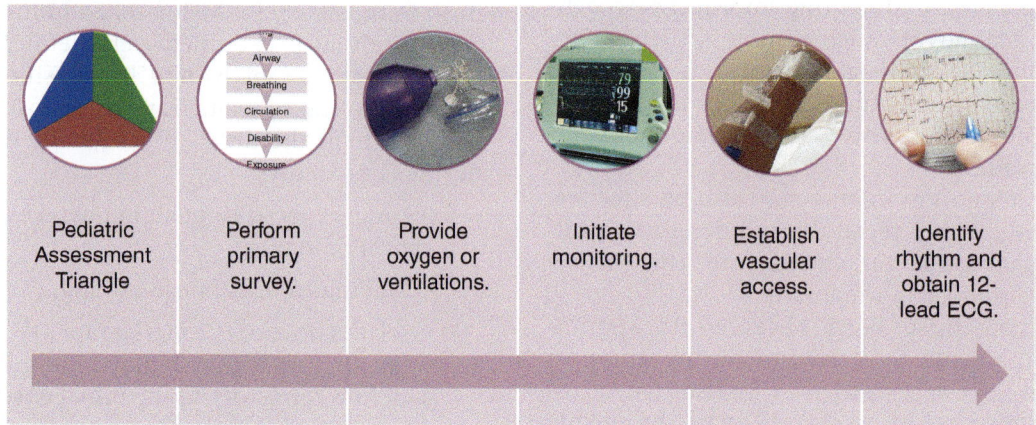

**Figure 6-2** Prehospital management of SVT should follow these steps.

A. Used with permission of the American Academy of Pediatrics, Pediatric Education for Prehospital Professionals, © American Academy of Pediatrics, 2000; B. Jones & Bartlett Learning.; C. © Jones & Bartlett Learning. Courtesy of MIEMSS.; D. © bymuratdeniz/E+/Getty Images; E. © natnaree sangkaew/Shutterstock; F. © diy13/Shutterstock.

VT is relatively uncommon in infants and children. It is most often precipitated by hypoxia or hypoperfusion. This rhythm may degrade into pulseless VT, ventricular fibrillation (VF), and ultimately, asystole if not treated aggressively.

Causes of VT other than hypoxia and hypoperfusion are shown on **Table 6-5**.

> Tricyclic antidepressant overdose is a relatively common cause of QT prolongation and ventricular tachycardia. Typically, infants or children will ingest this medication through an unintended medication misadventure or overdose. Early administration of sodium bicarbonate 1 mEq/kg IV early in the course of treatment can be lifesaving.

VT can be monomorphic or polymorphic. There are two possible algorithms to follow with VT: stable and unstable. Treatment is highly dependent on the stability of the patient. Patient stability is judged *primarily* on the presence or absence of cardiopulmonary compromise.

The initial steps for management of VT include history, physical exam, and assessment. Oxygenation and ventilation should be optimized. Cardiac monitor should be applied and IV access should be obtained. Once the rhythm has been identified as VT, proceed with treatment based on the stability of the patient.

### Stable Ventricular Tachycardia

In patients with tachycardia with a QRS duration of ≥0.09 seconds and no evidence of cardiac compromise, you should presume that they have stable VT. When the rhythm is regular and a monomorphic QRS is present, consider using adenosine to aid in differentiation between stable VT and SVT. The dosing for adenosine is the same as for SVT:

- 0.1 mg/kg rapid IV push followed by an appropriate flush
  - Maximum initial dose is 6 mg.
- A second dose of 0.2 mg/kg rapid IV push followed by an appropriate flush may be administered if the patient is refractory to the initial dose.
  - Maximum second dose is 12 mg.

**Table 6-5** Selected Causes of Ventricular Tachycardia

| Condition | Predisposing Factors |
|---|---|
| Long QT syndrome | Congenital<br>- Familial or genetic long QT syndrome<br>Acquired<br>- Medications,* including but not limited to:<br>  - Ondansetron<br>  - Certain antipsychotics<br>  - Antidysrhythmics<br>  - Certain antibiotics<br>  - Antihistamines |
| Electrolyte disturbances | Dialysis<br>Renal failure<br>High-dose albuterol<br>Insulin administration, particularly in diabetic ketoacidosis<br>Diuretic therapy<br>Anorexia nervosa with purging behaviors |
| Toxic exposure or ingestion | Organophosphate poisoning<br>Arsenic |
| Environmental factors | Hypothermia |
| Structural or conduction issues | Recent history of cardiac surgery or previously corrected congenital heart disease |
| Infection | Recent history of viral infection which may lead to myocarditis<br>Bacterial infection leading to endocarditis |

*It is not necessary to remember all of these drugs, as the list is exhaustive. It is important to take an in-depth history screening for use or unintentional exposure to these medications.

© Jones & Bartlett Learning.

- In some cases, a third dose may be administered, but only per local protocols.

Consult online medical direction as needed and initiate rapid transport.

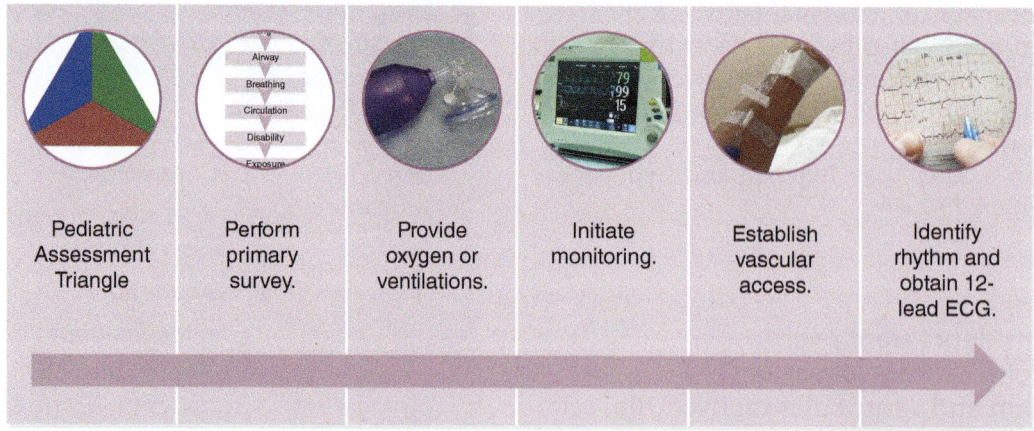

| Pediatric Assessment Triangle | Perform primary survey. | Provide oxygen or ventilations. | Initiate monitoring. | Establish vascular access. | Identify rhythm and obtain 12-lead ECG. |

**Figure 6-3** Prehospital management of ventricular tachycardia should follow these steps.

A. Used with permission of the American Academy of Pediatrics, Pediatric Education for Prehospital Professionals, © American Academy of Pediatrics, 2000; B. Jones & Bartlett Learning.; C. © Jones & Bartlett Learning. Courtesy of MIEMSS.; D. © bymuratdeniz/E+/Getty Images; E. © natnaree sangkaew/Shutterstock.; F. © diy13/Shutterstock.

## Unstable Ventricular Tachycardia

Patients with hemodynamic instability should be synchronized cardioverted without delay (**Figure 6-3**). Unstable VT with a pulse is a rhythm with a high risk of deteriorating into pulselessness and cardiac arrest. Sedation may be considered, but only in circumstances where it will not delay care or cause hemodynamic instability.

The appropriate energy dosage for synchronized cardioversion is as follows:

- 0.5–1 J/kg initial dosage
- Increase to 2 J/kg for subsequent attempts

Amiodarone and lidocaine are commonly used antidysrhythmics for this condition. The current literature does not demonstrate superiority of one agent over the other. Factors impacting the decision regarding which agent should be used include availability, practitioner comfort, and medical control preference. Additionally, patients with a known history of VT may already be on a daily antidysrhythmic. This information is important to pass on to medical control, because they may want to pursue treatment that can supply an additive or synergistic effect when combined with the therapy that the patient is already on.

> Any patient without a pulse should be treated using the appropriate arm of the pulseless arrest algorithm. Specifics of this will be discussed later.

### VT TREATMENT PEARLS

- When antidysrhythmics are used, follow current AHA guidelines or local protocols.
- Obtain a 12-lead ECG before and after cardioversion, if possible.
- Carefully monitor hemodynamic status throughout transport, and be prepared to respond quickly to pulseless arrest, as patients are prone to cardiovascular decline and/or cardiac arrest.

## CASE STUDY

## Case 1

### Dispatch

It is 0430, and you and your partner are dispatched to a 12-month-old female with a fever who "won't stop crying." The dispatch location is a two-story single-family home. It is a spring morning and the outside temperature is 77°F (25°C).

### Case Questions

- What are your initial concerns?
  - A fussy child with a fever is a nonspecific complaint and could include numerous diagnoses on your differential list.

- Consider appropriate personal protective equipment (PPE).
- Based on the dispatch information, what is the possible differential diagnosis for this patient?
  - Viral illness (COVID-19, influenza, respiratory syncytial virus [RSV])
  - Dehydration
  - Maltreatment/nonaccidental trauma
  - Intussusception
  - Cardiac dysrhythmia
  - Ingestion or poisoning

## Initial Observations

The parent is standing outside her vehicle, with the child inside, secured in her car seat. As you approach the scene appears safe. The mother tells you the patient has been inconsolable all night. She felt warm and the mother is concerned she has a fever. They have just completed a drive around the block in an effort to calm the patient.

- Pediatric Assessment Triangle (**Figure 6-4**)
  - Appearance
    - Alert, active, inconsolable
  - Work of breathing
    - **F**laring not present
    - **R**etractions not present
    - **A**udible airway sounds—no abnormal sounds noted on initial observation
    - **P**ositioning—actively crying without tripoding or active airway positioning
- Circulation
  - Appropriate skin color with no signs of poor perfusion

### Case Questions

- Based on your initial impression, is this patient "Quick" or "Not Quick"?
  - This patient has no signs of hemodynamic or respiratory compromise.
  - Currently the patient is "Not Quick."
  - Remember, the patient priority can change as you proceed with the history and physical exam.

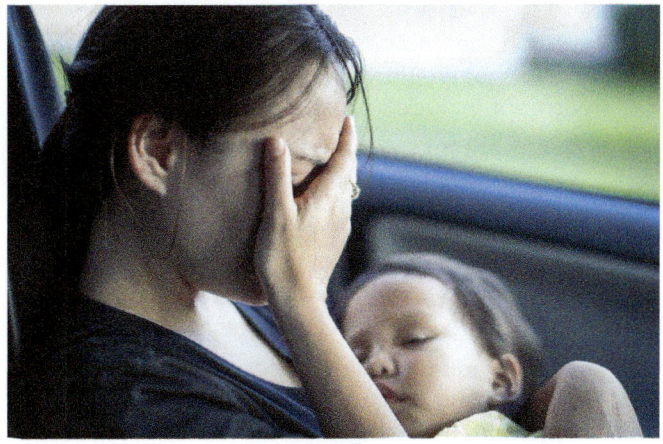

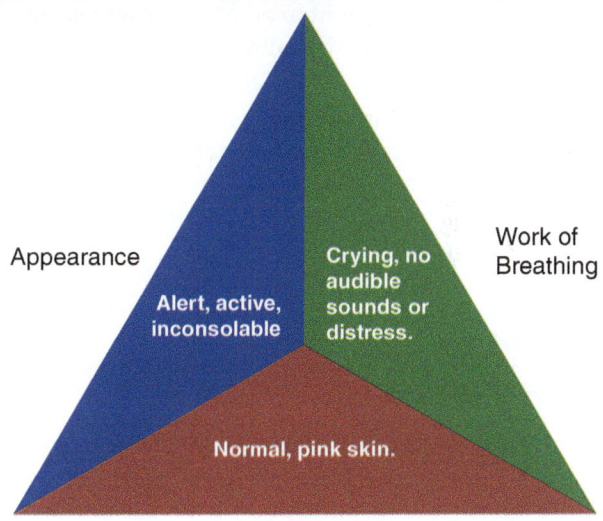

**Figure 6-4** You are called to a 12-month-old fussy child with a fever.

A. Used with permission of the American Academy of Pediatrics, Pediatric Education for Prehospital Professionals, © American Academy of Pediatrics, 2000; **B.** © christinarosepix/Shutterstock.

## Primary Survey

The primary survey for this patient reveals the following:

**X**—No bleeding found

**A**—The airway is open and patent. The patient is crying loudly with no concerning audible airway noises.

**B**—Rapid with good rise and fall of the chest. The lungs are clear bilaterally.

**C**—Peripheral pulses are intact and strong. The skin is warm and well perfused. Capillary refill is less than 2 seconds.

**D**—Alert; Glasgow Coma Scale (GCS) score is 15 (E4, V5, M6).

**E**—The patient is sitting in car seat of vehicle. No abnormalities noted on exposure; however, the patient feels warm to the touch and you suspect she has a fever.

- Based on the findings noted in the primary survey, what would your initial interventions and treatment include?
  - Treatment for this patient should initially focus on measures necessary to calm her.
  - Calming the patient will reduce cardiac and respiratory demand.
  - In patients with fever, reducing temperature can aid in improving cardiac and respiratory status.
    - Fever reduction can be accomplished by optimizing environmental factors. This includes removing excessive clothing and moving the patient to an environment where the temperature is controlled and appropriate.
    - Administration of antipyretic medications such as acetaminophen or ibuprofen will help lower temperature. Make sure to ask parents when the last time was they administered these medications, and consult local protocols.

## Detailed Assessment

### History Taking

After moving the patient into the ambulance, you begin to ask additional questions about the history for this patient while your partner takes measures to control her temperature.

**OPQRST:**

- **O**nset: The condition appeared rapidly, over the course of the past 6 hours.
- **P**rovocation/palliation: The parents are not aware of any factors that make her condition worse or better.
- **Q**uality: Unable to assess
- **R**adiation: Unable to assess
- **S**everity: Unknown
- **T**iming: 6 hours

**SAMPLER:**

- **S**igns/symptoms: The patient lost her appetite the evening before this occurred. She did not eat well and vomited once after dinner. She has been very fussy and inconsolable. She has been warm to the touch.
- **A**llergies: No known allergies to medications, foods, or the environment
- **M**edications: Her parents gave her an appropriate dose of acetaminophen 4 hours prior to your arrival.
- **P**ast medical history: None

- **L**ast oral intake: 1900 the evening before
- **E**vents leading up to the emergency: She has not been sleeping all night and crying continuously. Her parents called the on-call nurse line at her pediatrician's office, who advised them to call 911.
- **R**isk factors: Possible infection

### Vital Signs

As you were discussing the history, the patient was attached to the monitor and the following vital signs were obtained (**Figure 6-5**):

**Heart rate:**

- 229 beats/min
- The ECG appears to show narrow complex tachycardia without P waves.
- This is significantly elevated and may be a result of her irritability or the cause of it.

**SpO$_2$:**

- 95% on room air (RA)
- This patient is saturating well, however supplemental oxygen may aid in cardiac demand by increasing the partial pressure of oxygen available in the blood.

**ETCO$_2$:**

- 34 mm Hg
- The patient is mildly hypocarbic as a result of the tachypnea and crying.

**Respiratory rate:**

- 50 breaths/min
- Febrile patients may have tachypnea in an effort to meet metabolic demand and aid in active cooling.

**Blood pressure:**

- 96/53 mm Hg
- The patient's blood pressure is intact; however, it is likely she is compensating.

**Temperature:**

- 99.1°F (37.3°C)
- Fever may be contributing to the tachycardia.
- Febrile illnesses can lower the threshold for going into SVT in patients with an underlying conduction abnormality.

**Blood glucose:**

- 94 mg/dL

**Weight:**

- 10 kg per length-based tape estimation

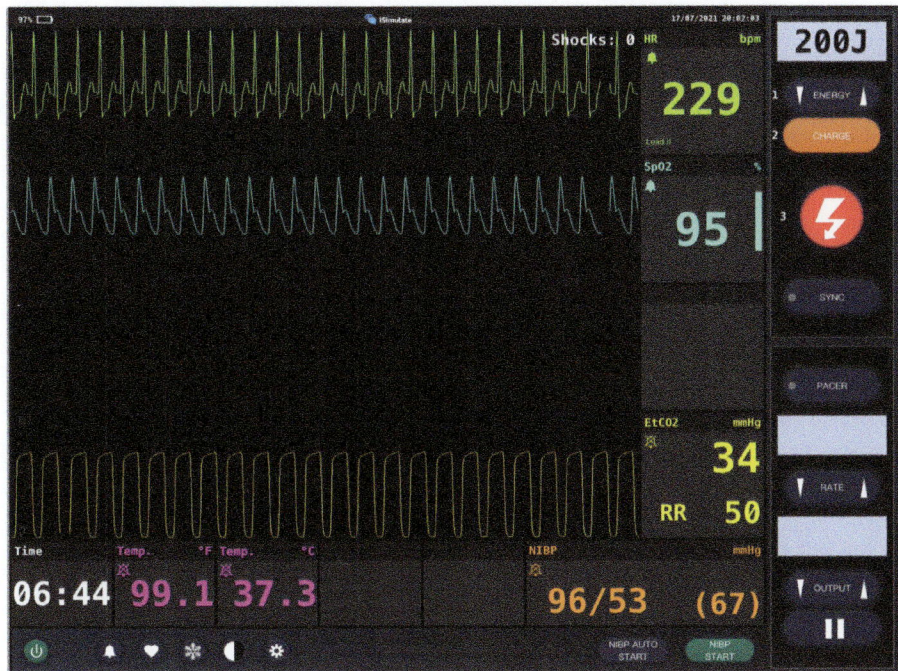

**Figure 6-5** The patient's vital signs indicate she is tachypneic.

Courtesy of iSimulate.

The patient is a previously healthy 12-month-old female with approximately 6 hours of fever and inconsolability. Her ECG shows a narrow complex tachycardia with rate >220 and no P waves, consistent with SVT. She is currently hemodynamically stable with mild respiratory distress (tachypnea).

## Detailed Exam

### HEENT (Figure 6-6):

- **H**ead: Moist mucous membranes
- **E**yes: PERRL; tears present
- **E**ars: Unremarkable
- **N**ose: Mucus present
- **T**hroat: Unremarkable

### Chest, heart. and lungs:

- Pulses: Peripheral pulses palpable and rapid
- Cardiac auscultation: Regular rate and rhythm; unable to adequately assess for murmur, rub, or gallop due to rapid rate
- Lung auscultation: The lungs are clear to auscultation bilaterally. The breath sounds are equal.
- Chest exam: Chest wall movement is symmetric. There is no injury noted to the chest on visual inspection.

### Neurologic:

- Neurovascular status intact

### Abdomen and pelvis:

- Soft and nontender. Bowel sounds are present and normal.

### Extremities:

- Upper extremities: Unremarkable
- Lower extremities: Unremarkable

### Back:

- Unremarkable

## Treatment

The initial treatment for this patient should focus on basic life support (BLS) measures to optimize oxygenation and hemodynamics. Applying oxygen to a patient who is tachypneic and tachycardic is not unreasonable, even in the setting of oxygen saturations greater than 94% on room air. Blow-by oxygen administration may be considered if the patient is unable to tolerate a nasal cannula or mask ventilation. Placing the patient in a position of comfort and minimizing distress by allowing them to remain with a caregiver whenever possible is also appropriate. Vagal stimulation with noninvasive maneuvers should also be considered.

When advanced life support and critical care resources are available, vascular access should be obtained. Febrile patients with rapid respiratory and pulse rates are prone to dehydration from insensible losses and will likely benefit from an appropriate fluid bolus.

**Detailed Physical Exam**

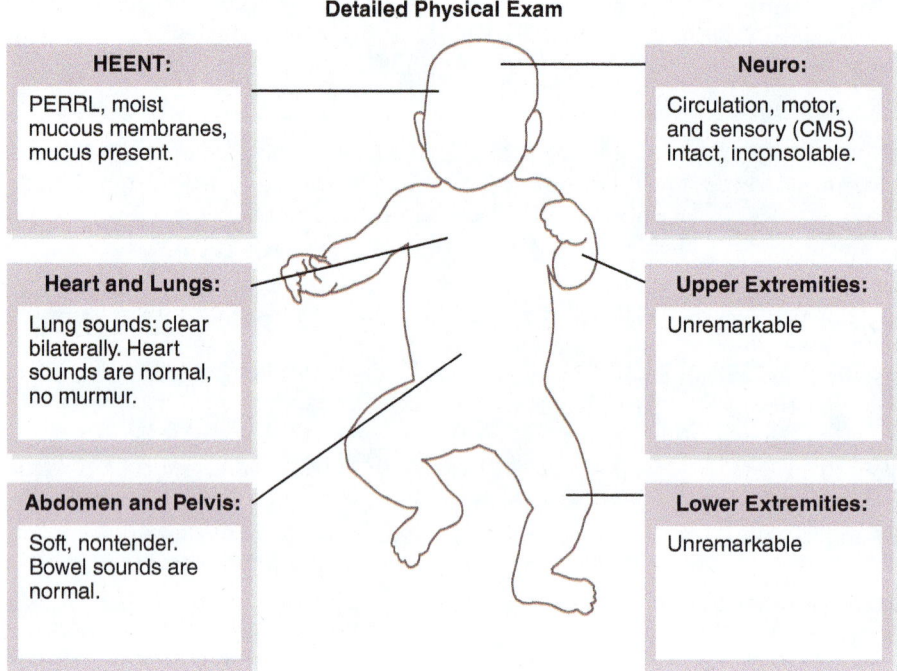

**HEENT:**

PERRL, moist mucous membranes, mucus present.

**Heart and Lungs:**

Lung sounds: clear bilaterally. Heart sounds are normal, no murmur.

**Abdomen and Pelvis:**

Soft, nontender. Bowel sounds are normal.

**Neuro:**

Circulation, motor, and sensory (CMS) intact, inconsolable.

**Upper Extremities:**

Unremarkable

**Lower Extremities:**

Unremarkable

**Figure 6-6** Would you consider a head-to-toe assessment or toe-to-head assessment in this child?

© Jones & Bartlett Learning.

Adenosine administration may be considered if calming the child or vagal maneuvers do not improve heart rate. Refer to the steps described earlier in this chapter for specifics on adenosine use and administration. Consider synchronized cardioversion if the child decompensates.

Transport the patient to the closest most appropriate facility. Practitioners should be prepared for rapid decompensation. Discuss with your partner en route to the call what steps you may take if the patient decompensates during transport. The management strategy will largely be based off local protocols, guidelines, and available resources.

## Ongoing Management

Physical exam for this patient does not suggest signs of cardiac overload or failure. Vascular access is obtained and a 200 mL normal saline bolus is administered (20 mL/kg). No signs of volume overload were present during or after this bolus.

After initiating vagal maneuvers, the patient's heart rate decreases to approximately 140 beats/min. The patient calms down, and you are now able to obtain a blood pressure of 88/56 mm Hg (stable). The patient's respiratory rate decreases to 30 breaths/min and the ETCO$_2$ increases to 36 mm Hg.

## Case Questions

- Where is the most appropriate treatment destination and why?
  - This patient should be transported to the closest appropriate pediatric-ready facility, preferably one with cardiology and cardiac intensive care resources.
- Can you safety transport this patient in your ambulance?
  - The patient was secured safely to the cot.
- Will you allow a parent to ride in the ambulance?
  - Allowing a caregiver to ride with the child and assist in providing care can help to limit the patient's distress, which will help reduce cardiac demand. The mother was allowed to ride with the EMS crew and was restrained to the bench seat.

## CASE WRAP-UP

Diagnosis: Supraventricular tachycardia

On arrival to the hospital the patient was in stable condition. She was admitted to the floor for close observation on telemetry. She had no further episodes of SVT and was discharged with close follow-up care to be provided by her pediatrician and a pediatric cardiologist.

SVT is the most common pathologic rhythm disturbance requiring treatment in children. Practitioners should be prepared to perform basic and advanced therapies for this rhythm disturbance. Many patients will remain stable and require minimal intervention; however, in some cases rapid deterioration may occur.

Transport to a facility with access to pediatric cardiology resources is important and should be performed when practical.

## Bradycardia

Bradycardia is a heart rate that is abnormally low for age (**Figure 6-7**). Not all bradycardia is pathologic. In some cases, patients may have a resting heart rate that is below the lower limit of normal and still maintain adequate peripheral perfusion. This is common in athletes and physically fit individuals, and in some children during sleep.

Common pathologic causes of bradycardia are summarized in **Table 6-6**.

Overall management of symptomatic bradycardia is directed at identifying and treating the underlying cause. In cases where the underlying cause cannot be managed, direct pacing of the heart may be necessary.

### Common Findings in Bradycardia

Children with bradycardia often have a history of fussiness, lethargy, irritability, or poor feeding. Some infants may have apnea spells leading to bradycardia, particularly if born prematurely. Older children may describe feeling of lightheadedness, weakness, syncope, and dyspnea. It may be difficult to determine the patient's complaint, as children may be unable to verbalize to caregivers what they are experiencing.

Altered mental status is a late sign and indicates that the brain is not getting enough blood flow to adequately oxygenate the tissues. Hypotension and shock may be present in patients with altered mental status secondary to bradycardia.

In patients with altered mental status or seizures, elevated ICP should be considered on the differential, particularly in the presence of elevated blood pressure. Altered mental status with bradycardia, hypertension, and seizure activity should be considered elevated ICP until proven otherwise. This requires rapid transport and likely neurosurgical intervention to resolve.

### Bradycardia Treatment

As with all cardiac rhythm disturbances, the treatment is determined primarily by the patient's clinical

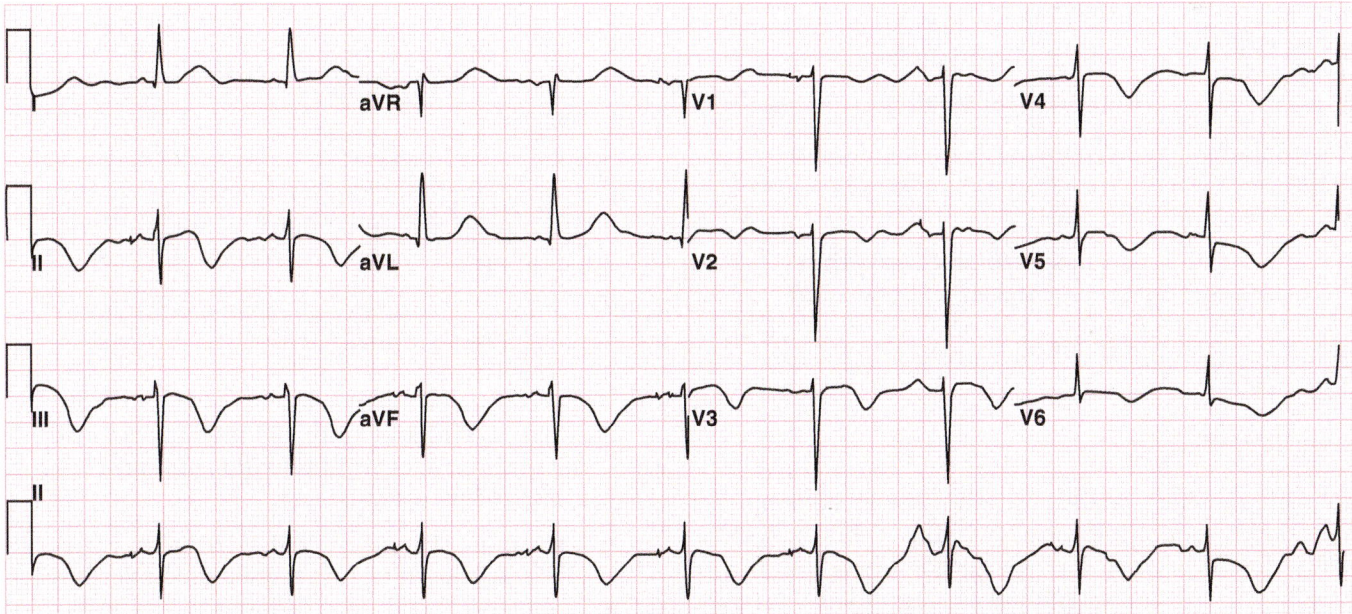

**Figure 6-7** ECG showing bradycardia, although not all bradycardia is pathologic.

**Table 6-6** Pathologic Causes of Pediatric Bradycardia

| Cause | Precipitating Factors |
|-------|----------------------|
| Hypoxia | <ul><li>Hypoventilation</li><li>Airway obstruction</li><li>Drowning</li><li>Suffocation</li><li>Breath-holding spells</li></ul> |
| Vagal stimulation | <ul><li>Intubation or airway visualization</li><li>Insertion of supraglottic airway</li><li>Deep suctioning</li><li>Sudden exposure to cold</li><li>Pain</li><li>Valsalva</li></ul> |
| Electrolyte disturbance | <ul><li>Renal failure</li><li>Toxic ingestion</li><li>Eating disorders</li><li>Laxative or diuretic use/abuse</li></ul> |
| Hypothermia | <ul><li>Environmental</li><li>Infants and neonates left exposed during exam and transport</li></ul> |
| Elevated intracranial pressure | <ul><li>Head injury</li><li>Obstructive hydrocephalus</li><li>Intracranial bleed</li></ul> |
| Overdose or ingestion | <ul><li>Overdoses that affect breathing may lead to bradycardia due to hypoxia</li><li>Ingestion of antidysrhythmic medications</li></ul> |
| Conduction disturbance | <ul><li>Heart block</li><li>Myocarditis</li></ul> |

© Jones & Bartlett Learning.

status (**Figure 6-8**). Stable patients should be monitored closely and transported without delay. Practitioners should prepare for rapid decompensation and be ready to provide resuscitation as appropriate.

In patients who are unstable, the initial steps for treating bradycardia are similar to those of other cardiac rhythm disturbances. Airway and ventilation should be optimized as hypoxia is by far the most common cause of bradycardia in children. In patients with a pulse less than 60 beats/min who have altered level of consciousness and other signs of poor perfusion, cardiopulmonary resuscitation (CPR) with high-quality chest compressions should be initiated while attempting to identify and treat reversible causes.

Once oxygenation, ventilation, and circulation have been addressed, the patient should be placed on a cardiac monitor. IV peripheral access should also be obtained (intraosseous [IO] access can be considered in a conscious patient who is ill or decompensating). A 12-lead ECG should be obtained, if possible, but do not delay emergency care in an unstable patient to accomplish this.

Once these actions have been taken, practitioners should begin to work through and address the following potential reversible causes:

- Hypoxia
  - Optimize ventilation and oxygenation.
- Hypovolemia
  - Provide isotonic crystalloid boluses.
- Hypoglycemia
  - Provide IV dextrose.
- Increased vagal tone
  - Remove or address any vagal stimuli.
- Hyperkalemia
  - Sodium bicarbonate 1 mEq/kg IV/IO
  - Calcium gluconate 50 mEq/kg IV/IO
- Acidosis
  - Address hypoventilation or other respiratory causes.
  - Sodium bicarbonate 1 mEq/kg IV/IO may be appropriate in some cases, such as toxic ingestion or overdose—consult online medical control.
- Hypothermia
  - Optimize environmental factors to promote normal temperature.
- Overdose
  - Attempt to identify any potential ingestion or overdose agent and provide appropriate antidote when available.
  - Naloxone 0.1 mg/kg IV/IO/IM/IN should be given in known or suspected opioid overdose.
  - Calcium channel and beta blocker overdoses may respond favorably to:
    - Calcium gluconate 20 mg/kg IV/IO

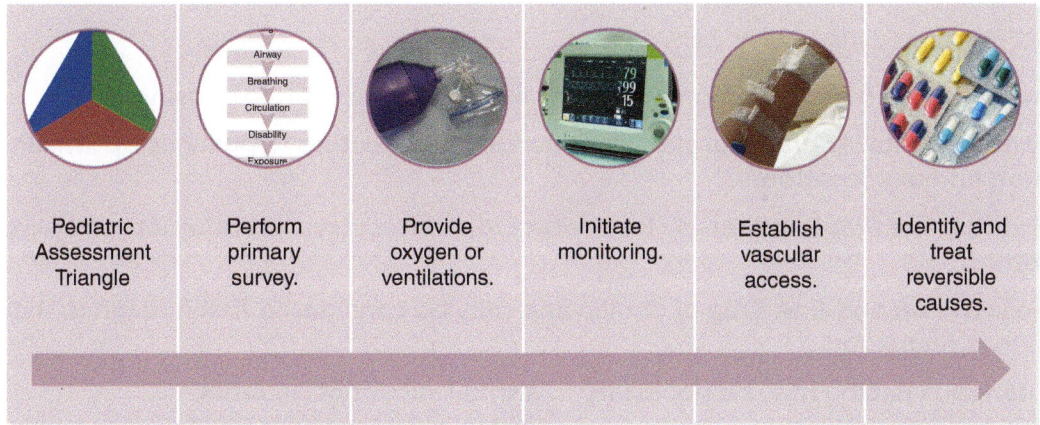

**Figure 6-8** The management steps for pediatric bradycardia.

A. Used with permission of the American Academy of Pediatrics, Pediatric Education for Prehospital Professionals, © American Academy of Pediatrics, 2000; **B.** Jones & Bartlett Learning.; **C.** © Jones & Bartlett Learning. Courtesy of MIEMSS.; **D.** © bymuratdeniz/E+/Getty Images; **E.** © natnaree sangkaew/Shutterstock; **F.** © nokwalai/Shutterstock.

- Glucagon 0.1 mg/kg IV/IO
- Epinephrine infusion 0.1 mcg/kg/min to support hemodynamic status

■ Provide information to receiving facility so they can have appropriate medications ready to treat overdose when appropriate.

### Epinephrine

Epinephrine is the preferred first-line agent in the treatment of bradycardia refractory to BLS interventions. The appropriate dose is 0.01 mg/kg IV/IO every 3 to 5 minutes. When the prefilled code-dose syringes with a concentration of 0.1 mg/mL are used, this works out to 0.1 mL/kg of the prefilled solution. Always check your math and confirm appropriate dose and volume calculation prior to administration.

Emergency treatment for pediatric bradycardia differs from adult bradycardia in that the initial drug of choice for pediatric bradycardia is epinephrine. A major exception is when the bradycardia is secondary to known or suspected increased vagal tone. Atropine is particularly effective at resolving cases of bradycardia due to increased vagal tone and may be considered before epinephrine administration when the clinical picture warrants. Examples include patients who have just had deep nasopharyngeal suctioning or patients who have just had laryngoscopy performed.

### Atropine

Atropine may be given in pediatric bradycardia when there is suspicion that increased vagal tone is the underlying cause. The dose for atropine is 0.02 mg/kg IV/IO. This dose may be repeated once in 3 to 5 minutes. The minimum dose is 0.1 mg, and the maximum single dose is 0.5 mg. Additional doses should be discussed with online medical direction prior to administration.

### Transcutaneous Pacing

All of the interventions discussed up to this point primarily increase sinoatrial (SA) node rate. In cases where conduction between the SA node and the ventricles is disrupted, delayed, or dissociated, SA node rate increase may not translate into increased ventricular rate.

Situations where transcutaneous pacing should be considered include the following:

- High-grade heart block, regardless of origin (second degree and above)
- AV conduction abnormalities encountered after cardiac surgery
- Patients with SA node denervation status post cardiac transplantation

If the underlying electrical activity is nonperfusing, pacing is not indicated and the patient should be treated using the pulseless electrical activity (PEA) arm of the pulseless arrest algorithm.

Pacing is not considered standard treatment for pulseless electrical activity and generally is only indicated in patients with underlying electrical activity that is triggering perfusing beats.

## BRADYCARDIA TREATMENT PEARLS

- Stable bradycardia may be benign in healthy individuals who are perfusing well.
- Treatment for unstable bradycardia should focus on correcting hypoxia by optimizing ventilation and oxygenation.
- Epinephrine is the first-line therapy for bradycardia refractory to ventilation and oxygenation optimization.
- Atropine is the second-line drug of choice and may be considered first line when increased vagal tone is suspected.
- Transcutaneous pacing may be necessary in a small subset of patients.

## CASE STUDY

### Case 2

#### Dispatch

You and your partner are responding to a 7-year-old female described as "drowning, unresponsive" at a river park. It is 1730 on a Saturday evening. The outside temperature is 94°F (34.4°C).

#### Case Questions

- What are your initial concerns?
  - Depending on the setting of this river park, scene safety may be an issue. Consider additional resources such as law enforcement and/or specialized rescue.
  - Based on the dispatch information, this situation has a high probability of being a cardiac arrest, and you and your partner should prepare as if that is the case. It would be helpful to preplan actions, interventions, and medications, if possible. You and your partner should also consider what transport destination is appropriate, and whether an alternative method of transport such as air medical may be indicated for this patient.
- Based on the dispatch information, what are the possible differential diagnoses for this patient?
  - In addition to the fact that this patient has likely experienced a submersion injury (drowning), other possible injuries and conditions should be considered.

- Seizure disorder
  - If the patient has a history of seizure disorder, it is possible that a seizure preceded the drowning and could be contributing to altered level of consciousness and depressed respiratory drive.
- Cardiac dysrhythmia
  - If the patient has an underlying cardiac abnormality, cardiac dysrhythmia could have preceded the drowning and led to altered level of consciousness and submersion injury.
- Trauma
  - If the patient was diving into the water, the possibility of head and spinal trauma should be considered. If there is any question as to whether this may have occurred or not, such as in an unwitnessed drowning event, c-spine precautions should be applied.
- Ingestion
  - It is possible the patient intentionally or unintentionally ingested a substance that caused depressed level of consciousness and led to drowning.
- Anaphylaxis
  - If the patient has an allergy to insect stings or bites, or significant food allergy, the possibility of anaphylaxis leading to drowning should be considered in the appropriate clinical context.

## Initial Observations

As you pull up to the scene it appears there are no immediate safety concerns. A bystander waves you over to the patient. You see a 7-year-old female lying supine on the ground with a life vest around her waist. There is no visible movement. A family member is being coached through hands-only CPR by the 911 dispatcher.

- Pediatric Assessment Triangle (**Figure 6-9**)
  - Appearance
    - Unresponsive
  - Work of breathing
    - The patient is apneic and there is no visible respiratory effort.
  - Circulation
    - The patient is pale and dusky with cyanosis present.

A family member states, "We were swimming in the river and she suddenly disappeared!" According to the bystander, the child was found downstream entangled in tree roots and other debris. She was "blue and not breathing" when she was pulled up onto the riverbank.

## Primary Survey

The primary survey for this patient reveals the following:

**X**—No bleeding noted

**A**—Open and patent

**B**—Apneic with no visible respiratory effort

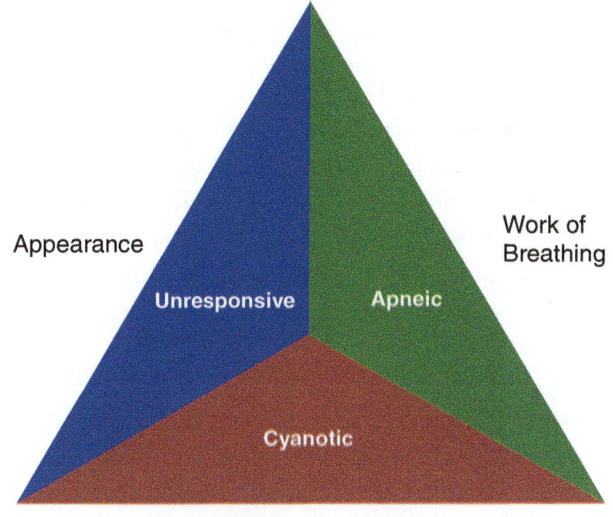

**Figure 6-9** In this patient all three sides of the Pediatric Assessment Triangle are concerning.

- What other considerations do you have now based on the initial information you have received?
  - This patient could also have multiple traumatic injuries as a result of being pulled down the river. Appropriate trauma precautions should be taken and a thorough secondary assessment should be performed when appropriate, but only if time permits.

- Based on your initial impression, is this patient "Quick" or "Not Quick"?
  - This patient is "Quick."
  - She is pulseless, apneic, and has signs of poor peripheral perfusion. There is also a high probability that she has suffered traumatic injuries.
  - Even when patients are "Quick," a thorough history and assessment is still important. There are critical interventions that need to be efficiently performed prior to initiating transport to the hospital. Taking a "load and go" approach without performing critical interventions may decrease the odds of survival for this patient.
  - In addition to high-quality CPR and other important BLS interventions, careful attention should be paid to maintaining normothermia in this patient. Hypothermia could exacerbate underlying pathology and lead to poor survival chances.
    - Use warmed fluids for resuscitation (if available).
    - Optimize the temperature in the transport environment.
    - Patients who are wet should be dried as much as possible to prevent evaporative heat loss.
    - With the exception of during exam and treatment, the patient should be kept covered as much as possible to preserve body heat.

**C**—No palpable peripheral or central pulses. Skin is cold, wet to the touch, and mottled with cyanosis present.

**D**—Unresponsive; GCS 3 (E1, V1, M1).

**E**—Lying supine on the ground

## Case Questions

- Based on the findings noted in the primary survey, what would your initial interventions and treatment include?

  - Initial treatment for this patient should focus on high-quality CPR and other BLS interventions to address hypoxia and absent perfusion.

  - Intubation is a high-risk, low-frequency occurrence in pediatric patients. If adequate ventilation can be achieved with bag-valve mask (BVM) techniques, delaying the insertion of an advanced airway until return of spontaneous circulation (ROSC) has been achieved is reasonable.

  - If the patient is in a "can't ventilate, can't oxygenate" situation, then advanced airway insertion may be necessary to address hypoxia and hypoventilation.

## High-Quality CPR

Pediatric cardiac arrest requires effective delivery of BLS care. When ventilations and compressions are delivered in a choreographed manner, the efficacy of each individual intervention is maximized.

The most effective strategy for resuscitating pediatric patients is to address both oxygenation and perfusion. For this reason, once trained medical professionals are present, the use of hands-only CPR is not recommended, because it does not address hypoxia. Although adults may be suffering from underlying poor cardiac function which leads to arrest, most children have strong healthy hearts, and addressing hypoxia while supporting circulation will often correct cardiac arrest.

### Compression Rates

The appropriate compression-to-ventilation ratio for infants and children is as follows:

- 30:2 when single-rescuer CPR is being performed
- 15:2 when two-rescuer CPR is being performed

## Detailed Assessment

### History Taking

While other crew members address ventilation and perfusion, you begin to obtain a history, reveling the following:

**OPQRST:**

- **O**nset: Approximately 30 minutes ago
- **P**rovocation/palliation: Unknown

- **Q**uality: None
- **R**adiation: None
- **S**everity: Unknown
- **T**iming: 30 minutes

**SAMPLER:**

- **S**igns/symptoms: Unresponsive, apneic, hypothermic
- **A**llergies: No known allergies to medications, foods, or the environment
- **M**edications: None
- **P**ast medical history: None
- **L**ast oral intake: Snack at 1600
- **E**vents leading up to the emergency: Fell into fast moving river
- **R**isk factors: None

## Vital Signs

As you were obtaining the history, the patient was attached to the monitor and the following vital signs were obtained (**Figure 6-10**):

**Heart rate:**

- 42 beats/min
- Weak and thready

**SpO$_2$:**

- The SpO$_2$ probe was unable to detect a reliable waveform.
- This is likely a result of poor perfusion and cold extremities.

**ETCO$_2$:**

- 54 mm Hg (with assisted ventilations)
- The elevated ETCO$_2$ is the result of poor gas exchange and the inability to adequately remove trapped carbon dioxide in the lungs.
- In patients with pulseless arrest the observed ETCO$_2$ during CPR may be low, as poor perfusion fails to deliver carbon dioxide to the lungs where it can be exchanged at the level of the alveoli.
- Patients with a sudden rise in ETCO$_2$ during CPR are likely experiencing a sudden increase in cardiac output and may have ROSC.
- This patient has bradycardia, inadequate circulation, and per resuscitation guidelines for bradycardia, compressions should continue until signs of perfusion improve and the pulse is above 60 beats/min.

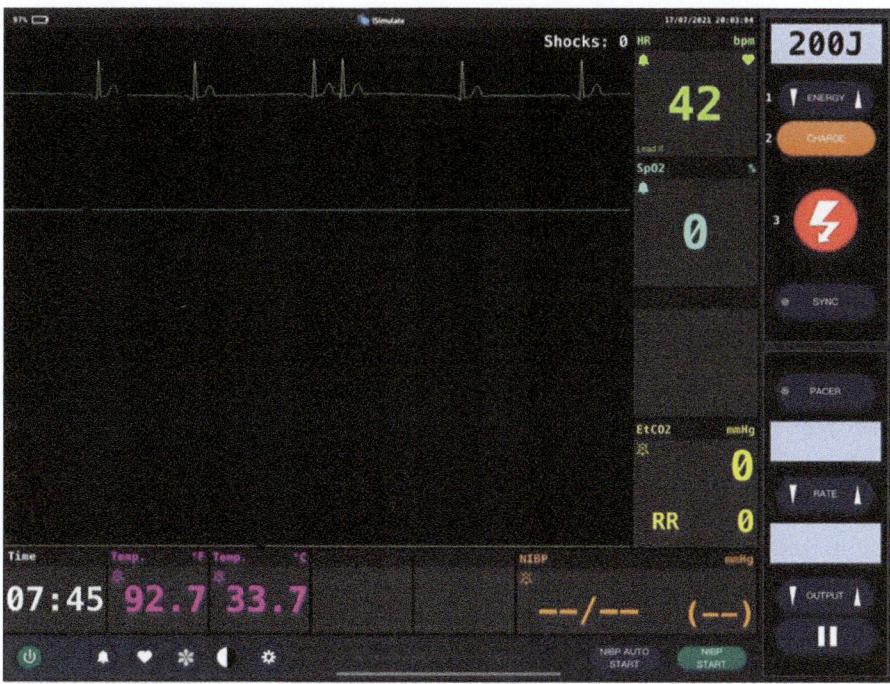

**Figure 6-10** The monitor display shows the patient's vital signs.
Courtesy of iSimulate.

**Respiratory rate:**

- 0 breaths/min

- The key to improving this patient's perfusion and increasing her pulse is to address the apnea.

- 100% oxygen should be administered via BVM or with an advanced airway when indicated.

**Blood pressure:**

- Unable to obtain

- This is likely due to hypoperfusion and movement with CPR.

**Temperature:**

- 92.7°F (33.7°C)

- This is classified as mild hypothermia.

- Addressing hypothermia will increase this patient's chances for survival.

**Blood glucose:**

- 121 mg/dL

- Blood glucose levels during acute episodes of stress will often be elevated.

- If this patient's blood glucose was observed to be low, it must be addressed to rule it out as a potential cause or exacerbating factor in the arrest.

**Weight:**

- Estimated weight of 25 kg based on length-based tape

The patient is a previously healthy 7-year-old female found in full arrest after freshwater submersion injury with unknown down time and high probability of associated traumatic injury. Hands-only bystander CPR was being performed on arrival of EMS personnel. The patient is responding poorly to BLS care and continues to be bradycardic with poor perfusion and gas exchange, as indicated by clinical exam and exhaled ETCO$_2$ observation. She has associated hypothermia.

Care for this patient should include the following:

- Continued CPR

- Optimization of ventilation and oxygenation to address hypoxia and hypercapnia

- Medication administration as appropriate
  - Includes epinephrine and atropine for treatment of bradycardia

- Strategies to improve temperature and prevent further heat loss
  - Patient compartment should be warm.
  - Keep patient covered as much as possible.
  - Use warmed IV fluids.

- Rapid transport to the closest appropriate facility once initial BLS stabilization has taken place

## Detailed Exam

### HEENT (Figure 6-11):

- **H**ead: Small abrasion to the forehead
- **E**yes: PERRL, sluggish
- **E**ars: Unremarkable
- **N**ose: Unremarkable
- **T**hroat: Unremarkable

### Chest, heart, and lungs:

- Pulses: Weak and thready, bradycardic
- Cardiac auscultation: Normal, no murmur
- Lung auscultation: Bilateral rhonchi heard during BVM ventilation
- Chest exam: No visible trauma

### Neurologic:

- Unresponsive

### Abdomen and pelvis:

- Soft, nontender, no apparent fracture
- Abdomen is nondistended.

### Extremities:

- Upper extremities: Cold and mottled
- Lower extremities: Cold and mottled

### Back:

- No visible injury

## Ongoing Management

After approximately 2 minutes of high-quality CPR and ventilation with 100% oxygen, you are no longer able to palpate a pulse.

As you are loading the patient into the ambulance your partner obtains an IO in the left lower extremity and hangs a 20 mL/kg bolus of warmed normal saline. You are able to cover the patient with warmed blankets, with the chest exposed for continued delivery of high-quality compressions.

## Cardiac Arrest

There are two arms to the cardiac arrest algorithm: shockable and non-shockable. 93.5% of pediatric patients will be in a non-shockable rhythm (i.e., PEA or asystole). That is the case for the patient in this scenario. As discussed before, the primary treatment for any cardiac arrest patient is rapid initiation of high-quality CPR and addressing the underlying cause—most often hypoxia in pediatrics.

### Non-Shockable Rhythms

#### Pulseless Electrical Activity

PEA is a non-shockable rhythm. It is a clinical condition where there is organized electrical activity that is

**Detailed Physical Exam**

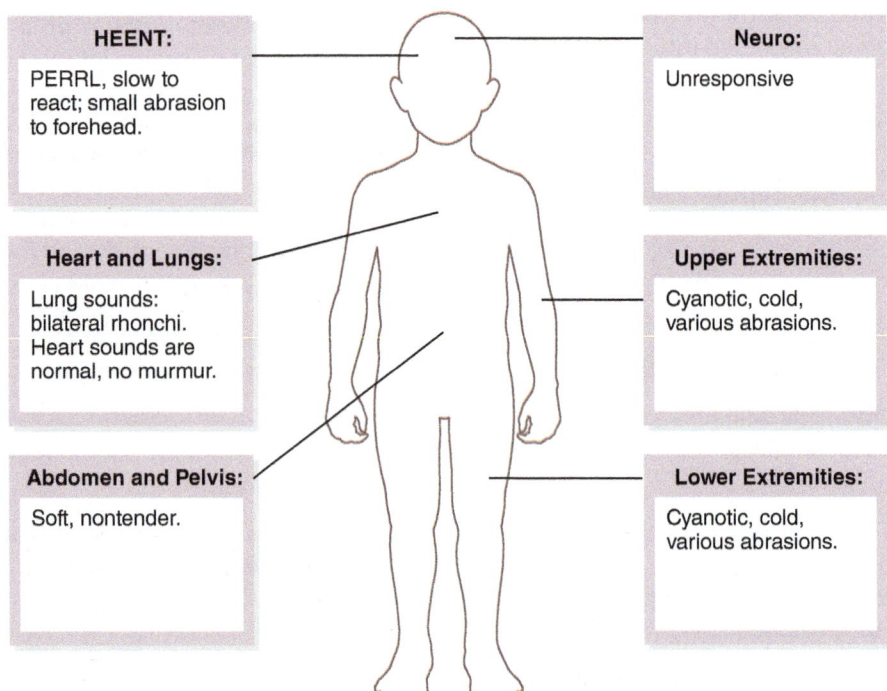

**HEENT:**
PERRL, slow to react; small abrasion to forehead.

**Neuro:**
Unresponsive

**Heart and Lungs:**
Lung sounds: bilateral rhonchi. Heart sounds are normal, no murmur.

**Upper Extremities:**
Cyanotic, cold, various abrasions.

**Abdomen and Pelvis:**
Soft, nontender.

**Lower Extremities:**
Cyanotic, cold, various abrasions.

**Figure 6-11** Absence of spontaneous respirations is noted during secondary survey.

## EPINEPHRINE

Expert opinions vary regarding administration of vasoactive medications to patients with hypothermia. The general consensus guidelines recommend the following:

- Hold epinephrine until core body temperature is 86°F (30°C) or above.
  - Once temperature is above this range, administer the standard dose of epinephrine.
  - The time interval between doses may be extended. Most clinicians will transition to every 6 to 8 minutes between doses.
  - Continue rewarming the patient.

Pearls:

- Excessive epinephrine administration should be avoided in hypothermic patients.

- It is generally not recommended to administer more than three doses until the temperature has been corrected to a normothermic range (95°F or 35°C or above).

- Always follow local protocols and guidelines.

- Establish contact with medical control early to optimize care.

- Patients are considered to be "actively drowning" until they receive positive-pressure ventilation.

- Providing airway support with BVM early will improve patient outcomes.

## Case Questions

- What is the most appropriate treatment destination and why?
  - This patient should be transported to a pediatric tertiary care center with pediatric critical care capabilities if possible. If this is not practical via ground transport, then air transport should be considered if the patient is stable enough. Most air medical transport programs will not transport patients in active arrest, as high-quality CPR is not generally achievable in the aircraft cabin.
  - Ideally, the transport destination for this patient will have extracorporeal membrane oxygenation (ECMO) capabilities in order to provide rewarming and heart-lung support for the submersion injury. When possible, allow the parent to ride with their child.
- Can you safely transport this child in the ambulance?
  - This patient should be transported on a rigid board to allow for effective chest compressions.
- Will you allow the parent to ride in the ambulance?
  - The parent rode restrained in the front seat with the EMS crew.

capable of producing a perfusing rhythm with no palpable pulse or signs of adequate perfusion (**Figure 6-12**). This is what makes PEA distinct from pulseless VT of VF (both of which are shockable). VF and VT are not generally associated with adequate perfusion, whereas bradycardia, sinus rhythm, or tachycardia may produce perfusion in the setting of adequate myocardial function.

PEA has a poor overall prognosis unless the underlying cause is addressed.

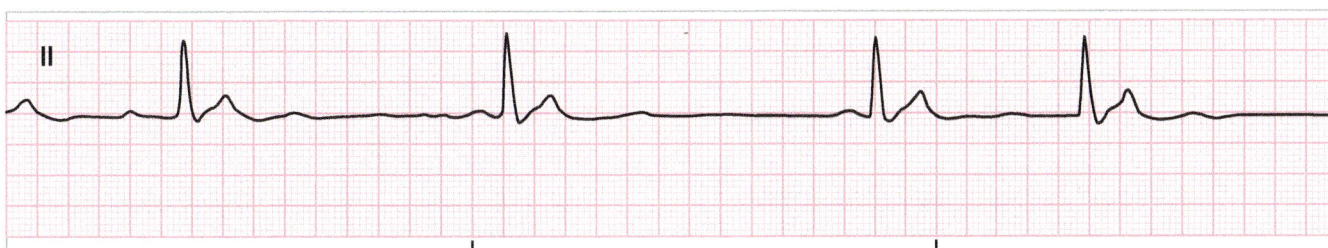

**Figure 6-12** Pulseless electrical activity is a clinical situation, not a specific dysrhythmia.

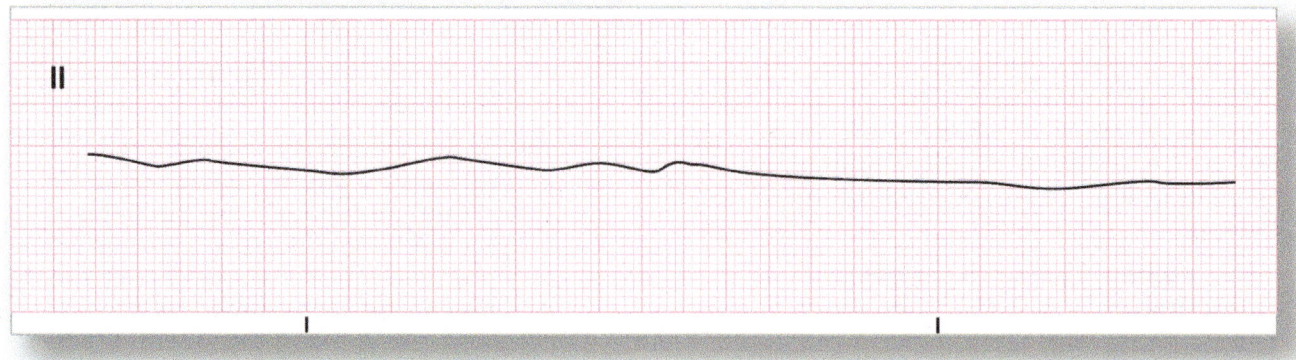

**Figure 6-13** Asystole reflects an absence of ventricular electrical activity. It is also known as ventricular standstill.

From Arrhythmia Recognition: The Art of Interpretation, courtesy of Tomas B. Garcia, MD.

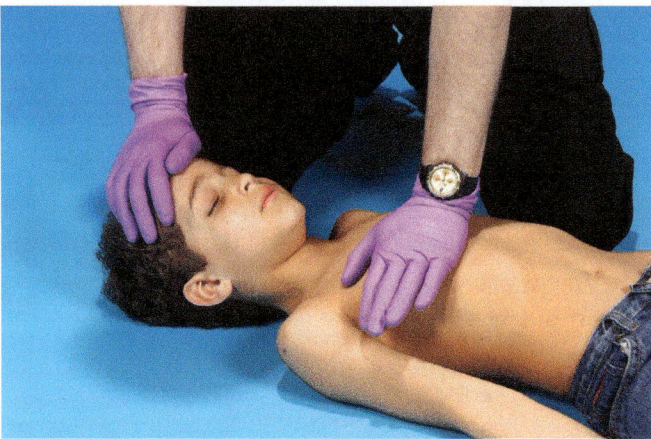

**Figure 6-14** Asystole and PEA are both non-shockable rhythms. In these patients, immediately begin choreographed CPR with assisted ventilations.

© Jones & Bartlett Learning.

## Asystole

Asystole is the absence of ventricular electrical activity (**Figure 6-13**). It may not always have a flat line or complete absence of electrical activity. In some cases there will be random electrical discharges that are not associated with cardiac activity as the few remaining viable myocardial cells depolarize and die. Asystole also has poor outcomes in pediatric patients. It is an end-of-life rhythm and rarely survivable unless an identifiable cause is quickly addressed.

## Non-Shockable Rhythm Treatment

The following steps are necessary to treat non-shockable arrest:

- Begin high-quality choreographed CPR (**Figure 6-14**).
- Attach the monitor and assess the rhythm.
  - Specific identification is not as important as determining whether it is shockable or not.

### HS AND TS

The causes of PEA and asystole can be remembered using the Hs and Ts memory aid:

- **Hypovolemia**
- **Hypoxia**
- **Hydrogen ion imbalance (acidosis or alkalosis)**
- **Hypoglycemia**
- **Hypo/hyperkalemia**
- **Hypothermia**
- **Thrombosis (coronary or pulmonary)**
- **Tension pneumothorax**
- **Tamponade**
- **Toxins**

Utilizing this memory aid can help the practitioner recall and work through possible causes of PEA and asystole.

- Obtain vascular access as rapidly as possible. (IO is likely the most efficient option when available.)
- Administer the appropriate weight-based dose of epinephrine every 3 to 5 minutes.
  - 0.01 mg/kg IV/IO
    - This works out to 0.1 mL/kg IV/IO of 1:10,000 concentration
- Identify and treat reversible causes using the Hs and Ts memory aid.

- Continue 2-minute cycles of CPR, and reassess.
  - Pause compressions and switch compressors every 2 minutes.
  - Analyze rhythm.
  - Resume compressions if necessary.
  - Shock when appropriate.
  - Administer medications when appropriate.
  - You can use the following cadence to recall the appropriate order of action:
    - Compressions, monitor, medication.
- Shift algorithms for appropriate treatment as patient condition evolves.
- Consider local protocols for patient disposition.

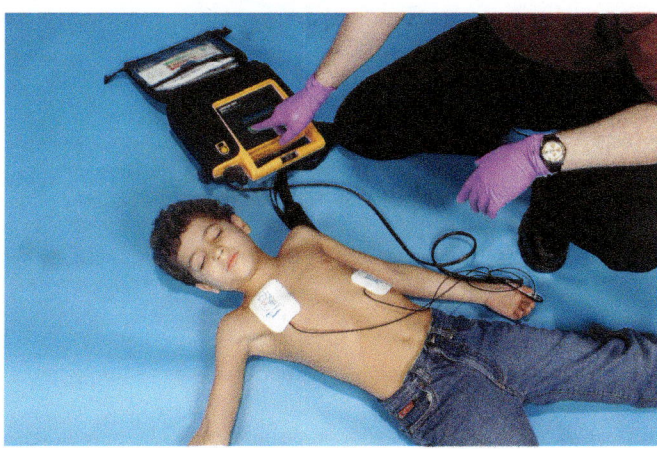

**Figure 6-15** For patients with shockable rhythms, start with choreographed CPR and then deliver a shock at 2 J/kg.

© Jones & Bartlett Learning.

## Shockable Rhythms

### Pulseless Ventricular Tachycardia and Ventricular Fibrillation

VF and pulseless VT are shockable rhythms (**Figure 6-15**). They are rarely the presenting arrest rhythms in pediatric patients, with a few exceptions. VF is a completely disorganized rhythm with no identifiable ECG waves (**Figure 6-16**). It represents quivering of the ventricles and no perfusing cardiac activity. Pulseless VT may be regular or irregular (**Figure 6-17**). It is a wide complex tachycardia, as described previously. Ventricular contraction may be absent or so rapid that there is inadequate time of systole and diastole, resulting in pulseless arrest.

### Shockable Rhythm Treatment

The following steps are necessary to treat shockable arrest:

- Begin high-quality choreographed CPR.
- Attach the monitor and assess the rhythm.
  - Specific identification is not as important as determining whether it is shockable or not.
- Deliver initial shock at 2 J/kg as early in the arrest as possible.
- Obtain vascular access as rapidly as possible. (IO is likely the most efficient option when available.)
- Administer the appropriate weight-based dose of epinephrine every 3 to 5 minutes.
  - 0.01 mg/kg IV/IO
    - This works out to 0.1 mL/kg IV/IO of 1:10,000 concentration.

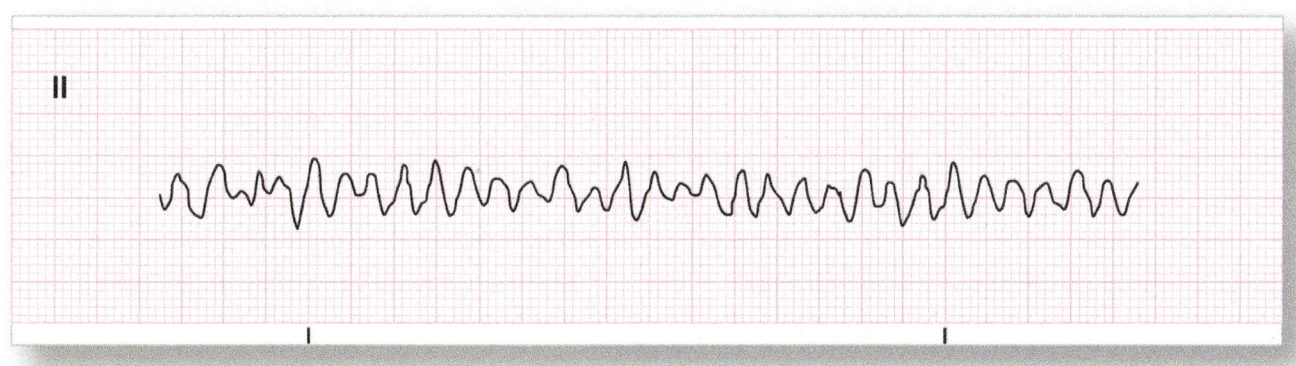

**Figure 6-16** Ventricular fibrillation is a ventricular dysrhythmia during which there is no organized depolarization of the ventricles.

From Arrhythmia Recognition: The Art of Interpretation, courtesy of Tomas B. Garcia, MD.

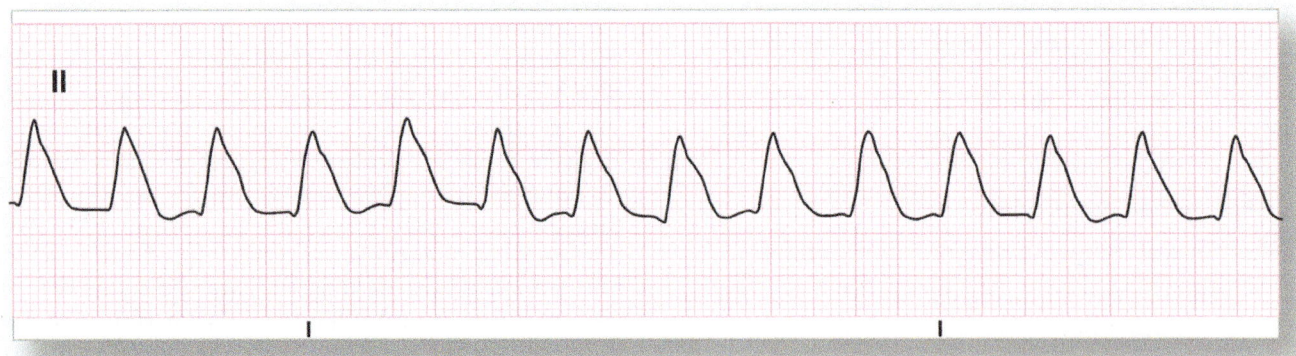

**Figure 6-17** Pulseless ventricular tachycardia occurs when ventricular contractions are replaced with rapid, ineffective contractions.

From Arrhythmia Recognition: The Art of Interpretation, courtesy of Tomas B. Garcia, MD.

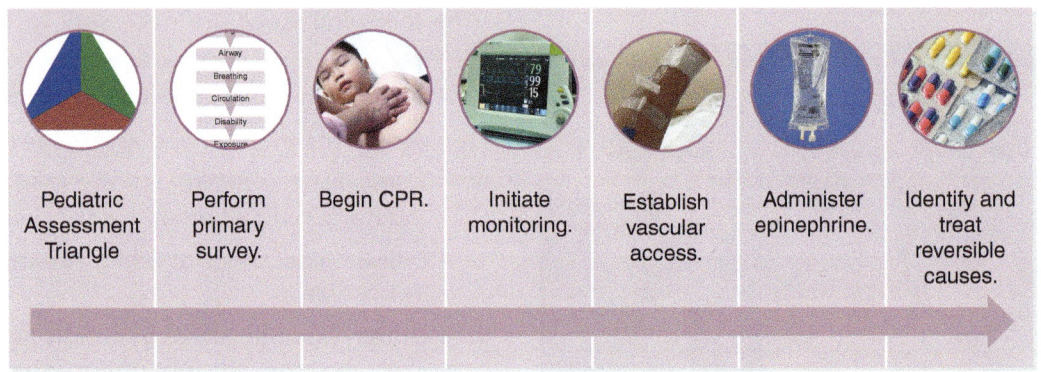

| Pediatric Assessment Triangle | Perform primary survey. | Begin CPR. | Initiate monitoring. | Establish vascular access. | Administer epinephrine. | Identify and treat reversible causes. |

**Figure 6-18** Prehospital management of pediatric patients in cardiac arrest should follow these steps.

A. Used with permission of the American Academy of Pediatrics, Pediatric Education for Prehospital Professionals, © American Academy of Pediatrics, 2000; **B & F.** Jones & Bartlett Learning.; **C.** © parinoi/Shutterstock.; **D.** © bymuratdeniz/E+/Getty Images; **E.** © natnaree sangkaew/Shutterstock; **G.** © nokwalai/Shutterstock.

- Administer an antidysrhythmic after epinephrine administration.
  - Amiodarone 5 mg/kg IV/IO every 3 to 5 minutes for a maximum of three doses.
    - Maximum initial dose is 300 mg.
    - Maximum second and third doses are 150 mg.
  - Lidocaine 1 mg/kg IV/IO loading dose is also appropriate.
    - Studies have indicated there is no evidence of either lidocaine or amiodarone being superior in pulseless arrest.
- Continue 2-minute cycles of CPR, and reassess.
  - Pause compressions and switch compressors.
  - Analyze rhythm.
  - Resume compressions if necessary.
  - Shock when appropriate.
  - Administer medications when appropriate.

- You can use the following cadence to recall the appropriate order of action:
  - Compressions, monitor, medication
- Shift algorithms for appropriate treatment as patient condition evolves.
- Consider local protocols for patient disposition.

## Cardiac Arrest Summary

The key steps to treating pulseless arrest are as follows (**Figure 6-18**):

- Begin immediate high-quality, choreographed CPR.
- Ensure adequate ventilation and oxygenation.
- Apply a cardiac monitor.
- If cardiac monitor is not available, use an automated external defibrillator (AED), and defibrillate any shockable rhythm as soon as possible.
  - Early and rapid defibrillation is one of the most important interventions is shockable arrest.

- In persistent arrest that is refractory to defibrillation, epinephrine should be administered within the first 10 minutes of losing a pulse when possible.
- Reversible causes should be identified and treated as soon as possible.
- Attempt to obtain a focused history when possible, with attention to family history of sudden cardiac death, ventricular dysrhythmias, or known genetic or cardiac abnormalities.

## Case Progression

As you are preparing to transport the patient, she is getting progressively more difficult to ventilate with basic maneuvers, and there is copious, frothy, blood-tinged

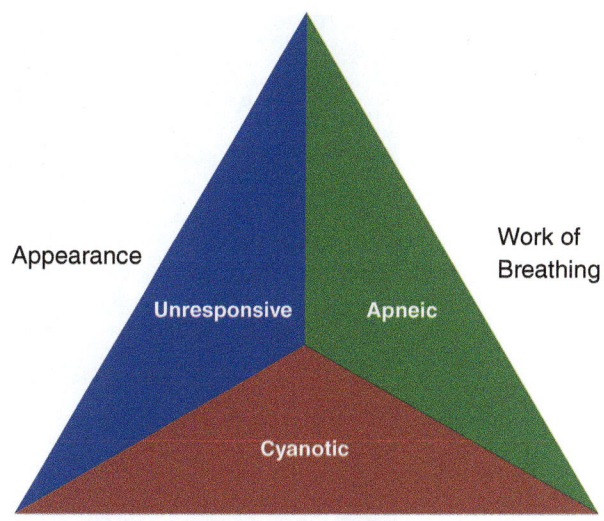

**Figure 6-19** Reassessment of this patient shows that all three sides of the Pediatric Assessment Triangle are still nonreassuring.

Used with permission of the American Academy of Pediatrics, Pediatric Education for Prehospital Professionals, © American Academy of Pediatrics, 2000.

sputum being produced from the mouth and nose. You make the decision to intubate prior to transport. You successfully intubate the patient and initiate transport to the tertiary care pediatric hospital 25 minutes away. You reassess the patient and find the following:

- Pediatric Assessment Triangle (**Figure 6-19**)
  - Appearance
    - Unresponsive
  - Work of breathing
    - Apneic
  - Circulation
    - Dusky, mottled, and cyanotic

The repeat primary survey reveals:

**X**—No bleeding found

**A**—Intubated

**B**—Assisted

**C**—Absent brachial pulses, cyanotic, cold to the touch, dry

**D**—GCS 3 (E1, V1, M1)

**E**—Lying on EMS stretcher

Repeat vital signs show the following:

**Heart rate:**

- 48 beats/min
- No palpable pulses, indicating the patient is in PEA (**Figure 6-20**)

## CARDIAC ARREST TREATMENT PEARLS

- **The initiation of high-quality, choreographed CPR is essential.**
- **Early defibrillation in shockable rhythms is lifesaving.**
- **Early identification of reversible causes (Hs and Ts) is essential in non-shockable arrest.**
- **Overall survival for pediatric cardiac arrest is less than 10%.**
  - **3.7% for infants**
  - **9.8% for children**
  - **16.3% for adolescents**
- **Vascular access (IV or IO; IV preferred) with fluid and medication administration were associated with improved survival rates.**
- **Advanced airway attempts were not associated with improved survival in cases where basic airway management was effective.**
- **Other than epinephrine, amiodarone, and lidocaine, when appropriate, the routine use of additional drugs such as sodium bicarbonate and calcium gluconate has been shown to decrease survival overall, unless specifically indicated in toxicologic overdose.**

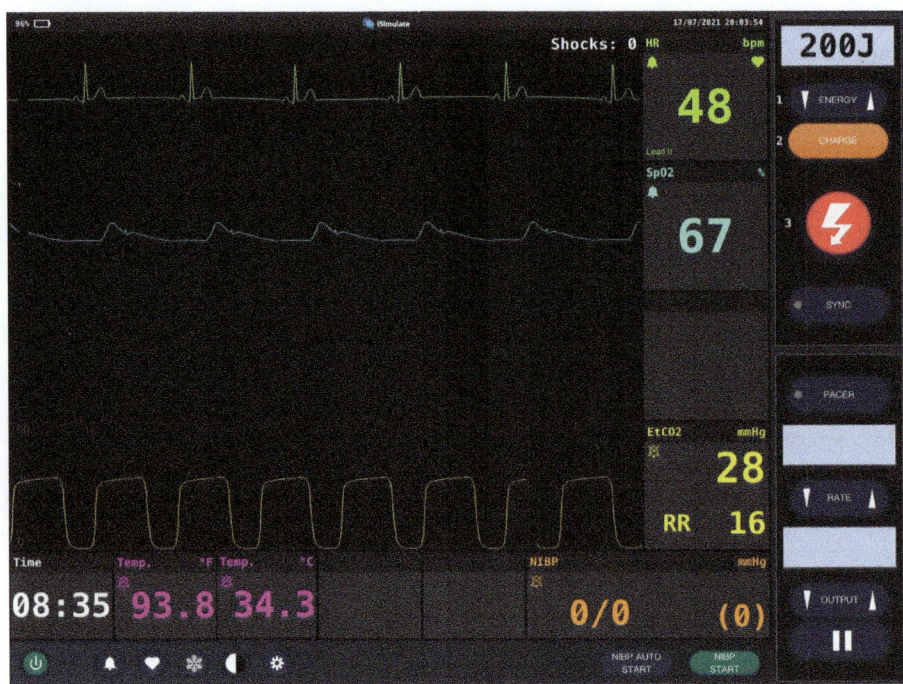

**Figure 6-20** Vital signs indicate the patient is in PEA.
Courtesy of iSimulate.

**SpO₂:**

- 67% with 100% $FiO_2$

**ETCO₂:**

- 28 mm Hg
- This indicates that the patient's perfusion is getting worse and less carbon dioxide is being transported to the lungs for exhalation, despite the fact that it is building up in the bloodstream.

**Respiratory rate:**

- 16 breaths/min assisted
- No spontaneous ventilations observed

**Blood pressure:**

- Unable to obtain

**Temperature:**

- 93.8°F (34.3°C)

**Blood glucose:**

- 97 mg/dL

## Treatment

The overall care provided to this patient up to this point included high-quality, choregraphed CPR, advanced airway insertion, perfusion support with IV fluids, rewarming with fluids and environmental controls, and appropriate drug administration for resuscitation.

Continued care during transport should be focused on optimizing ventilation and perfusion by transitioning to continuous compressions and ventilating the patient at approximately 20 breaths/min now that there is an advanced airway in place. Continued administration of vasoactive drugs as indicated by protocol is appropriate.

Advanced notification for the receiving facility is critical. Some facilities may have eCPR capabilities in which the patient can be placed on ECMO while resuscitation is underway. This can be lifesaving.

## ROSC Considerations

When patients achieve ROSC, it is imperative that practitioners respond aggressively to support oxygenation and perfusion in order to maintain it.

Many patients will achieve return of circulation with inadequate respiratory effort, so it is important to continue to ventilate and oxygenate these patients.

Vital signs should be obtained immediately with attention to blood pressure. Blood pressure optimization is the key to protecting neurologic function. Fluid boluses and vasoactive infusions should be used to support circulation and perfusion. Push-dose pressors may be used while setting up vasoactive infusions.

$ETCO_2$ should be maintained above 20 mm Hg, targeting a range of 25–35 mm Hg.

## Compassionate Options for Pediatrics (COPE)

Approximately 16,000 pediatric patients suffer from cardiac arrest annually in the United States. EMS personnel should take steps to increase their level of comfort discussing end-of-life situations with parents when resuscitation efforts appear futile. Self-care and critical incident stress debriefing is also important for prehospital practitioners, especially when incidents involve pediatric patients.

Depending on the protocols and guidelines where you work, care for pediatric cardiac arrest patients may continue until transferred at the hospital or death is called in the field. This will depend on policy and circumstances.

EMS personnel may be the individuals responsible for telling parents and caregivers that their child has died. COPE is a project that provides EMS personnel with the tools to approach pediatric death and dying scenarios before, during, and after the encounter. The main focus is to alleviate personal secondary trauma leading to PTSD among all individuals involved with the pediatric death.

COPE will assist EMS personnel with the guidance to communicate and comfort families. It also provides EMS personnel with a better understanding of self-care for prehospital practitioners. More on COPE can be found on the Emergency Medical Services for Children Innovation and Improvement Center website: https://emscimprovement.center/news/cope -compassionate-options-pediatric-ems/.

## CASE WRAP-UP

Diagnosis: Drowning, PEA

The patient was transported to the pediatric tertiary care center where she was still noted to be in PEA. She was refractory to additional rewarming efforts and required eCPR and initiation of ECMO for rewarming and heart/lung support. She was transferred to the PICU where she was eventually rewarmed. Her lungs recovered while on ECMO and she was eventually weaned off

cardiac and respiratory support over the next 4 weeks. While she survived her submersion injury, the prolonged downtime resulted in significant neurologic deficit. She was transferred to a long-term inpatient rehabilitation facility where she participates in multiple therapies to maximize her remaining function. She continues to show modest improvement with aggressive physical, occupational, speech, and cognitive therapies.

## CASE TAKEAWAY POINTS

Drowning is the leading cause of death in pediatric patients between ages 1 and 4 years, and it is the third-leading cause of death in all patients younger than 14 years.

Drowning often results in non-shockable arrest (PEA or asystole), thus choreographed CPR with ventilations

should be performed. Prehospital management should focus on oxygenation, ventilation, and perfusion. Hypothermia is a common finding and should be rapidly corrected.

## LESSON WRAP-UP

Understanding the differences between pediatric and adult ECGs allows for proper interpretation and identification of dysrhythmias. It is also critical to remember that cardiac events in children are most often caused by respiratory failure, not underlying dysfunctions of the heart, and therefore treatment should focus on restoring oxygenation and hemodynamics.

Pediatric dysrhythmias can be broadly classified as too fast, too slow, or not enough.

Postresuscitation care (both prehospital and in-hospital) is key for reducing neurologic deficit post arrest. Maintenance is blood pressure is imperative, as is ensuring adequate oxygenation.

EMS practitioners should take advantage of training opportunities to learn therapeutic communication and self-care when dealing with pediatric death and dying.

## REFERENCES

Barranco F, Lesmes A, Irles JA, et al. Cardiopulmonary resuscitation with simultaneous chest and abdominal compression: comparative study in humans. *Resuscitation.* 1990;20(1):67-77. doi:10.1016/0300-9572(90)90088-v

Bronzetti G, Brighenti M, Mariucci E, et al. Upside-down position for the out of hospital management of children with supraventricular tachycardia. *Int J Cardiol.* 2018;252:106-109. doi:10.1016/j.ijcard.2017.10.120

Calhoun AW, Sutton ERH, Barbee AP, et al. Compassionate options for pediatric EMS (COPE): addressing communication skills. *Prehosp Emerg Care.* 2017;21(3):334-343. doi:10.1080/10903127.2016.1263370

Cheng A, Duff JP, Kessler D, et al. Optimizing CPR performance with CPR coaching for pediatric cardiac arrest: a randomized simulation-based clinical trial. *Resuscitation.* 2018;132:33-40. doi:10.1016/j.resuscitation.2018.08.021

Crosson J, Hanash C. Emergency diagnosis and management of pediatric arrhythmias. *J Emerg Trauma Shock.* 2010;3(3):251. doi:10.4103/0974-2700.66525

Lee J, Yang W-C, Lee E-P, et al. Clinical survey and predictors of outcomes of pediatric out-of-hospital cardiac arrest admitted to the emergency department. *Sci Rep.* 2019;9(1):7032. doi:10.1038/s41598-019-43020-0

Lewis J, Arora G, Tudorascu DL, Hickey RW, Saladino RA, Manole MD. Acute management of refractory and unstable pediatric supraventricular tachycardia. *J Pediatr.* 2017;181:177-182.e2. doi:10.1016/j.jpeds.2016.10.051

McBride ME, Marino BS, Webster G, et al. Amiodarone versus lidocaine for pediatric cardiac arrest due to ventricular arrhythmias. *Pediatr Crit Care Med.* 2017;18(2):183-189. doi:10.1097/pcc.0000000000001026

Saul JP, Scott WA, Brown S, et al. Intravenous amiodarone for incessant tachyarrhythmias in children. *Circulation.* 2005;112(22):3470-3477. doi:10.1161/circulationaha.105.534149

Tijssen JA, Prince DK, Morrison LJ, et al. Time on the scene and interventions are associated with improved survival in pediatric out-of-hospital cardiac arrest. *Resuscitation.* 2015;94:1-7. doi:10.1016/j.resuscitation.2015.06.012

Topjian AA, Raymond TT, Atkins D, et al. Part 4: pediatric basic and advanced life support; 2020 American Heart Association Guidelines for Cardiopulmonary Resuscitation and Emergency Cardiovascular Care. *Circulation.* 2020;142(16 Suppl 2):S469–S523. https://cpr.heart.org/en/resuscitation-science/cpr-and-ecc-guidelines/pediatric-basic-and-advanced-life-support

Vega RM, Kaur H, Edemekong PF. Cardiopulmonary arrest in children. PubMed. Updated October 9, 2021. Accessed June 23, 2020. https://www.ncbi.nlm.nih.gov/books/NBK436018/

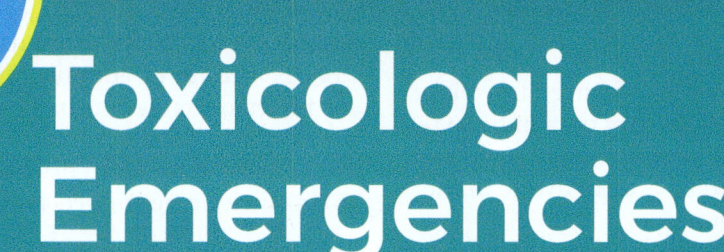

# CHAPTER 7

# Toxicologic Emergencies

## LESSON OBJECTIVES

- Review the different routes of toxic exposure and the age groups at risk for exposure.
- Differentiate between intentional and unintentional exposure.
- Discuss management of pediatric patients of toxic exposure using the Pediatric Assessment Triangle (PAT) and XABCDE.
- Identify common signs and symptoms associated with toxic exposure along with their treatment.
- Understand when and how to notify poison control.

## Introduction

In 2018, over 44% of calls to U.S. poison control centers involved children younger than 6 years. In that same year, approximately 6% of calls were for children ages 6 to 12 years. This means that over half of calls to poison control centers involve children 12 years and younger. The vast majority (85%) of these cases were observed at home without the need to contact emergency medical services (EMS) or go to the hospital.

Toxic exposures can be divided into intentional and unintentional categories. Intentional toxic exposures include suicide attempts and recreational ingestion. Intentional exposure is defined by the patient's intent to take the substance to lead to a desired result—whether that be intoxication, enhanced performance, or some other effect. This is in contrast to a toddler who ingests a laundry detergent pod, for example. Even though the toddler intended to ingest the substance, they were not doing so with an intended outcome—in this case the exposure would be classified as unintentional. It is typically teens and adults who have intentional exposure. Although teens account for less than 10% of exposures, they have significantly higher mortality.

Unintentional exposure involves ingestion or exposure to a substance without intended effect. As mentioned earlier, although some infants and toddlers will purposefully ingest a substance, they rarely have an intent in mind, and therefore the vast majority of infant and toddler toxic exposure is classified as accidental.

Carbon monoxide poisoning, insecticide exposure, and a toddler ingesting a household cleaning product or medication are all examples of unintentional exposure. In the United States, 76.7% of all exposures are classified as unintentional, with nearly 100% of exposures in children younger than 6 years classified as unintentional.

## Routes of Exposure

There are four primary routes of exposure, as follows:

- Ingestion
- Inhalation
- Absorption
- Injection

### Ingestion

Ingestion accounts for 83.5% of toxic exposures in the United States. This route involves taking the substance into the oropharynx and swallowing it. The degree of systemic distribution after ingestion varies based on the substance. Some substances will have rapid upper gastrointestinal (GI) absorption, whereas others will have limited absorption until they hit the small intestine. As such, the onset of symptoms can vary widely with ingestion—from seconds to hours or days after ingestion.

## Inhalation

Inhalation involves the toxic substance traveling through the air and into the respiratory tract of the patient. This can be a life-threatening issue for both the patient and first responders if they are not aware of the environmental hazard on arrival.

Toxic gases are divided into three categories, shown in **Table 7-1**.

## Absorption

Many substances can be absorbed through the skin and subsequently be distributed to tissues within the body. Organophosphate fertilizers are an example of an absorbed poison. The common scenario is a farmer who has been fertilizing a field without proper chemical protective clothing or a child who has walked barefoot in a recently fertilized area. Insecticides can also be absorbed.

## Injection

Injection of a substance directly into the circulatory system is a common route for both legal and illicit substances. Many of the drugs used in EMS involve injection as a route of administration. The onset of action for injected toxins is usually very rapid. There may be a noticeable local site reaction or "track marks" that are present in frequent drug users. Commonly injected toxins include heroin, cocaine, and anabolic steroids.

# Assessment of Toxic Exposures

A detailed history is one of your most valuable tools when assessing pediatric patients who may have ingested a toxic substance. Because most pediatric toxic exposures are unintentional, the patient may not be able to tell you what they ingested. Interviewing the parents for what types of substances are present will provide valuable information (**Figure 7-1**). Once a substance is identified or suspected, use the mnemonic TART to help remind you what questions should be asked and what information is critical to gather.

| Table 7-1 Toxic Gas Classification | |
|---|---|
| Simple asphyxiants | Displace oxygen and result in less oxygen available for inhalation |
| | Examples include nitrogen, methane, and carbon dioxide |
| Chemical asphyxiants | Impede oxygen transport to the cells and tissues of the body |
| | Examples include carbon monoxide and cyanide |
| Irritants/corrosives | Cause direct damage to the lung tissues, resulting in decreased ability for oxygen to cross the alveolar capillaries into the bloodstream |
| | Examples include chlorine and phosgene gases |

© Jones & Bartlett Learning.

**TART**

T—Toxin

A—Amount

R—Route

T—Time

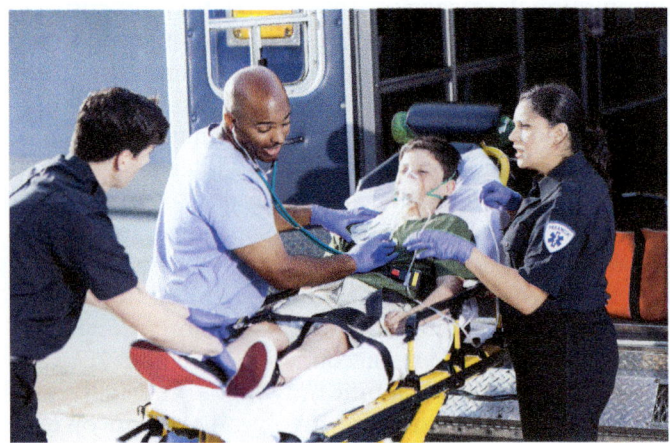

**Figure 7-1** A patient interview may provide valuable information about what was ingested.

© kali9/E+/Getty Images.

**T** stands for toxin. Attempt to get the name of the toxin. Taking a photo of the label to show emergency department staff may be safer and more effective than transporting the container itself. Also, identify the type of substance. Was it a pill, liquid, capsule, patch, or some other formulation? This can help determine how rapidly a substance might be absorbed.

**A** stands for amount. The amount can be represented in multiple ways. In the case of a liquid, try to determine the amount ingested in milliliters or ounces. Terms such as "half a bottle" are meaningless without context. The concentration of the liquid is important to note when dealing with medicines. Try to identify how many milligrams of a substance are contained in each milliliter of liquid. In the case of pills, it is important to identify both the suspected number of pills, and the strength of each pill. Sertraline, for example, comes in 25-, 50-, and 100-mg pills. Simply stating that the patient took 10 pills is less helpful than stating that the patient ingested ten 50-mg pills.

**R** stands for route. The route of exposure is important as it helps identify how rapidly a substance may be absorbed, along with what effects might be present. Inhaled chlorine gas will have different effects than ingested chlorine bleach solution. The route of exposure also helps determine what mechanism of detoxification or what type of antidote may be necessary to reverse the harmful effects of the substance.

**T** stands for time. Timing of the first exposure and the length of exposure for certain substances helps determine what treatments are necessary and effective. For example, carbon monoxide can be treated with hyperbaric therapy; however, this method is most effective when provided within a specific time frame from the initial exposure.

# Common Substances

In children younger than 6 years, the most common toxic exposure is cosmetics or personal care products. Examples include mouthwash, shampoo or conditioner, baby oil, soaps, and nail polish. Cleaning substances are the next most common source of toxic exposure. Combined, cosmetics and personal care products along with cleaning substances account for nearly 25% of all chemicals to which children younger than 6 years are exposed (**Table 7-2**). Although analgesics (pain medications) are third on the list of common exposures, they are the substances that lead to the greatest number of fatal incidents of toxic exposure (followed by fumes/gases/vapors; **Table 7-3**).

Prehospital practitioners should be aware of "one pill can kill" substances. These are substances for which even small exposures, one pill or only a few milliliters,

**Table 7-2** Most Common Causes of Toxic Exposures in Children Younger Than 6 Years

| Substance | Percentage |
|---|---|
| Cosmetics and Personal Care Products | 12.1% |
| Cleaning Substances | 10.7% |
| Analgesics | 9.0% |
| Foreign Bodies | 6.9% |
| Topical Preparations | 4.7% |
| Antihistamines | 4.6% |
| Vitamins | 4.3% |
| Dietary Supplements/Herbals | 4.1% |
| Pesticides | 3.6% |
| Gastrointestinal Preparations | 2.6% |

© Jones & Bartlett Learning.

**Table 7-3** Most Common Causes of Poisoning Deaths in Children Younger Than 6 Years

| Substance | Percentage |
|---|---|
| Analgesics | 20.5% |
| Fumes/Gases/Vapors | 16.7% |
| Unknown Drugs | 8.0% |
| Antihistamines | 6.4% |
| Cardiovascular Drugs | 5.7% |
| Batteries | 4.9% |
| Cleaning Substances | 3.4% |
| Stimulants/Street Drugs | 3.4% |
| Alcohols | 2.7% |
| Antidepressants | 2.7% |

© Jones & Bartlett Learning.

can cause fatal effects. The list of substances that can cause lethal consequences is long; however, the mnemonic ABC GET MOM, shown in **Table 7-4**, can aid prehospital practitioners in recalling some of the most common examples.

**Table 7-4** Exceptionally Dangerous Toxic Exposures

| | |
|---|---|
| **A** | Antimalarial medications such as quinine, chloroquine, and hydroxychloroquine can have fatal effects in small amounts if ingested by children. Many of these substances have QT prolonging properties and can lead to fatal arrhythmias. |
| **B** | Beta blockers are some of the most prescribed blood pressure medications in the United States and are present in many households. These medications can cause severe bradycardia, hypotension, and life-threatening hypoglycemia in children. |
| **C** | Clonidine and calcium channel blockers |
| **G** | Glyburide or other sulfonylureas used to treat diabetic patients |
| **E** | Ethylene glycol (antifreeze) |
| **T** | Tricyclic antidepressants (TCAs) |
| **M** | Methanol (nail polish remover) |
| **O** | Opioids (hydromorphone or other narcotic pain medications) |
| **M** | Methyl salicylates (oil of wintergreen) |

© Jones & Bartlett Learning.

# Button Battery Ingestion

The incidence of button battery ingestion is on the rise. The number of toys and devices that use these as a source of power has been steadily increasing in the past two decades. Young children tend to put anything and everything in their mouth, and button batteries represent a significant hazard if ingested. Children younger than 6 years account for the majority of button battery ingestions. Adverse outcomes are more common in children younger than 4 years. This is likely because these children are less able to adequately describe their symptoms and may not understand how to tell caregivers that they ingested a battery when asked.

Serious injury can occur in as little as 2 hours after the ingestion of a button battery. Localized tissue destruction to the mucosal lining of the GI tract, vocal cord destruction, and acute hemorrhage are all possible.

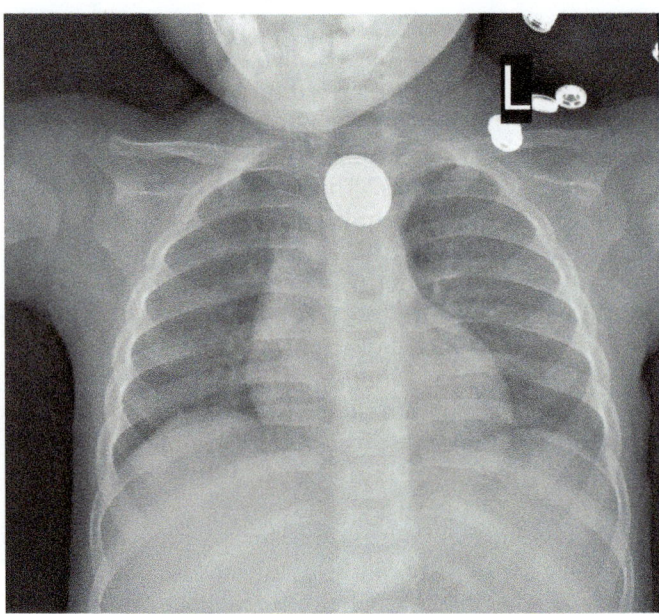

**Figure 7-2** This image shows a button battery lodged in the esophagus of a young child. Note the faint line near the outer edge. This characteristic differentiates a button battery from other circular metal objects such as coins.

Case courtesy of Dr Yair Glick, Radiopaedia.org, rID: 52187.

Heavy metals can also be absorbed into the bloodstream and deposited in tissues as the button battery transits the GI tract. These metals can lead to neurologic dysfunction and may remain in the tissues for decades.

The most dangerous area for a button battery to lodge is the esophagus, where it will cause local tissue destruction that can potentially compromise the airway (**Figure 7-2**). All children who ingest or are suspected of ingesting a button battery must be evaluated in the emergency department where x-rays can be obtained to determine the battery's location.

If the button battery passes into the stomach, the passage is usually uneventful, but the patient should be observed in the hospital to ensure that the object does in fact pass. Serial x-rays may be necessary to track the progress of the battery. Although most children who ingest a button battery have an uneventful course, 10% may have severe consequences, typically isolated to the GI tract.

# Illicit Substance Abuse

Adolescents are the most common pediatric users of illicit substances (**Figure 7-3**). They tend to gravitate toward inexpensive and easily accessible substances. Alcohol is at the top of this list. More than 1 in 4 children between ages 12 and 17 years admits to the use of alcohol at some point. Marijuana is also a commonly abused illicit substance. The frequency of marijuana use is increasing as many states across the country have legalized

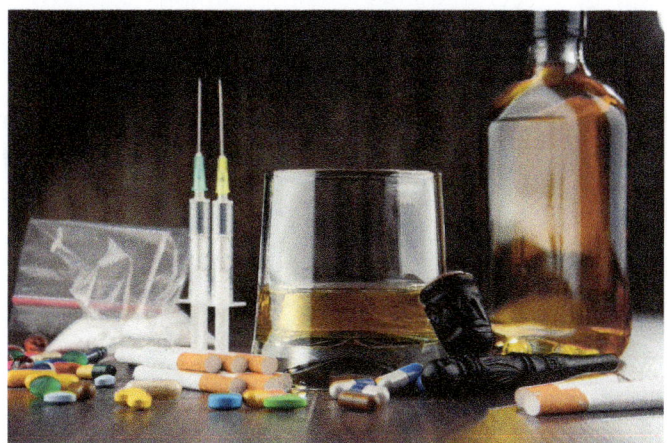

**Figure 7-3** Adolescents may consume or use alcohol, cigarettes, or other illicit substances.
© monticello/Shutterstock.

| Table 7-5 Hazardous Material Identification Methods | |
| --- | --- |
| **Formal** | **Informal** |
| Placards or identification signage | Odors <br> ■ Rotten eggs (hydrogen sulfide) <br> ■ Almonds (cyanide) <br> ■ Garlic (arsenic, organophosphates) |
| Bills of lading | Visual inspection |
| Identification codes or numbers | Carrying method (barrels vs. boxes, etc.) |
| Chemical detection and testing equipment | |

© Jones & Bartlett Learning.

adult consumption. The growth of vaping and electronic cigarette devices is also leading to increased marijuana usage, because these devices can be easily hidden and clues such as clothing smelling of smoke are absent.

Inhalants are also a commonly abused substance among teens and can be household items such as spray paints, permanent markers, glues, and correction fluid. Hallucinogens such as kratom and synthetic stimulants found in bath salts are also popular targets for abuse. These substances are easily accessible and, in many cases, legal for adults to use, meaning that they are commonly found in the home.

When approaching the patient who may have overdosed, it is important to use caution. These situations can often involve safety risks for prehospital practitioners, such as unintentional exposure to unknown chemicals and belligerent patients or bystanders.

It is important to know the organizations within your jurisdiction that can help individuals who suffer from addiction. EMS can be an important player in redirecting adolescents with addiction toward the resources they need to break the cycle of drug abuse.

# Scene Safety

Safety is always the primary concern when responding to any call. Calls involving potential toxin exposure, overdose, or hazardous materials present a unique set of safety considerations. The call may come in as a behavioral emergency, because the patient may be under the influence of toxins that alter their behavior and judgment. Violence is possible, as patients who have been exposed to toxins may be unpredictable. When addressing patients with a behavioral emergency, toxin exposure should be on the differential diagnosis, although you must always first rule out a medical cause for altered mental status.

Any patient who has attempted suicide, no matter how mild or severe the case, should be evaluated in the emergency department. Practitioners should attempt to collect evidence of toxin exposure, including any bottles, bags, or containers. Plants that are the suspected exposure medium should be transported if it can be done so safely. In cases where it is unsafe to transport some of the evidence you see, photographs may be helpful if departmental policy allows. Make sure to abide by Health Insurance Portability and Accountability Act (HIPAA) privacy standards any time photographs or items contain confidential patient information.

When dealing with a hazardous material (HazMat) scene, identifying the agent is important to determine scene safety and management. Identification methods can be both formal and informal. See **Table 7-5** for further information about hazardous material identification methods.

HazMat scenes should be secured and EMS personnel should wait from a safe distance. Know what resources you can mobilize, such as a HazMat team, to help respond to the incident. Attempt to identify the number of patients and have EMS resources ready for when the scene is made safe or when the patients have been decontaminated and transported to the triage area. Use a loudspeaker or shout to tell victims to remain where they are and not approach until they have been decontaminated. Make sure hospitals have advance notice of the HazMat incident in case any victims transport themselves. This way hospitals can take measures to make sure they do not become a secondary HazMat incident.

## Poison Control

There are 55 regional poison control centers in the United States. These centers provide professional help and resources both to the public and to healthcare professionals who may be treating patients (**Figure 7-4**). The call takers are often nurses or other healthcare professionals with access to medical toxicology physicians and resources. They provide expert advice and treatment recommendations over the phone. They will open a file for the encounter and provide follow-up advice as the case progresses.

You do not need to know the exact substance when contacting poison control. In many cases the medical toxicologist can provide advice based on the toxidrome (set of symptoms and presentation) alone, although knowing the substance is incredibly helpful.

Pharmacists may also be present in poison control centers and can help with guiding treatment for specific medication overdoses and adverse reactions.

The universal number for poison control in most U.S. jurisdictions is 1-800-222-1222.

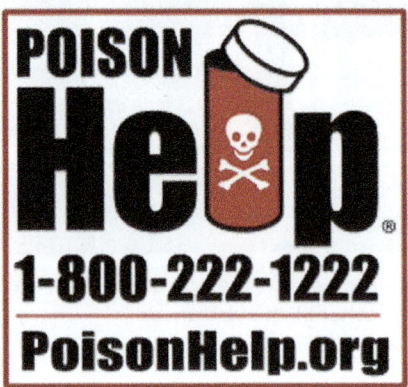

**Figure 7-4** In the United States, the American Association of Poison Control Centers has a 24-hour hotline.

## CASE STUDY

### Case 1

#### Dispatch

You and your partner are dispatched to the local middle school for a 13-year-old male who has developed a sudden onset altered level of consciousness (LOC), dizziness, headache, palpitation, and chest tightness. It is a mild spring afternoon. The weather is clear and the outside temperature is 78°F (25.5°C).

#### Case Questions

- What are your initial concerns?
  - The initial concerns for this patient include altered LOC with palpitations and chest tightness. The dizziness and headache are also concerning. Altered LOC is always concerning in any patient. It can indicate inadequate oxygenation to the brain or potential intoxication from any number of substances.
- Based on the dispatch information, what are the possible differential diagnoses for this patient?

- Based on the dispatch information, the differential diagnosis for this patient includes:
  - Seizure
  - Cerebrovascular accident (CVA)
  - Hypoglycemia
  - Trauma
  - Infection
  - Ingestion
  - Hazardous materials exposure

Make sure to assess the scene carefully for any clues such as drug paraphernalia, prescription medications, or signs that there may have been an exposure to a toxic substance. Be aware that some schools have dangerous chemicals in their science labs that can produce noxious gases when combined.

#### Initial Observations

When you arrive on the scene, you are flagged down by the principal who escorts you to the nurse's office

The patient answers when you call his name and is somewhat coherent. He appears sleepy and will occasionally laugh at nothing in particular. The principal states that the child's teacher called for assistance when the patient was not acting right in class. She indicated that he was in "lala land."

## Case Questions

- Based on your initial impression, is this patient "Quick" or "Not Quick"?

  - Altered level of consciousness is always a medical emergency, although based on the PAT, this patient is not "Quick." There are many potential medical and behavioral causes for what is happening to this patient. You have time to ask questions to determine which are highest on your differential.

- Have you identified any possible red flags?

  - Red flags include altered LOC and pale skin. This patient requires additional work-up by a physician in a hospital. This includes laboratory screening, possible imaging, and other diagnostic tests.

## Primary Survey

The primary survey for this patient reveals the following:

  **X**—No bleeding found

  **A**—Open, patent, and clear

  **B**—Respirations equal and nonlabored

  **C**—Pulses are strong and regular. The capillary refill time is brisk. The skin is warm, pale, and dry.

  **D**—The patient is sleepy but easily arousable. Glasgow Coma Scale (GCS) is 15 (E4, V5, M6).

  **E**—Ate lunch approximately 45 minutes prior to going to class

## Case Questions

- Based on the findings noted in the primary survey, what would your initial interventions and treatment include?

  - The patient is overall stable currently. Treatment should be focused on maintaining an open and patent airway and ensuring that he does not develop any respiratory or circulatory compromise. This involves careful assessment and reassessment.

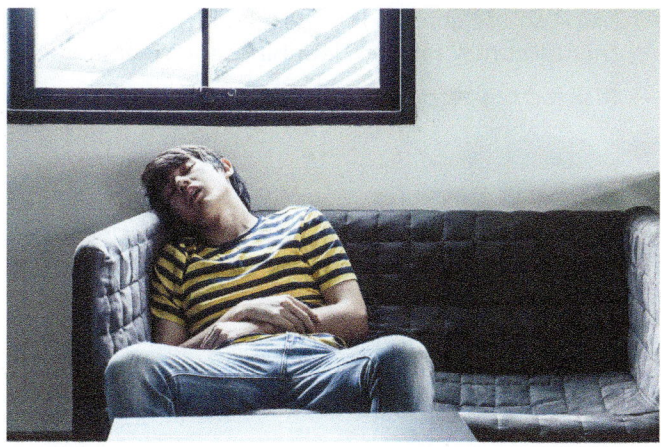

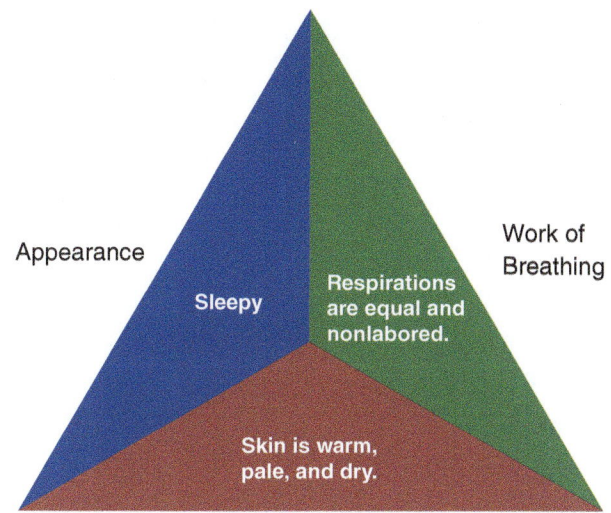

Appearance

Work of Breathing

Sleepy

Respirations are equal and nonlabored.

Skin is warm, pale, and dry.

Circulation to Skin

**Figure 7-5** A 13-year-old male with altered level of consciousness.

A. © Momentum Fotograh/Shutterstock; B. Used with permission of the American Academy of Pediatrics, Pediatric Education for Prehospital Professionals, © American Academy of Pediatrics, 2000.

where the student is located. She informs you that the parents have been called.

- Pediatric Assessment Triangle (**Figure 7-5**)

  - Appearance

    - Sleepy, but arousable

  - Work of breathing

    - **F**laring not present

    - **R**etractions not present

    - **A**udible airway sounds not present

    - **P**ositioning not present

  - Circulation

    - Skin warm, pale, and dry

## Detailed Assessment

### History Taking

As your partner attaches the monitor, you begin to take a detailed history.

**OPQRST:**

- **O**nset: Sudden
- **P**rovocation/palliation: None
- **Q**uality: None
- **R**adiation: None
- **S**everity: 0/10
- **T**iming: 15 minutes

**SAMPLER:**

- **S**igns/symptoms: Altered mental status, dizziness, headache, palpitations, and a feeling of chest tightness
- **A**llergies: No known allergies to medications, foods, or the environment
- **M**edications: None
- **P**ast medical history: None
- **L**ast oral intake: Ate lunch with friends approximately 45 minutes ago. He states that one of his friends gave him a brownie that his sister made.
- **E**vents leading up to the emergency: After lunch he went to class and had a sudden onset of palpitations, chest tightness, headache, altered mental status, random laughing, and sleepiness.
- **R**isk factors: None

### Vital Signs

As you were discussing the history, the patient was attached to the monitor and the following vital signs were obtained (**Figure 7-6**):

**Heart rate:**

- 70 beats/min
- This is within normal range.

**SpO₂:**

- 99% on room air (RA)

**ETCO₂:**

- 40 mm Hg

**Respiratory rate:**

- 18 breaths/min

**Blood pressure:**

- 116/68 mm Hg

**Temperature:**

- 98.2°F (36.8°C)

**Blood glucose:**

- 94 mg/dL

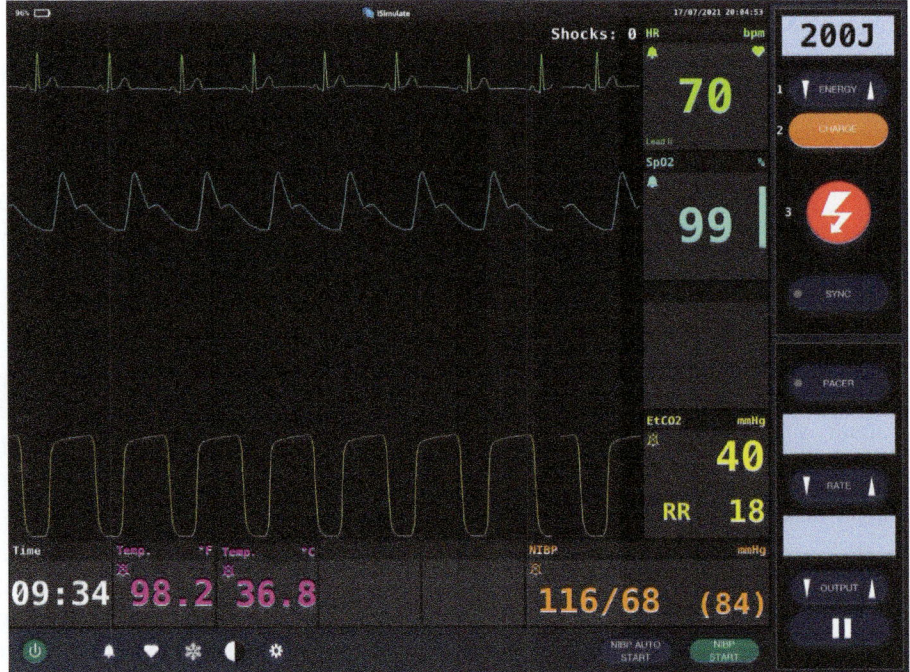

**Figure 7-6** The monitor shows reassuring vital signs for this patient.

Courtesy of iSimulate.

This patient has very stable vital signs, which is reassuring when there is an altered level of consciousness.

> If chest pain is present, it is reasonable to obtain a 12-lead electrocardiogram and possibly cardiac markers to assess myocardial ischemia or infarction.

This is a 13-year-old male with no past medical history presenting with acute-onset altered level of consciousness, palpitation, headache, and chest tightness in proximity to eating lunch where he was provided a homemade brownie from a friend. His vital signs are reassuring and do not support infectious etiology or hypoglycemia. He is currently stable but at risk for decompensation given his altered level of consciousness.

## Detailed Exam

**HEENT (Figure 7-7):**

- **H**ead: Unremarkable
- **E**yes: PERRL, unremarkable
- **E**ars: Unremarkable
- **N**ose: Unremarkable
- **T**hroat: Unremarkable

**Chest, heart, and lungs:**

- Pulses: Palpable in all extremities
- Cardiac auscultation: Regular rate and rhythm with no rubs, gallops, or murmurs auscultated
- Lung auscultation: Clear bilaterally with good aeration
- Chest exam: Symmetric chest rise

**Neurologic:**

- Neurovascular status intact. Sleepy but easily arousable. Alert and oriented to person, place, time, and event.

**Abdomen and pelvis:**

- Soft and nontender. Bowel sounds are normal.

**Extremities:**

- Upper and lower extremities: Unremarkable

**Back:**

- Unremarkable

## Treatment

The primary treatment for this patient will be supportive care and data gathering to find out what he may have ingested. Practitioners should be prepared for rapid deterioration and possible respiratory or circulatory compromise.

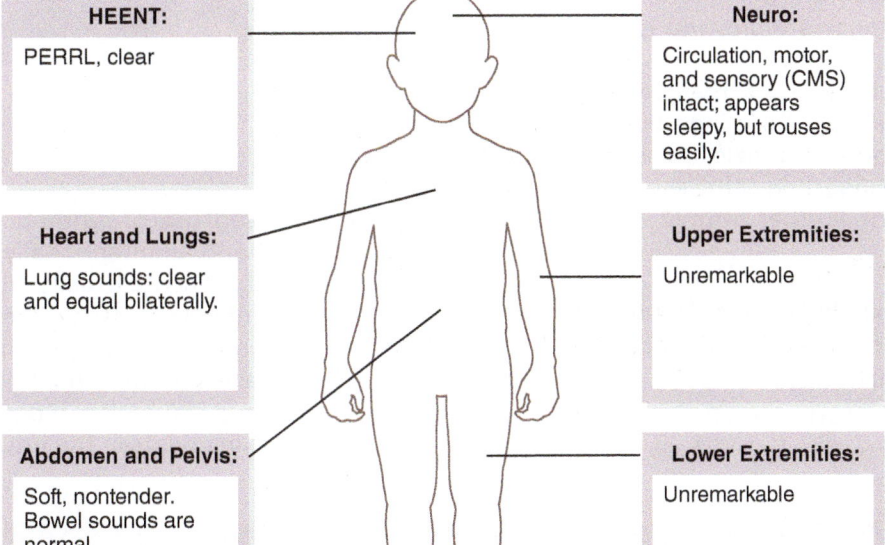

**Detailed Physical Exam**

**HEENT:**
PERRL, clear

**Heart and Lungs:**
Lung sounds: clear and equal bilaterally.

**Abdomen and Pelvis:**
Soft, nontender. Bowel sounds are normal.

**Neuro:**
Circulation, motor, and sensory (CMS) intact; appears sleepy, but rouses easily.

**Upper Extremities:**
Unremarkable

**Lower Extremities:**
Unremarkable

**Figure 7-7** The patient's detailed exam is reassuring.
© Jones & Bartlett Learning.

The differential for this patient is narrowed by the fact that the onset was acute and there are no signs of infection. His blood glucose level is normal and there was no witnessed seizure activity. His behavior is not consistent with classic postictal state. There is no evidence of trauma and his neurologic exam is nonfocal, which speaks against CVA. Ingestion rises to the top of the differential list for this patient.

## Ongoing Management

The patient is loaded into the ambulance and remains stable during transport. You ask the principal to ask the students the patient ate lunch with if there is a possibility that he ingested any drugs or other substances.

### Case Questions

- What is the most appropriate treatment destination?
  - You decide to transport the patient to the local pediatric hospital for additional work-up.
- Can you safely transport this child in your ambulance?
  - You contact his mother by cell phone, and she provides verbal consent to treat him. She says she will meet him there in approximately 1 hour.

## CASE WRAP-UP

Diagnosis: Ingestion of a brownie that had marijuana in it (edible)

Shortly after you drop the patient off, dispatch tells you that the principal has called. You call her back and she informs you that the patient's friends admitted to providing him a brownie laced with marijuana (**Figure 7-8**). You go back into the emergency department to inform the physician of this information. As you do so, the nurse approaches and informs you that the patient's urine toxicology screen is positive for marijuana, confirming the diagnosis.

Marijuana ingestion and intoxication, both intentional and unintentional, are growing issues as more states legalize the substance. Children may present with atypical symptoms after marijuana ingestion, making diagnosis difficult. Toxic ingestion is largely a diagnosis of exclusion in the field unless the patient openly admits to the ingestion or the evidence of ingestion is readily present. Further complicating the issue

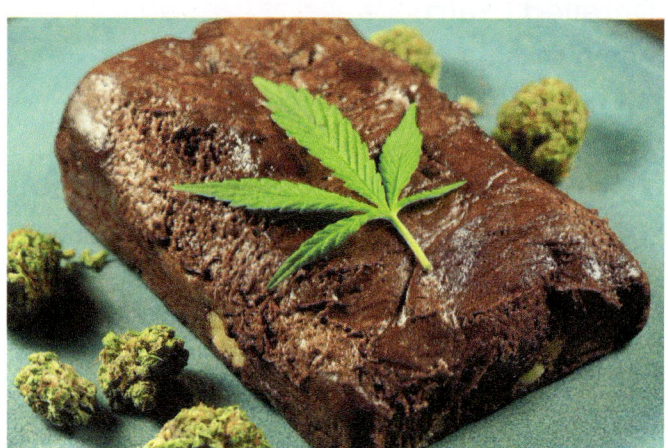

**Figure 7-8** Marijuana ingestion can be intentional or unintentional.
© Atomazul/Shutterstock.

is the increased use of synthetic cannabinoids, both intentionally and unintentionally, and the increased adverse effects of acute toxicity and withdrawal.

The patient in this case was monitored for approximately 12 hours and discharged once he was back at his neurologic baseline. The school now has a more comprehensive drug education program in place to help prevent these incidents in the future.

> **Patients with toxic ingestion should also be screened for coingestion, especially if electrolyte abnormalities or QTc or QRS prolongation is noted on ECG.**

## CASE TAKEAWAY POINTS

The etiology of altered mental status in children is one of the most difficult diagnoses to arrive at. In most cases definitive diagnosis will not be made in the field; however, the clues obtained by first responders can aid personnel at the hospital in clinching the diagnosis.

The treatment for marijuana intoxication is symptomatic management. The extent of management has numerous factors, including the age of the individual and the amount of cannabis ingested.

Ingestion is a diagnosis of exclusion however, and all possible medical causes should be addressed and explored before simply stating that the patient has ingested a toxic substance. The clinical evidence should support that ingestion is the most likely cause.

## CASE STUDY

## Case 2

### Dispatch

You and your partner respond to a single-family residence for a 3-year-old male for possible toxic ingestion (**Figure 7-9**). Dispatch reports that the caller stated the patient is lethargic. It is a warm summer afternoon. The air temperature is 82°F (27.8°C).

### Case Questions

- What are your initial concerns?
  - As discussed previously, any patient with altered level of consciousness is a significant concern.
- Based on the dispatch information, what is the possible differential diagnosis for this patient?
  - For the 3-year-old in this case, the differential diagnosis includes ingestion, glucose abnormalities, environmental emergencies, and nonaccidental trauma, to name a few. A careful assessment of the scene and a thorough history will be necessary to diagnose and treat this patient.

### Initial Observations

As you arrive on scene, the mother frantically approaches the ambulance. She informs you that her son was playing in his grandmother's room this afternoon and she found him holding an open bottle of "heart pills."

- Pediatric Assessment Triangle
  - Appearance
    - Fatigued and lethargic
  - Work of breathing
    - **F**laring not present
    - **R**etractions not present
    - **A**udible airway sounds not present
    - **P**ositioning not present
  - Circulation
    - Skin warm and dry

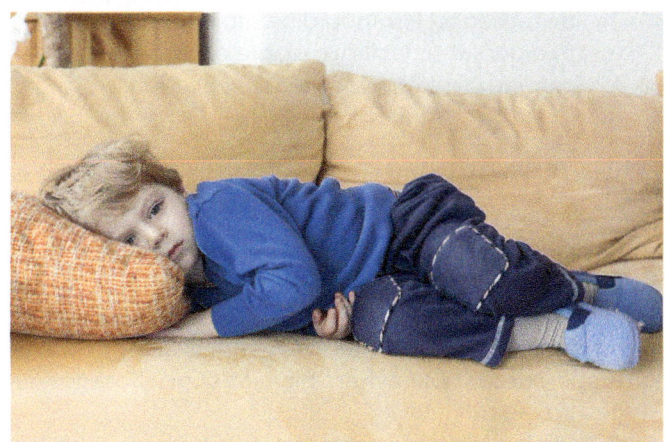

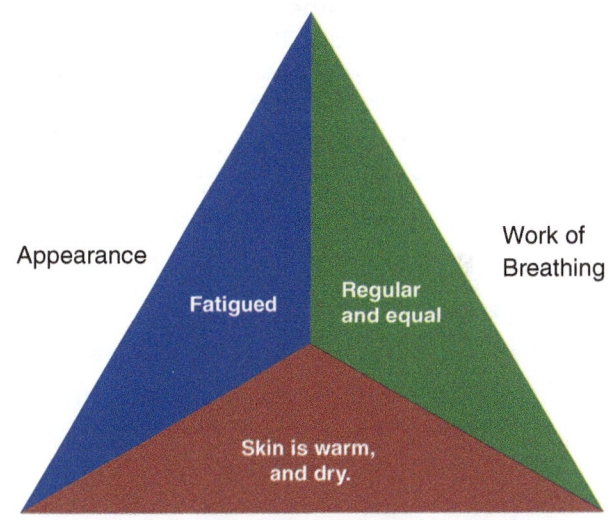

Appearance — Fatigued

Work of Breathing — Regular and equal

Circulation to Skin — Skin is warm, and dry.

**Figure 7-9** A lethargic 3-year-old with possible toxic ingestion.

The mother hands you a pill bottle with the following label: "Digoxin 0.25 mg tablets. Quantity 60." You count 10 pills left in the bottle. The grandmother says she refilled the prescription 10 days ago and thinks there were approximately 40 left after she took her morning dose. The child was unattended for a considerable amount of time before being discovered, and the mother estimates it could have been up to 90 minutes ago when he ingested the medication.

## Case Questions

- Based on your initial impression, is this patient "Quick" or "Not Quick"?

  - This patient is "Quick." The altered level of consciousness and large volume of digoxin ingested make him particularly susceptible to rapid decompensation due to cardiac rhythm disturbance. He should be rapidly transported to a pediatric facility capable of advanced cardiac life support and detoxification.

## Digoxin Toxicity

Digoxin is a cardiac glycoside commonly used in the treatment of cardiac dysrhythmias. The typical signs of toxicity include cardiac rhythm disturbance, neurologic impairment, and GI upset. Although children are more resistant to the cardiotoxic effects of digoxin, they are still susceptible when high enough dosages are ingested.

Pediatric patients present predominantly with bradycardia or heart block rather than ventricular dysrhythmias that are seen in adults. The treatment is largely the same as it is in adults, with dosages adjusted for weight.

Digoxin is in the category of "one pill can kill" drugs.

## Primary Survey

The primary survey for this patient reveals the following:

**X**—No bleeding found

**A**—Open and patent

**B**—Rapid respirations, lungs clear bilaterally

**C**—Strong, slow radial pulses palpated, with extra beats present. Capillary refill time is brisk. Skin is warm and dry.

## Case Questions

- Based on the findings noted in the primary survey, what would your initial interventions and treatment include?

  - The initial treatment for this patient is to support airway, breathing, and circulation. A cardiac monitor should be applied and intravenous (IV) access obtained. Poison control should be contacted to provide additional guidance if time permits. Do not delay transport to discuss the case with poison control.

- Have you identified any red flags?

  - Bradycardia is a red flag in this case.

**D**—GCS is 15 (E4, V5, M6). The patient is alert, fatigued, and irritable. He has had three episodes of nonbloody emesis.

**E**—Lying on the couch

## Detailed Assessment

### History Taking

As your partner applies the monitor and obtains IV access, you begin to take a detailed history.

**OPQRST**:

- **O**nset: Sudden
- **P**rovocation/palliation: None
- **Q**uality: None
- **R**adiation: None
- **S**everity: None
- **T**iming: Approximately 90 minutes ago

**SAMPLER**:

- **S**igns/symptoms: Lethargy, irritability, and bradycardia
- **A**llergies: No known allergies to medications, foods, or the environment
- **M**edications: None
- **P**ast medical history: None
- **L**ast oral intake: Ate breakfast approximately 3 hours ago, has vomited three times in the last 30 minutes
- **E**vents leading up to the emergency: Playing unsupervised in the grandmother's bedroom. Found with an open bottle of digoxin.
- **R**isk factors: Age and unsupervised play around medications that are not stored properly

### Vital Signs

As you were discussing the history, the patient was attached to the monitor and the following vital signs were obtained (**Figure 7-10**):

**Heart rate:**

- 40 beats/min
- This is bradycardic for this patient. Pediatric resuscitation guidelines generally recommend starting cardiopulmonary resuscitation (CPR) for a pulse less than 60 beats/min. In this case, the patient has signs of adequate perfusion and is maintaining well. If signs of poor perfusion

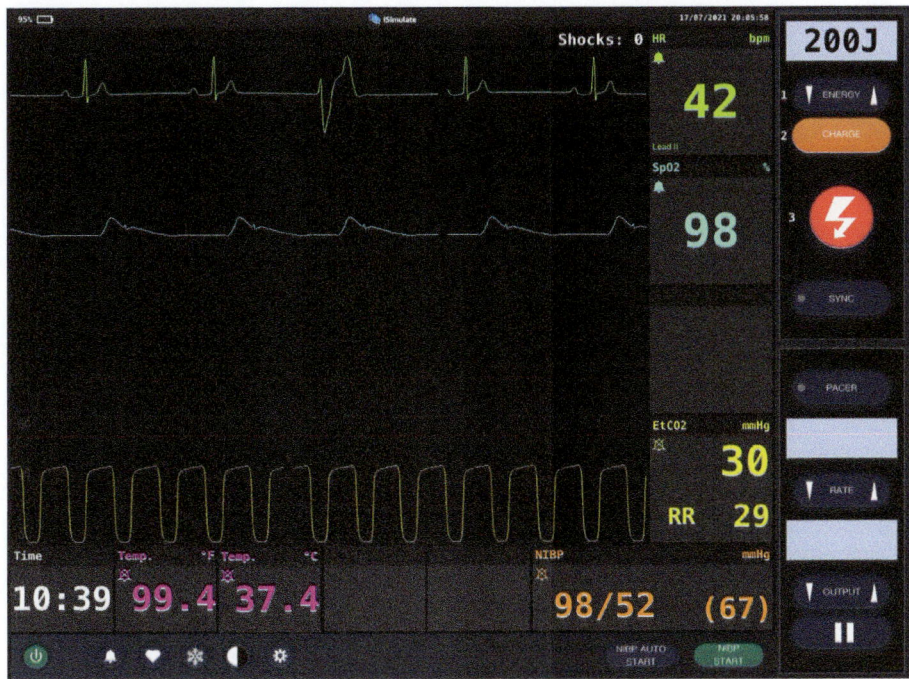

**Figure 7-10** This patient's vital signs are consistent with digitalis toxicity.
Courtesy of iSimulate.

or unconsciousness develop, resuscitation with compressions should commence.

- You note a first-degree AV block on the monitor.

**SpO₂:**

- 98% RA

**ETCO₂:**

- 30 mm Hg

**Respiratory rate:**

- 29 breaths/min

**Blood pressure:**

- 98/52 mm Hg

- This is adequate and indicates that compressions are not necessary for this patient.

**Temperature:**

- 99.4°F (37.4°C)

**Blood glucose:**

- 84 mg/dL

The vital signs here are consistent with digoxin toxicity. As mentioned earlier, pediatric patients are more susceptible to bradydysrhythmias and heart block than adults.

This is a 3-year-old male with no significant past medical history presenting with altered mental status, bradycardia, and first-degree heart block with adequate perfusion in the setting of ingesting approximately thirty 0.25-mg digitalis pills. He is currently hemodynamically stable but at risk for acute circulatory and respiratory decompensation as the result of his drug ingestion (**Figure 7-11**).

## Detailed Exam

**HEENT:**

- **H**ead: Unremarkable
- **E**yes: PERRL, unremarkable
- **E**ars: Unremarkable
- **N**ose: Unremarkable
- **T**hroat: Unremarkable

**Chest, heart, and lungs:**

- Pulses: Peripheral pulses palpable in all extremities
- Cardiac auscultation: Bradycardic rate, extra beats, no murmurs present
- Lung auscultation: Clear bilaterally with good aeration
- Chest exam: Symmetric rise

**Neurologic:**

- Neurovascular status intact, patient is lethargic and irritable but easy to arouse.

**Abdomen and pelvis:**

- Soft, nontender. Bowel sounds are normal.

**Detailed Physical Exam**

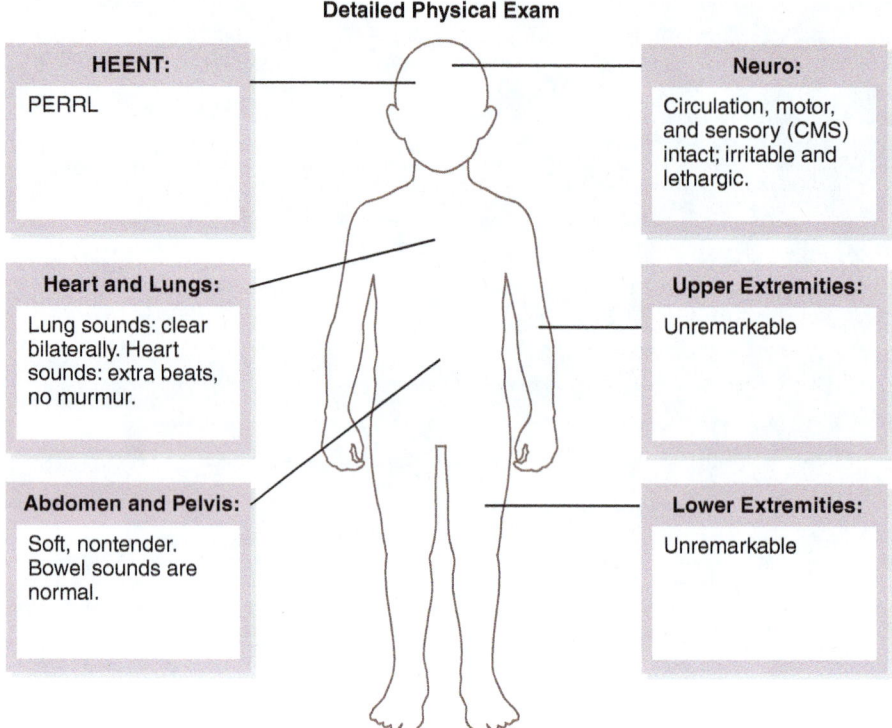

**HEENT:**

PERRL

**Neuro:**

Circulation, motor, and sensory (CMS) intact; irritable and lethargic.

**Heart and Lungs:**

Lung sounds: clear bilaterally. Heart sounds: extra beats, no murmur.

**Upper Extremities:**

Unremarkable

**Abdomen and Pelvis:**

Soft, nontender. Bowel sounds are normal.

**Lower Extremities:**

Unremarkable

**Figure 7-11** The secondary survey did not reveal anything of further concern for this patient.

© Jones & Bartlett Learning.

**Extremities:**

- Upper extremities: Unremarkable
- Lower extremities: Unremarkable

**Back:**

- Unremarkable

## Treatment

This patient should be emergently transported to the closest pediatric facility. Rapid deterioration is possible, so practitioners should reassess constantly and be prepared. Careful cardiac monitoring to detect any evolution of the first-degree AV block with bradycardia is also necessary.

Atropine for this patient would have minimal effect as the SA node is not fully associated with the ventricles due to evolving heart block. Transcutaneous pacing could potentially send the patient into a lethal dysrhythmia.

The definitive management for this patient involves administration of digoxin-specific antibodies that will scavenge digoxin form the bloodstream and neutralize it. These medications are not readily available for EMS or critical care transport; however, most major hospitals should have them on the formulary.

## Ongoing Management

The patient's mental status was reassessed and remained the same throughout transport. Likewise, there was no deterioration of the heart block or cardiac rhythm. IV therapy and fluid bolus were administered.

## Case Questions

- What is the most appropriate treatment destination and why?

  - You and your partner load the patient for rapid transport to the closest pediatric specialty facility. You call ahead to the receiving facility make sure they are aware the patient has digoxin toxicity so they can prepare to provide appropriate therapy.

- Can you safely transport this child in your ambulance?

  - The patient was safely restrained to a pediatric securing device on the stretcher. The mother was allowed to ride in the front seat.

## CASE WRAP-UP

Diagnosis: Digoxin toxicity

At the hospital, the patient remained lethargic and bradycardic. He was admitted to the cardiac intensive care unit and observed for further cardiac compromise while digoxin-binding antibody was administered, and serial digoxin levels were trended (**Figure 7-12**). He was discharged after 48 hours and instructed to follow up with his pediatrician and has now established with a pediatric cardiologist. Social services visited the patient's home and provided the mother with resources for safe medication storage to help prevent this from occurring in the future.

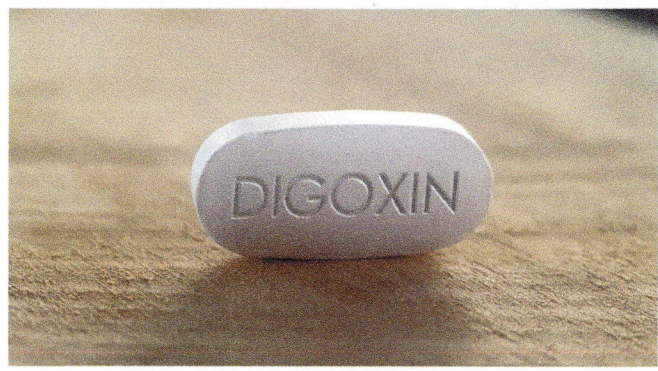

**Figure 7-12**  Digoxin is a commonly used cardiac glycoside medication.
© Sonis Photography/Shutterstock.

## CASE TAKEAWAY POINTS

Digoxin is derived from the foxglove plant. It was classically used for edema treatment and is one of the most commonly used cardiac glycoside medications. It is used as an inotrope for the improvement of systolic function in patients with congestive heart failure and as an atrioventricular (AV) nodal blocking agent in patients with atrial tachycardia dysrhythmias. Knowing how and why this drug might be used can help to determine if individuals in the home may be prescribed this medication and increase your index of suspicion that the pediatric patient may have ingested this substance.

## LESSON WRAP-UP

Careful history and thorough examination are necessary to aid in the diagnosis of pediatric ingestions. The TART acronym can help practitioners recall what questions are important when obtaining a history from a patient who has suffered an ingestion. The appropriate treatment for toxic exposures requires rapid recognition, and identification of the specific substance is very helpful in definitive care planning.

It is important to know what resources are available in your region to help with ingestion cases. Knowing which hospitals have toxicology capabilities and advanced therapy modes such as dialysis and extracorporeal membrane oxygenation (ECMO) can be lifesaving for patients who require these treatments while recovering from their ingestion.

## REFERENCES

Burns C, Burns R, Sanseau E, et al. Pediatric Emergency Medicine Simulation Curriculum: marijuana ingestion. *MedEdPORTAL*. 2018;14:10780. doi:10.15766/mep_2374-8265.10780

Cooper ZD. Adverse effects of synthetic cannabinoids: management of acute toxicity and withdrawal. *Curr Psychiatry Rep*. 2016;18(5):52. doi:10.1007/s11920-016-0694-1

Cummings ED, Swoboda HD. Digoxin toxicity. In: StatPearls [Internet]. Treasure Island, FL: StatPearls Publishing. Updated Oct 13, 2019. Accessed December 22, 2021. https://www.ncbi.nlm.nih.gov/books/NBK470568/

Dire D. Disk Battery Ingestion. Medscape. January 29, 2020. Accessed December 22, 2021. https://emedicine.medscape.com/article/774838-overview

Gummin DP, Mowry JB, Spyker DA, et al. 2018 Annual Report of the American Association of Poison Control Centers' National Poison Data System (NPDS): 36th annual report. *Clin Toxicol (Phila)*. 2019;57(12):1220-1413. doi:10.1080/15563650.2019.1677022

National Capital Poison Center. Poison statistics. Accessed December 22, 2021. https://www.poison.org/poison-statistics-national

National Model EMS Clinical Guidelines. National Model. January 2019. Accessed December 22, 2021. https://nasemso.org/wp-content/uploads/National-Model-EMS-Clinical-Guidelines-2017-PDF-Version-2.2.pdf

Wang GS, Hoyte C. Common substances of abuse. *Pediatr Rev*. 2018;39(8):403-418. doi:10.1542/pir.2017-0267

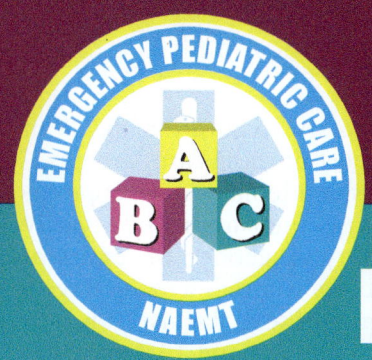

# CHAPTER 8

# Pediatric Maltreatment

## LESSON OBJECTIVES

- Discuss the epidemiology of pediatric maltreatment.
- Describe the different forms of maltreatment.
- Identify a possible victim of maltreatment.
- Gather an appropriate history.
- Provide an appropriate level of care.
- Interact professionally with caregivers.

## Introduction

Pediatric maltreatment is both a medical diagnosis and a crime. The legal definition of maltreatment may vary between jurisdictions; however, the medical diagnosis can be broadly defined as physical or emotional injury to a child as a direct result of actions taken by a parent or caregiver. Emergency medical services (EMS) professionals and emergency department staff are often the first medical practitioners to evaluate the victims of child abuse.

Multiple mechanisms of abuse fall under the broad term *pediatric maltreatment*. Some forms of abuse, such as physical injury, may be easier to recognize. Other forms, such as neglect or medical child abuse (e.g., Munchausen by proxy), may be more nuanced and difficult to identify. All medical practitioners who treat ill and injured children must maintain an index of suspicion for maltreatment as recognition is the first step to preventing further harm to the child.

## Types of Child Maltreatment

**Table 8-1** defines the major categories of maltreatment. The perpetrator of maltreatment is generally defined by statute as a parent, guardian, or caretaker.

| Table 8-1 Types of Pediatric Maltreatment | |
| --- | --- |
| Physical abuse | When a parent, guardian, or caretaker injures or allows the injury of a child younger than 18 years. |
| Emotional abuse | A consistent pattern of behavior interfering with the normal social and psychological development of a child. |
| Sexual abuse | Engagement in any sexual activities with a dependent, allowing others to engage in sexual activities with a dependent, or forcing a dependent to engage in sexual activities. |
| Child neglect | Failure to provide for the basic social, medical, or emotional welfare of a child that results in significant harm or imminent risk of harm to that child. |

© Jones & Bartlett Learning.

**Figure 8-1** breaks down the overall incidence of each form of maltreatment. Many children have more than one form of abuse inflicted upon them, which

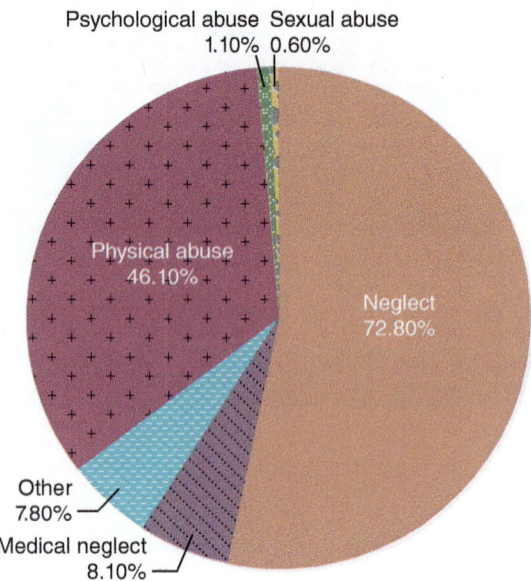

Psychological abuse 1.10%  Sexual abuse 0.60%

Physical abuse 46.10%

Neglect 72.80%

Other 7.80%

Medical neglect 8.10%

**Figure 8-1** There are different forms of maltreatment and some children experience more than one kind.

© Jones & Bartlett Learning.

is why the individual categories add up to more than 100%. It is also important to consider that the statistics only reflect the volume of reported and proven child abuse. It is suspected that a large amount of abuse goes unreported or unrecognized. When the abuse is ultimately discovered, it may have been occurring for a significant period of time.

The most common form of maltreatment is neglect, accounting for over half of child abuse cases. Recent data suggest that in fatal cases of child abuse, 72.8% of victims suffered from neglect and 46.1% suffered physical abuse, either exclusively or in combination with another type of maltreatment.

> **Although neglect is the most common form of maltreatment overall, victims often suffer from multiple forms of abuse.**

# Epidemiology, Demographics, and Risk Factors

The risk for child abuse decreases with age, although the manner of abuse changes as children get older. The risk for maltreatment is highest in children younger than 1 year (it is more than double the rate for any other age).

Children younger than 3 years account for 28.7% of child abuse victims, and most of these cases are physical abuse. Although males and females have approximately the same risk of abuse, the pattern and severity of abuse does appear to vary by gender. Males are at highest risk for physical abuse, whereas females have a significantly higher incidence of sexual abuse. It is estimated that overall, 25% of females and 10% of males have experienced some form of sexual abuse prior to 18 years of age. This information may be incomplete, however, as the actual rate of male sexual abuse may be higher due to nondisclosure. Males are at higher risk of severe physical abuse resulting in death. Regardless of the gender and age variation, it is clear that child maltreatment is a serious and widespread problem.

> **Children younger than 3 years are at the highest risk for child abuse and maltreatment.**

Child abuse is carried out by one or both biologic parents in 91.7% of cases. In 40% of cases the mother was the sole perpetrator of abuse, compared to 21.7% of cases in which the father was the sole perpetrator. Other perpetrators included the unmarried partner of the parent, relatives, siblings, clergy, school staff, and foster parents.

The factors that put children at risk for child abuse and maltreatment are complex. In most cases, no single factor is responsible for predisposing a child to risk of abuse; rather, it is a complex interplay between the environment, caregiver, and child that sets up a "perfect storm" leading to episodes of abuse. These factors have been categorized and listed in **Table 8-2**.

The factors in Table 8-2 are important to consider but should not be the sole basis for suspecting abuse or neglect in a child. Cases of abuse and neglect occur across all demographics; therefore, the index of suspicion should always be present regardless of the perception that a social situation does not fit within the stereotypical pattern expected in cases of abuse.

# Red Flags for Abuse

As mentioned previously, abuse and maltreatment should always be considered when there is no clear explanation for the child's illness or injury. Certain circumstances may be "red flags" for abuse. These circumstances can often be observed when sizing up the scene, interacting with caregivers, and when interviewing and interacting with the patient.

**Table 8-2** Risk Factors for Child Abuse and Maltreatment

| Child | Environment | Caregiver |
|---|---|---|
| ▪ Age younger than 3 years<br>▪ Developmental delays<br>▪ Intellectual disabilities<br>▪ Medical complexity<br>▪ Behavior disorders such as attention deficit/hyperactivity disorder<br>▪ Unplanned or unwanted pregnancy<br>▪ Stepchild | ▪ Unrelated male caregiver in the household<br>▪ Domestic or intimate partner violence<br>▪ Family stressors (financial, marital, illness, job instability)<br>▪ Poverty<br>▪ Isolation from social support systems (no extended family or friends in close proximity) | ▪ Young or single parents<br>▪ Lower education<br>▪ History of alcohol or substance abuse<br>▪ History of depression or other psychiatric illness<br>▪ Limited knowledge of child development (unrealistic expectations of the child)<br>▪ Negative perception of behaviors that are developmentally normal for children<br>▪ History of abuse or neglect directed toward the caregiver |

© Jones & Bartlett Learning.

# Scene Size-Up

Prior to meeting the patient or the caregiver, prehospital practitioners should pay close attention to the scene. Consider the following points when performing a scene size-up:

- Does the overall appearance of the home look like a safe environment for children?
  - If the environment does not look safe, factual and objective documentation of specific unsafe conditions is helpful.
  - Are there open medications or illicit substances present?
  - Are there legal drugs (such as edible forms of tetrahydrocannabinol [THC]) that may be appealing to young children in areas accessible to children?
- Is the environment clean?
  - Cleanliness is different than general untidiness. Homes with children are often messy, but not necessarily unclean. Excessive amounts of trash, human or animal excrement, insects or rodents, piles of dishes and food waste, or other unsanitary conditions are indications that neglect may be taking place.
- Does the child appear to be groomed and clean?
  - Children can easily get dirty while playing, however, this is different than a child who has clearly not been bathed in many days.

- Do the children have an odor that indicates they may have been in soiled diapers or clothing for prolonged periods of time?
- Are there rashes or skin breakdown present that indicate that proper hygiene is not being maintained between diaper changes?
- What are the sibling interactions within the home?
  - Do the siblings appear scared or reluctant to engage with caregivers?
  - Take care not to confuse age-appropriate apprehension of strangers with fear.
- Are there other members in the house who appear to be injured?
  - While it is not appropriate to examine individuals other than the patient, taking a moment to observe for any outward signs of injury on other individuals in the home is appropriate.
  - When other people in the same household have injuries suspicious for abuse, it should raise the prehospital practitioner's suspicion that the patient may also be a victim of abuse.

# Caregiver Behavior

The first interaction most prehospital practitioners will have with the caregiver is during the initial history. If the patient is too young to provide their history, it is important to carefully and accurately document the history given by the caregiver. One sign that abuse may be present is an evolving or changing story provided by the caregiver to explain the medical condition or injury that is present. Documenting that a caregiver's story changed or evolved during the course of treating the patient is appropriate as long as it is done in an objective manner using the caregiver's own words in direct quotes as much as possible. Documentation should not editorialize, judge, or try to explain why the story is changing, rather it should keep an accurate record of the story the caregivers provide. This story will likely be compared to the history they give in the emergency department, and potentially, the narrative provided to law enforcement.

> **An evolving story for a child's injury or medical condition is suspicious for abuse. When the reported facts change to form a more plausible explanation, it is important to include this in your documentation.**

Children who can speak often are able to provide at least some portion of their medical history. The amount and reliability of this history varies with age. It is important to address the child when appropriate and ask them what happened. When the caregiver appears uncomfortable with this, does not allow the child to speak, or frequently interrupts or corrects the child, they may be trying to "control the narrative" to reduce or eliminate the suspicion of abuse. This can also occur in cases where one parent is the abuser, and they will not allow the other parent or caregiver to provide any history.

Some specific caregiver behaviors that should raise suspicion for abuse or maltreatment can be found in **Table 8-3**.

## Confronting Caregivers

In general, confronting caregivers or disclosing to them that there are concerns for abuse is not necessary in the prehospital setting. This can put prehospital practitioners at risk and may further endanger the child. Additionally, if the suspected abuser is aware that there is a concern for abuse, they may elope, making it difficult for law enforcement to find and question them.

## Child Behavior

Bonding between the child and caregiver is protective against abuse and maltreatment. Bonded children

| **Table 8-3** Concerning or Suspicious Caregiver Behaviors |
|---|
| Apathy or lack of concern toward the child or situation |
| Overreaction to the child's behavior or misconduct |
| Changing or evolving story to explain the injury or condition |
| Providing explanation that is out of proportion with the observed injuries |
| Intoxication |
| Over- or underreaction to the child's injury or illness |
| Speaking over the child or not allowing the child to provide any history |
| "Correcting" aspects of the child's story that may be perceived as incriminating |

© Jones & Bartlett Learning.

will seek comfort and reassurance from caregivers and loved ones, because they trust that those individuals will protect them. A child's ability to control emotions and cope with stress is largely dependent on having the social and emotional support that comes with adequately bonded relationships. When a child is under duress, they will become dysregulated.

Signs that may be suspicious for maltreatment can be separated into two categories: behavioral and physical. **Table 8-4** lists red flag behaviors and physical signs. This list is not comprehensive.

# Bruising in Children

Bruising is a common finding when examining a child; however, there are specific circumstances under which bruising should raise suspicion for possible maltreatment. The first question to consider is whether the bruising is located in an area that is prone to injuries. For example, bruising on the anterior shins in young ambulatory children is not unexpected when seen in the right age range and the bruising is consistent with incidental contact with objects while walking or running. On the other hand, a child with multiple linear or patterned bruises along the anterior or posterior lower legs, especially when the child is not ambulatory, is highly suspicious for abuse.

**Table 8-4** Signs Concerning for Abuse in Children

| Physical | Behavioral |
|---|---|
| ▪ Human bite marks | ▪ Apprehension around adults (out of proportion for age and development) |
| ▪ Unexplained burns | ▪ Fear or anxiety when other children cry |
| ▪ Rope burns or ligature marks | ▪ Behavioral extremes |
| ▪ Injuries that do not correspond to age-appropriate developmental milestones; e.g., injuries from rolling off an elevated surface in a child younger than 3 months old or falling injuries in nonambulatory children | ▪ Overly compliant |
|  | ▪ Soreness or moving awkwardly |
|  | ▪ A child who appears to be afraid to go home |
|  | ▪ Being described as overly prone to accidents by parents or caregivers |
| ▪ Bruises or fractures in various stages of healing | ▪ Wearing inappropriate clothing in an attempt to hide injuries |
| ▪ Severe injuries without a plausible explanation | ▪ History of running away |
| ▪ Patterned bruises (consistent with an object or device used to strike the child) | ▪ Overly emotional or apologetic reaction when an adult is upset with them |
|  | ▪ Aversion to physical contact or touch |
| ▪ Injuries located in areas that are unlikely to be injured in an unintentional manner | ▪ Violence or abusive language to their peers or smaller "weaker" children |
|  | ▪ Sexually expressive or explicit behavior |

© Jones & Bartlett Learning.

Prehospital practitioners should also consider whether the mechanism of injury that led to the reported injury is developmentally appropriate for the patient.

> **Bruising in nonambulatory children is uncommon and suspicious for abuse in the absence of plausible explanation. A common saying in pediatrics is: "If they ain't cruising, they shouldn't be bruising."**

In children younger than 1 year, bruises to the face, neck, and back are especially concerning (**Figure 8-2**). Examine closely for bruising to the ear lobes, which are commonly pinched or pulled during abusive episodes. Cauliflower ear, or hemorrhage on the pinna of the ear between the skin and cartilage, in children without a reported history of trauma to the area is commonly associated with abuse.

As children begin to progressively cruise then walk, injuries will become an expected part of that learning process. Younger children have larger heads and will often lead "headfirst" while ambulating. Falls during this stage of development (around age 1 year) tend to

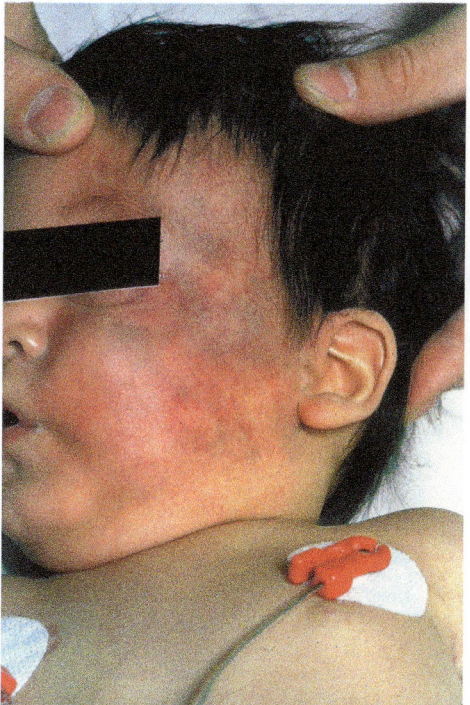

**Figure 8-2** In a nonmobile child, bruises to the face and neck are especially concerning.
Courtesy of Ron Dieckmann, MD, FAAP.

leave bruises and other soft-tissue injuries on the face and forehead. It is important to examine injuries closely and look for any patterns, such as finger or palm marks, to distinguish innocuous bruising from maltreatment.

As children approach age 4 years, bruising of the head and face due to discoordinated ambulation becomes less common. These children may still strike their head, but more often this is due to low clearance from counters, tables, or other objects. These types of injuries can lead to bruises and lacerations depending on the level of energy involved with the impact. Bruising to the bony prominences along the shins, knees, and elbows is common in children and occurs with increasing frequency as they begin to walk and play more independently. Children in this age range often have to climb up onto playground structures and other recreational equipment, leading to frequent incidental contact along bony prominences while playing.

Bruising that is located in areas that do not overlie bony prominences should raise concern for maltreatment if there is no associated plausible explanation. Bruising to the hands, buttocks, and abdomen are generally not associated with innocuous causes and are highly suspicious (**Figure 8-3**). When these bruises are large, located in multiple noncontiguous areas, and in various stages of healing, they are pathognomonic for abuse in the absence of a plausible explanation.

Bruising can also have multiple medical (nontraumatic) causes. Disruptions to normal coagulation and certain cancers can cause easy bleeding and bruising. Determining whether the bruising is unintentional, the result of a medical condition, or due to abuse does not need to be made in the field. Accurate documentation is critical, and this will aid physicians and investigators in determining whether the concern for abuse is warranted.

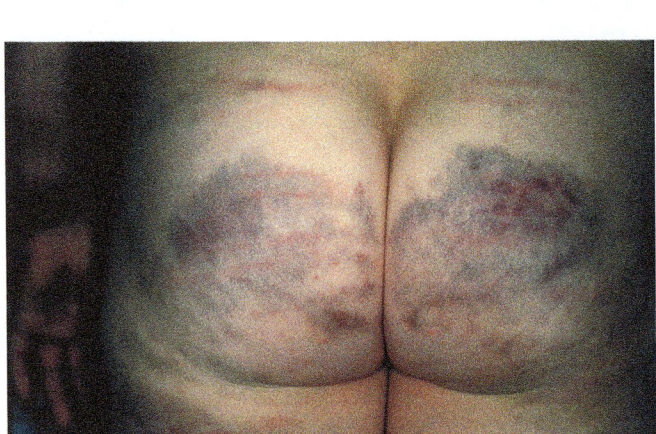

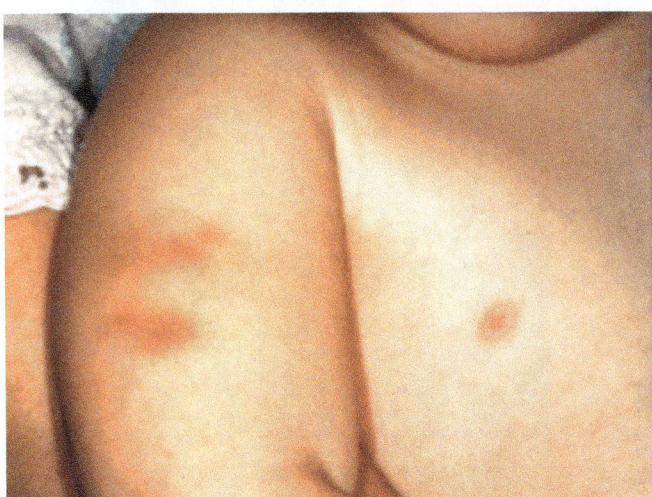

**Figure 8-3** Bruising to the arms or buttocks, as shown here, should raise concerns for abuse, especially in the context of a nonplausible explanation.

**A.** Courtesy of Ron Deickmann, MD, FAAP.; **B.** Courtesy of the American Academy of Pediatrics.

## TEN-4 FACES P

When assessing a child with bruising or soft tissue injuries, the mnemonic TEN-4 FACES P can be helpful for recalling red flag injuries that may be associated with abuse (**Figure 8-4**):

- In children **4 years** or younger, bruising to the **Trunk, Ears, or Neck** is suspicious.

- Any bruising or injury in a child **4 months** or younger is suspicious.

The FACES P mnemonic can be added to help healthcare practitioners remember additional areas where injuries are not typically associated with accidental causes:

- **Frenulum**
- **Auricular area**
- **Cheek**
- **Eyes**
- **Sclera**

In addition, any injury with a **Pattern** (resembles on object, palm, or fingers) is concerning for abuse.

All of this information is relevant when there is no plausible explanation for the injury or condition encountered.

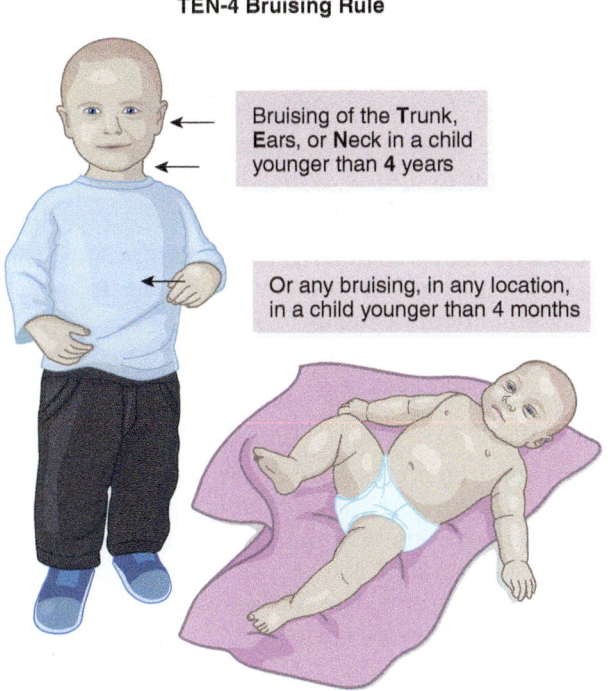

TEN-4 Bruising Rule

Bruising of the **T**runk, **E**ars, or **N**eck in a child younger than **4** years

Or any bruising, in any location, in a child younger than 4 months

**Figure 8-4** Practitioners can use the 10-4 FACES P mnemonic to consider the possibility of child maltreatment.

© Jones & Bartlett Learning.

## FRENULUM INJURIES

Injuries to the lingual or labial frenula, especially in nonambulatory patients who are bottle or spoon fed, are suspicious for an object being forced into the mouth. These objects could include a bottle, sippy cup, pacifier, straw, or finger. The tissues in this area are also susceptible to injury when the lips or tongue are pulled, or the cheeks are squeezed tightly into a "puckering" conformation during an episode of abuse.

This injury may be associated with innocuous causes in ambulatory children who fall while running with an object in their mouth, or who strike their head or face on a stationary object while running or falling.

## Pattern Marks

Injuries that resemble the pattern of an object are highly concerning for trauma caused by nonaccidental mechanisms. When there is not a plausible explanation

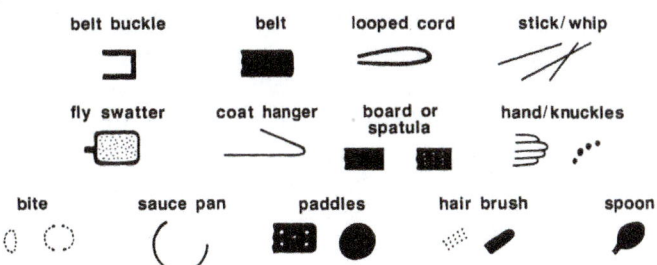

**Figure 8-5** Bruises or injuries with a patterned appearance may be indicative of maltreatment.

Reproduced from Johnson CF. Inflicted injury versus accidental injury. *Pediatr Clin North Am* 1990;37:803.

for how the injury occurred and a patterned bruise is present, maltreatment should be suspected.

Children who are struck with an open palm will often have a negative imprint of the hand on their skin. Capillaries between the fingers will break as blood is quickly pushed away from the point of impact into the surrounding tissues between the digits.

Cords and ropes will often leave sharp, linear striations along where they strike the child. Objects attached to the end of a cord, rope, or belt will often leave distinct imprints if they strike the skin.

Anytime there is a bruise or injury that has a patterned appearance, ask about it and document the caregiver's response in the patient history (**Figure 8-5**). Do not editorialize or offer an opinion on whether the explanation makes sense or sounds suspicious, simply document what was observed and said in a factual manner.

## Abusive Head Trauma

As mentioned previously, the highest risk period for children to suffer from maltreatment is during the first year of life. Although multiple forms of abuse occur in children younger than 2 years, abusive head trauma is the form of child abuse that most often leads to death or permanent disability. Abusive head trauma may be more widely known by the terminology shaken baby syndrome (SBS). This term has fallen out of use in favor of abusive head trauma, as the latter encompasses the multiple forms of injury that can occur during an episode of shaking.

Abusive head trauma has been a known form of maltreatment for as long as records and documentation of abuse have been kept. Data suggest that crying is most often the trigger for abusive head trauma episodes. There has been an increase in resources, education, and outreach for parents who may be dealing with a newborn or infant who is crying inconsolably, in an effort to reduce the incidence of abusive head trauma.

According to the National Center on Shaken Baby Syndrome, approximately 1,200 to 1,400 children per year are injured or die from abusive head trauma. The most common perpetrator is a parent or caregiver. The majority of abusers are men. When children survive abusive episodes, 80% will have some form of permanent brain damage or physical disability.

> **Crying and inconsolability combined with unrealistic expectations about appropriate developmental milestones can lead to outbursts of anger and episodes of abusive head trauma.**

The mnemonic PURPLE Crying has been used to help educate parents and caregivers about crying periods and what can be expected in infants **Table 8-5**.

| Table 8-5  PURPLE Crying | |
|---|---|
| P—Peak of crying | Crying periods may increase each week as the baby gets older, peaking around age 2 months, then declining in months 3 to 5. |
| U—Unexpected | Crying can come and go with no obvious provoking or palliating factors. |
| R—Resists soothing | Even when all of the baby's needs have been met, they may continue to cry without identifiable cause. |
| P—Pain-like face | The crying can be intense, and in some cases the baby may even look or act as if they are in pain or discomfort. |
| L—Long lasting | Babies can cry for as much as 5 hours per day or more in some cases. When babies are crying intensely, minutes can feel like hours. |
| E—Evening | Babies may cry more in the late afternoon or evening. |

Data from National Center on Shaken Baby Syndrome. PURPLE Crying. Accessed December 5, 2021. https://www.dontshake.org/purple-crying.

The injuries suffered during an episode of shaking occur secondary to multiple causes and are listed below:

- Shaking back and forth results in rapid acceleration and deceleration of the brain against the skull, leading to blunt trauma. This blunt trauma leads to diffuse axonal injury and swelling of the brain tissues.
- The back and forth shaking action disrupts the bridging vessels in the brain and leads to intracranial hemorrhage.
- Swelling within the brain, increased ocular pressure, and in some cases direct intentional injury to the eyes leads to retinal hemorrhages.
- When children are grasped during an abusive episode, the force required to hold onto them during the shaking will often lead to fractures. The most common fracture locations include the ribs and extremities. The cervical spine may be injured during severe episodes.
- Injuries to the internal organs such as the liver and pancreas may also occur.
- Blunt trauma to the head may be encountered if the patient's head is struck against a hard surface or if the abuser strikes the victim with an open palm or fist (**Figure 8-6**).

The signs of abusive head trauma are nonspecific. It is common for caregivers to call EMS or bring the patient to the emergency department with a vague and inconsistent story after an episode of abuse. They may say that the patient was in a normal state of health or feeling mildly ill with vague symptoms when they laid them down for a nap unattended. The caregiver may report that when they went to check on the child they were vomiting, not acting right, or unable to arouse them. A history of minor injury out of proportion with the exhibited symptoms, such as tripping and falling, rolling off the couch or changing table, or a sibling who fell on them may be described. The patient may present with the following signs or symptoms:

- Altered mental status (can be difficult to assess in an infant)
- Drowsiness, irritability, or difficult to arouse
- Seizures or spasms
- Decreased appetite
- Vomiting
- Posturing with the back arched and neck extended (a result of increased intracranial pressure leading to meningeal signs)

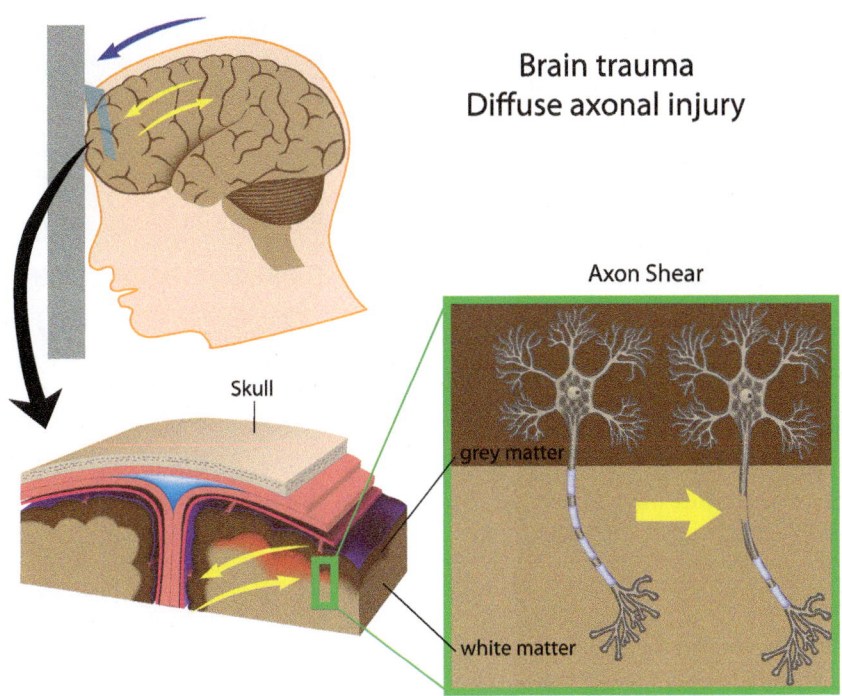

**Brain trauma**
**Diffuse axonal injury**

Axon Shear

Skull

grey matter

white matter

**Figure 8-6** Blunt force injury to the head may occur due to striking against a hard surface during episodes of abuse. Musculoskeletal injuries to the ribs and extremities may also occur due to the force exerted on the child while being held and shaken.

© Alila Medical Media/Shutterstock.

- Physical injury outside of the body may not be seen, but when it is present along with the additional signs, abuse should be strongly suspected.

The primary treatment for abusive head trauma is immediate treatment for any respiratory or circulatory compromise followed by managing symptoms of increased intracranial pressure. Prompt transport to a pediatric specialty center with physicians trained in trauma and neurosurgery is crucial.

# Burns

Burn injuries occur in children from both unintentional and intentional mechanisms. Intentional burns tend to be more serious, as children are forced into contact with the heat source. When a burn is unintentional, the child tends to recoil quickly away from the burn if they are developmentally able to do so. In rare cases, children may be unable to pull away or recoil from heat sources during unintentional injury, which may result in more serious burns. These situations are rare, and generally the story fits with the level of injury.

Thermal burns are caused by direct contact with high heat sources. This can occur when a patient places their hand on a hot stove or is forcefully dunked or submerged into a scalding hot liquid. A common source for unintentional thermal burn is in the kitchen when a hot item is touched or a vessel of hot liquid is pulled down from the counter or stove. Intentional thermal burns may occur from contact with cigarettes or in the bathtub when a patient is placed into bathwater that is too hot.

Electrical burns occur when a patient encounters an electricity source. Superficial injury occurs from direct contact in a similar fashion to a thermal burn, in addition to internal burn injury that can occur as the electricity courses through the body. In some cases, electrical burns will have an exit wound as well. A common cause of electrical burns in children is chewing on electrical cords. These children should be transported to the emergency department regardless of how stable they appear on initial exam. They require a cardiac workup and monitoring for arrhythmias.

Chemical burns occur when irritants contact the skin and lead to tissue destruction. Heat may or may not be involved. Household cleaning products, hair treatments, and medications being infused through intravenous (IV) lines are common causes of chemical burns. Practitioners should take caution to make sure they do not come into contact with the chemical and harm themselves. The first step in treatment of chemical burns is to remove the chemical and stop the burning process. Depending on the chemical involved and the amount present, high-level decontamination may be necessary.

When fumes are involved, use caution when transporting in enclosed spaces and do not take the patient into the hospital until decontamination has taken place.

When chemicals have been swallowed or forced into a patient's mouth, burning of the oral and esophageal structures can occur. Inhaled chemicals can lead to significant lung injury and chemical pneumonitis. Severe respiratory compromise may be present.

## Abusive Burns

Younger children tend to be the targets of abusive burns. Burns suffered from abuse tend to be more serious and can be full thickness in some cases. Submersion injuries into scalding hot liquid and intentional burning with cigarettes or other hot objects are two of the most common causes of intentional, abusive burns.

### Cigarette Burns

Contact burns from cigarettes tend to form uniform, circular injuries. They can be grouped (**Figure 8-7**) and located in areas that are not normally exposed in an attempt to hide the abuse (**Figure 8-8**). When children are unintentionally injured by cigarette burns, it tends to be from incidental contact on an exposed area that is momentary, such as when they are running or walking by a parent or caregiver who is holding a cigarette down at their side, resulting in a burn to the face or torso.

### Scald Burns

Burns from hot tap water are the most common forms of abusive and unintentional burn injury in children in the United States. Approximately 50% of all child abuse burns are caused by scald injuries. Most patients injured by scald injuries are younger than 2 years.

Accidental scald burns tend to involve the face, neck, and anterior chest. The most common mechanism is a vessel of hot liquid being pulled from an elevated surface down onto the patient or picked up and then spilled onto the anterior face, neck, and chest. These burns are typically most severe in the superior regions, and as the liquid trickles down, it tends to cool, resulting in less severe burns toward the inferior regions. There is often an "arrow down" pattern as the liquid cools and tapers to a point while running down the body. The margins of unintentional burns tend to be irregular. These burns tend to be less severe as the contact with the burning liquid is not excessive, as opposed to intentional submersion burns, where forced contact is prolonged.

A common mechanism for both intentional and unintentional scald burns is when a patient is placed into a tub with water that is too hot. When this action is unintentional, the burn is not usually full thickness

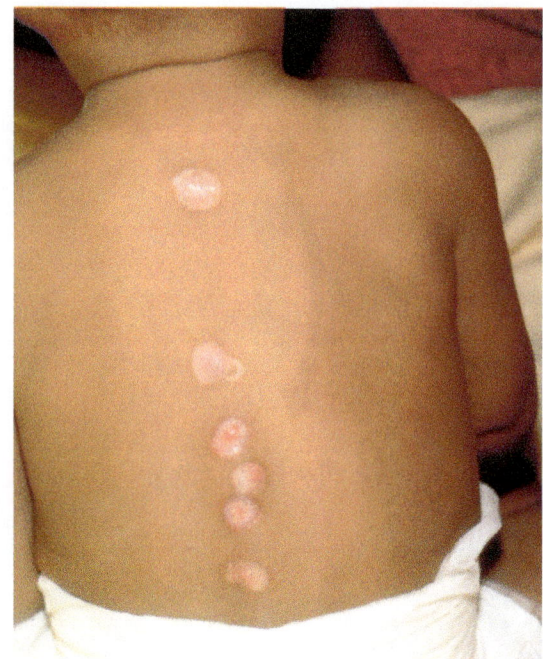

**Figure 8-7** This cluster of uniformly shaped burns is the result of intentional burning. Note how they are in a discrete area that can be hidden. This is a good example of a patterned burn that would be difficult to cause by unintentional mechanisms.
© Mediscan/Alamy Stock Photo.

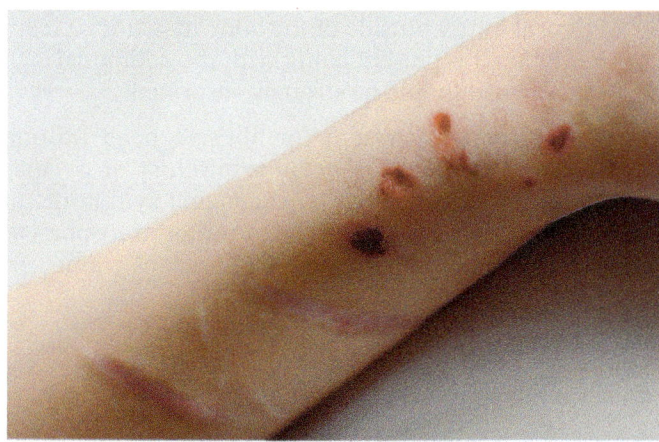

**Figure 8-8** The burns in this image are from a cigarette. Burns on areas of skin that are easily visible are less common as they cannot be easily hidden by the abuser.
© NataVilman/Shutterstock.

and the borders will be asymmetric and irregular. The patient is likely to pull their hand back or recoil immediately, limiting the exposure to the hot liquid.

When immersion burns are intentional, red flag signs may be present indicating that the nature of the injury was not accidental. When a child is intentionally dunked into a vessel of hot water, they will raise their legs, resulting in more severe burning to the buttocks

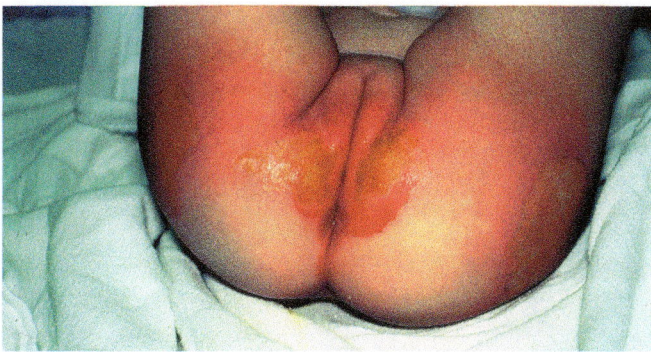

**Figure 8-9** Immersion scald burns are the most commonly inflicted burns. They usually involve the lower trunk, buttocks, perineum, arms, and legs. They can appear as "glove and stocking" burns or "donut" burns as in this image.

Courtesy of Ron Deickmann, MD, FAAP.

and perineum. If the buttocks come into contact with the bottom of the bathtub, this area may be spared and result in a donut-shaped burn, with a ring of severe burning surrounding a spared or mildly burned area. When extremities are forcefully placed into hot water, a "glove and stocking" pattern may be noted, with a sharp delineation present at the level where the extremity was held in the hot liquid (**Figure 8-9**). When the hand and arm are placed into a hot liquid, the patient will clench their fist and the palm will often be spared from severe burning. When these signs are present, the index of suspicion for abuse or intentional injury should be high.

The severity of submersion burns is impacted by multiple factors. The temperature of the liquid, duration of contact, and skin areas involved all influence the severity of the injury.

> Submersion burn injuries are common in the 1- to 4-year-old range and often happen in proximity to toilet training or accidents where the child has soiled themselves. Abusers will strip the child and wash them in hot water as punishment for having an accident. In some cases, cold water may be used and children can present with hypothermia.

# Pediatric Human Trafficking

Human trafficking is estimated to involve 21 million global victims every year. While this number may seem large, it likely does not reflect the true magnitude of the issue, as many victims of human trafficking go unreported. It is estimated that nearly a quarter of all human trafficking victims are children.

Human trafficking comes in many forms. Some examples of trafficking include the following:

- Prostitution
- Mail-order bride trade
- Child pornography
- Online sexual abuse and exploitation
- Performance in illegal sex venues catering to pedophiles
- Forced labor

Trafficking of child victims can be hard to spot, as the children may willingly travel with their abuser and not cry out for help. They may be manipulated into thinking that their abuser is actually a protector. The abuser often provides for the basic needs of the victims and may supply them with drugs or alcohol to keep them under their influence. Trafficking often involves threats to the safety of the child and the child's loved ones. The child may be convinced that if they seek help or try to escape, harm may come to their family.

The average age at which a victim enters the commercial sex industry is 12 to 14 years. Adolescents are often targeted because they have poor impulse control and may be easily manipulated with material goods or promises of popularity, fame, and money.

Teenagers who have run away from home or otherwise been separated from their family often lack the resources necessary to provide for their basic needs. This leaves them open to victimization in exchange for basic needs such as food and shelter. It is estimated that 9% to 28% of runaway or homeless teenagers have exchanged some form of sexual activity for items needed to survive. Abusers can then leverage this sexual activity against the victim to shame them, going so far as to threaten to divulge embarrassing information to the victim's family or friends. With the increased use of social media and cell phones capable of taking and sending images through text message, abusers can amass compromising photographs of their victims and then use this material to manipulate the victim into sending them more material or engaging in increasingly compromising and illicit acts.

Both males and females may be trafficked for forced labor and servitude. According to the U.S. Department of State, forced labor is the biggest sector of trafficking in the world. In some cases, when these victims agree to come to the United States, they are given false promises of work and education. However, the promised work conditions do not reflect the reality of the work they are forced to engage in when they arrive.

They often do not speak enough English to request help, and the adults they encounter may also be engaging in other illegal activities, and thus would be unlikely to help them even when the victim asks for help. Often these victims have their passports and identifying documents taken from them. They end up helpless and fully dependent on their abusers for survival.

Common red flags that should raise suspicion of human trafficking include the following:

- An individual with a child who is reluctant to let them speak to healthcare practitioners alone

- Inconsistent or nonsensical history

- Adolescents who do not know their address or how to get home, or who provide fake identifying information

- Unfamiliarity with the city or town in which they are located

- Unexplained absences from school or other social activities

- Work-related injuries

- Sexually expressive behavior

- Untreated chronic illnesses

- Sexually transmitted infection

- Trauma to the vagina or rectum

- Cigarette, iron, or acid burns

- History of abortions or miscarriages

- Tattoo or "brand" with an individual or organization's insignia

# Conditions Mistaken for Maltreatment

There are some common conditions of childhood that may be mistaken for bruising or other signs suspicious for abuse. Some of these conditions include the following:

- Congenital dermal melanocytosis (Mongolian spots)

- Coining (Cao Gio/Gua Sha/Kerikan)

- Cupping

## Congenital Dermal Melanocytosis

Congenital dermal melanocytosis (CDM), formerly known as Mongolian spots, are blue-grey lesions commonly seen on lumbosacral area, often just superior to

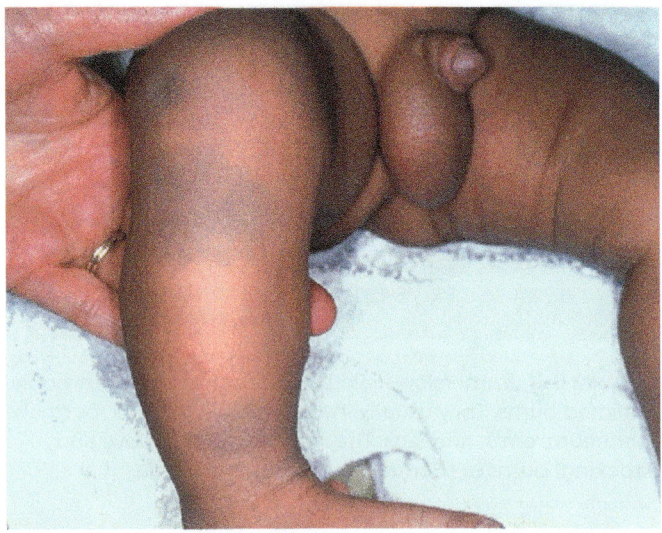

**Figure 8-10** CDM can be found on the back, shoulders, or extremities. Note the irregular borders and lack of pattern, favoring CDM over bruising secondary to abuse.
Courtesy of the American Academy of Pediatrics.

the buttocks (**Figure 8-10**). The lesions are the result of dermal melanocytes that have not dissipated after birth. These lesions are often present at birth and may initially darken, before ultimately fading over subsequent years. Typically, the lesions have faded completely by age 6 years. CDM is the most common pigmented lesion in newborns.

CDM appears with varying frequency based upon the ethnicity of the infant, as follows:

- Asian neonates: 80%–100%

- African American neonates: >90%

- Hispanic neonates: 46%–70%

- White neonates: <10%

The lesions of CDM typically have irregular borders and may not be uniform in color. They do not have a patterned appearance, which makes them distinct from bruising that has occurred as the result of being struck with a hand or other object. It is important to document these lesions in case questions arise later.

CDM is a benign condition. The lesions should not be painful to the touch and they tend to fade over a period of years, compared to bruising, which fades and changes over days to weeks.

## Coining (Cao Gio/Gua Sha/Kerikan)

Cao Gio (pronounced gow yaw), also known as coining, Gua Sha, or Kerikan, is practiced in some Southeast Asian cultures (Cambodia, Laos, Vietnam).

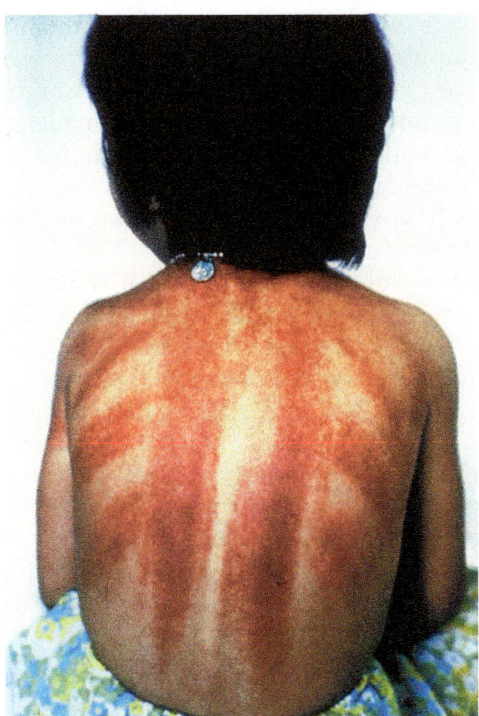

**Figure 8-11** These images demonstrate the varying appearance of coining based on the technique, timing, and location. Some techniques leave very light marking, while others can cause quite severe looking capillary breaks. Note the linear and chevron-shaped appearance on the back, which is classical for coining. These lesions are not tender to palpation and should not be actively bleeding.

Courtesy of the American Academy of Pediatrics.

The literal translation is "catch the wind." The Eastern medicine principle is that conditions such as cold, flu, headache, malaise, fever, fatigue, and other nonspecific illnesses can be caused by "bad wind" in the blood. Oil is applied to the skin in certain areas and then a coin, spoon, or other implement is stroked over those areas, as a form of dermabrasion, causing superficial capillary breakdown and increasing blood flow to the regions. In Eastern medicine, it is thought that this increased blood flow to the skin surface allows a gateway for the "bad wind" to escape. Although the lesions can look quite painful, they are in fact relatively painless and do not cause any physical damage or harm to the patient. In rare cases, when the practice is not carried out in accordance with traditionally accepted techniques and training, some patients may suffer burns or deeper bruising (**Figure 8-11**). This is not a common occurrence and does not reflect the intention of the therapy or the proper method for carrying out the treatment.

## Cupping

Cupping is an ancient Eastern medicine tradition similar to coining. The technique involves applying cups

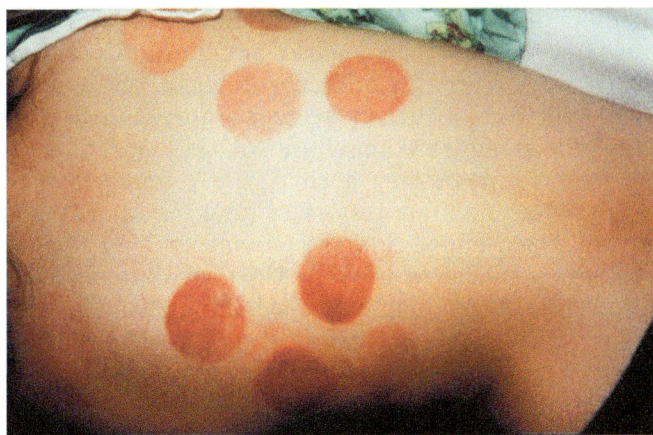

**Figure 8-12** Cupping is often used to treat sore muscles and is supposed to promote healing by removing negative forces and promoting circulation.

Courtesy of the American Academy of Pediatrics.

in such a manner that suction is created and a portion of the skin, soft tissue, and underlying muscle is pulled into the cup after a vacuum has been created. The concept is that the suction process promotes blood flow to the area, which can enhance circulation and recovery of the underlying tissues.

Two different methods are used to create suction. The more traditional method involves using a flame to heat the air inside the cup. It is then quickly applied to the skin, and as the air cools, a vacuum is created inside the cup, drawing in the skin and soft tissue. This method carries the risk of burn injury when not performed properly. An alternative method involves using modern cups that are manufactured with a connection on the top to which a vacuum pump can be applied. The pump is connected to the skin and the air is withdrawn, creating suction which draws in the skin and soft tissue. This is the more common method used today, although many practitioners still employ cupping with the traditional fire method.

Cupping has found increased popularity after the swimmer Michael Phelps was seen with markings caused by the practice at the 2016 Olympics. His trainer employed the method to aid in muscle recovery between races (**Figure 8-12**).

## History Taking

The initial history and detailed physical exam are the most important pieces of evidence the prehospital practitioner can obtain in a case of child maltreatment. History should be obtained from both the caregiver and the child when possible. Children should be interviewed separately from the parent when possible, with a chaperone in the room. In some cases, a family member may disclose that they have concern for abuse, but rarely will the actual abuser admit or disclose that abuse has occurred. Children younger than 3 years have limited ability to convey their history verbally and are at the greatest risk for abuse.

When interviewing a child, the primary goal is obtaining an accurate history of how the injuries occurred. Open-ended prompts provide the best opportunity to get detailed answers. The goal of the medical history is not to obtain a detailed account of abuse or maltreatment. Documentation should include verbatim statements in quotations when applicable. Detailed abuse history and additional questioning should be deferred to specially trained individuals with experience in forensic interviewing. In some cases, questions that are leading in nature have tainted child abuse investigations to the point where prosecution was made difficult or impossible.

## Mandated Reporting

A mandated reporter is an individual with a legal obligation to report suspected or confirmed cases of child abuse. Mandated reporters who do not report cases where a reasonable suspicion of abuse exists may be held criminally liable.

Most states require that only a reasonable suspicion of abuse needs to exist for reporting to occur. The job of investigating and proving whether abuse exists falls to the state after a report has been made, and prehospital practitioners are not responsible for performing any investigatory functions other than the initial history and physical examination that occurs while treating the patient.

When a child discloses abuse, it is important to control your emotions and listen without anger or disbelief. Open-ended questions such as, "Then what happened?" are helpful. Leading questions may retraumatize the child and contaminate the investigation. The currently accepted best practice is to conduct a "minimal fact interview" which includes what, where, when, and by whom. The victim's level of cognitive and emotional development will impact how effectively they may be able to answer these questions. When in doubt, obtain any medically necessary information, and allow Child Protective Services or law enforcement to conduct the remainder of the interview.

The role of EMS is to consider whether abuse has occurred, and when reasonable suspicion exists, to report that suspicion. Most states absolve mandatory reporters of potential liability when reports are made in good faith with the best interests of the patient in mind.

## CASE STUDY

### Case 1

#### Dispatch

You are dispatched to a private residence for a 3-month-old unresponsive female. It is a cool fall afternoon with an outside temperature of 56°F (13.3°C).

#### Case Questions

- What are your initial concerns?
  - This is an unresponsive pediatric patient. There is a high risk that respiratory and possibly cardiac arrest are present.
- Based on the dispatch information, what is the possible differential diagnosis for this patient?
  - The differential diagnosis for unresponsive pediatric patients is broad and includes both traumatic and medical causes. Some of the potential causes for unresponsive children include:

- Accidental ingestion or poisoning
- Trauma
- Hypothermia
- Sudden unexplained death
- Child abuse
- Seizures
- Hypoglycemia or other metabolic disturbance
- Hypovolemia and shock from gastrointestinal or traumatic losses

Scene assessment and awareness are critical in cases such as this. Pay close attention to possible substances that could have been ingested or the presence of objects that could have been aspirated. In this case the patient is 3 months old and not mobile, making it highly unlikely that the patient unintentionally ingested a substance or inhaled a foreign body unless it was left near the patient.

Carefully observe the caregiver behavior. Assessing the overall environment and interactions of the caregiver can help inform suspicion for potential abuse or criminal activity.

## Initial Observations

As you arrive on scene, a frantic couple rushes out to meet you, carrying the limp body of a 3-month-old female in their arms. They force her into your arms, yelling at you to help her. They continually repeat, "She isn't breathing, help her!" The child is limp, unresponsive, and has no obvious tone.

- Pediatric Assessment Triangle (**Figure 8-13**)
  - Appearance
    - Unresponsive
  - Work of breathing
    - The patient is agonal without adequate respiratory effort
    - **F**laring is not present
    - **R**etractions are not present
    - **A**udible airway sounds are not heard
    - **P**ositioning is limp and unresponsive
  - Circulation
    - Skin cyanotic with evidence of poor perfusion

The couple informs you that they are the girl's aunt and uncle. They have legal custody of the patient due to concern for parental drug use. They appear appropriately concerned and tell you that they laid her down to sleep in her portable playpen approximately 30 minutes ago. They heard a loud thump come from inside the room, and when they went to check on her, they found her on the floor crying and suspect she must have climbed out and possibly injured herself. When they picked her up, she vomited and then went limp. That is when they called 911 for assistance.

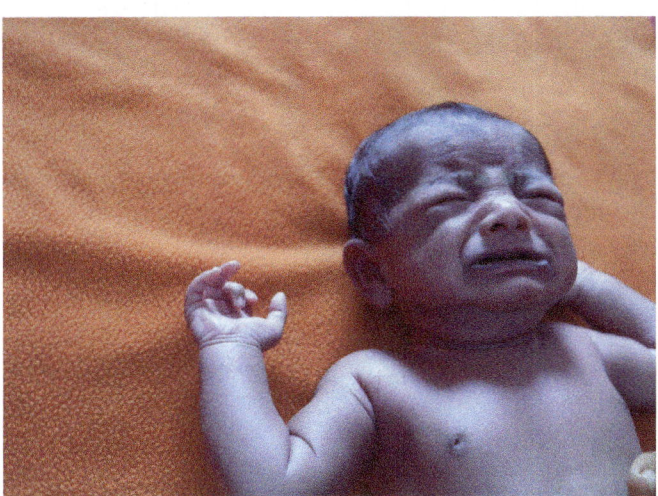

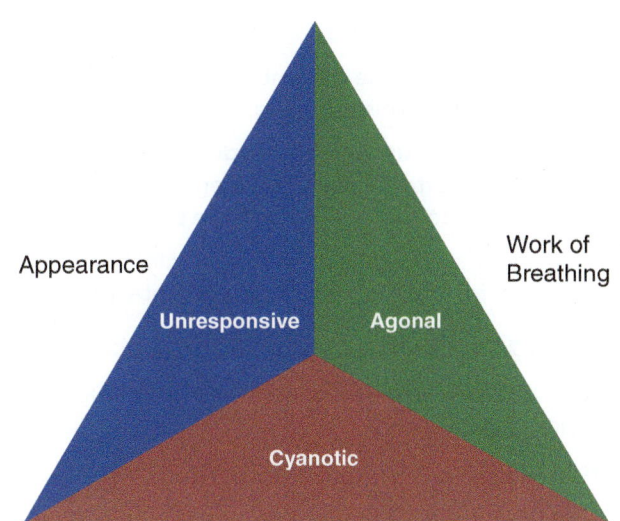

**Figure 8-13** The 3-month old child appears limp and floppy and is unresponsive.

## Case Questions

- Based on your initial impression, is this patient "Quick" or "Not Quick"?
  - This patient is "Quick." She is unresponsive with ineffective respiratory effort and signs of poor perfusion.
- Do any red flags for possible maltreatment exist?
  - The story that is being presented by the aunt and uncle is not plausible. It is not developmentally appropriate for a 3-month-old infant to climb out of a portable playpen and fall onto the floor, and the level of injury sustained from a low-level fall such as the one described would not result in trauma significant enough to cause sudden cardiopulmonary arrest.
- Does the couple's story sound credible?
  - No. Cruising, walking, and climbing are developmentally appropriate at 9 to 15 months or older.

- Falls from less than 3 feet are unlikely to result in serious injury.

- Falls from 3 to 6 feet are more likely to result in visible injury; however, the severity of those injuries is unlikely to be severe or life threatening in most cases. When a patient falls from a height of greater than 6 feet, serious injury becomes more likely.

- What are risk factors for child abuse?

  - Children in foster care are at higher risk of abuse and maltreatment. In this case, the caregivers are relatives of the biologic parents, and may have come from the same environment that led to drug abuse and the removal of the children.

## Primary Survey

The primary survey for this patient reveals the following:

**X**—No bleeding found

**A**—Open and patent

**B**—Agonal

**C**—Brachial pulses are absent, the skin is cyanotic.

**D**—The patient is unresponsive. Glasgow Coma Scale (GCS) score is 3 (E1, V1, M1).

**E**—In uncle's arms; bruise noted on patient's right upper arm

### Case Questions

- Based on the findings noted in the primary survey, what would your initial interventions and treatment include?

  - Initial treatment should focus on high-quality cardiopulmonary support.

  - Cardiopulmonary resuscitation (CPR) should be initiated immediately.

  - IV access should be obtained and a cardiac monitor should be applied.

  - Advanced airway placement should occur if time permits, otherwise continuing with basic airway management during the initial resuscitation is appropriate.

After approximately 10 minutes of CPR, return of spontaneous circulation (ROSC) is obtained, and the patient is intubated with a 3.5-mm endotracheal tube.

## Detailed Assessment

### History Taking

The aunt and uncle explain that the patient was in her normal state of health when they laid her down to take a nap. They heard a loud thud in the bedroom and came in to find her lying on the ground crying. They immediately picked her up to console her. She promptly vomited and went unresponsive. They immediately called 911. Additional history was obtained and documented as follows.

**OPQRST:**

- **O**nset: Sudden

- **P**rovocation/palliation: Unclear, they think she might have fallen out of the portable playpen

- **Q**uality: Unable to assess

- **R**adiation: Unable to assess

- **S**everity: Unknown

- **T**iming: Approximately 10 minutes prior to your arrival

**SAMPLER:**

- **S**igns/symptoms: Unresponsive, cyanotic, and pulseless

- **A**llergies: No known allergies to medications, foods, or the environment

- **M**edications: None

- **P**ast medical history: Born full-term. The patient had a viral upper respiratory infection a few weeks ago, but it fully resolved and she has been healthy since that time.

- **L**ast oral intake: The patient had a bottle of formula earlier this morning.

- **E**vents leading up to the emergency: The patient was in her portable playpen when they heard a loud thump and found her lying on the bedroom floor.

- **R**isk factors: Age, prior history of neglect resulting in removal from biologic parents (parental drug use)

### Vital Signs

Once ROSC was obtained, the following vital signs were obtained (**Figure 8-14**):

**Heart rate:**

- 158 beats/min

- The expected heart rate for a patient of this age is 100–160 beats/min

**SpO$_2$:**

- 99% on 100% FiO$_2$ via endotracheal tube

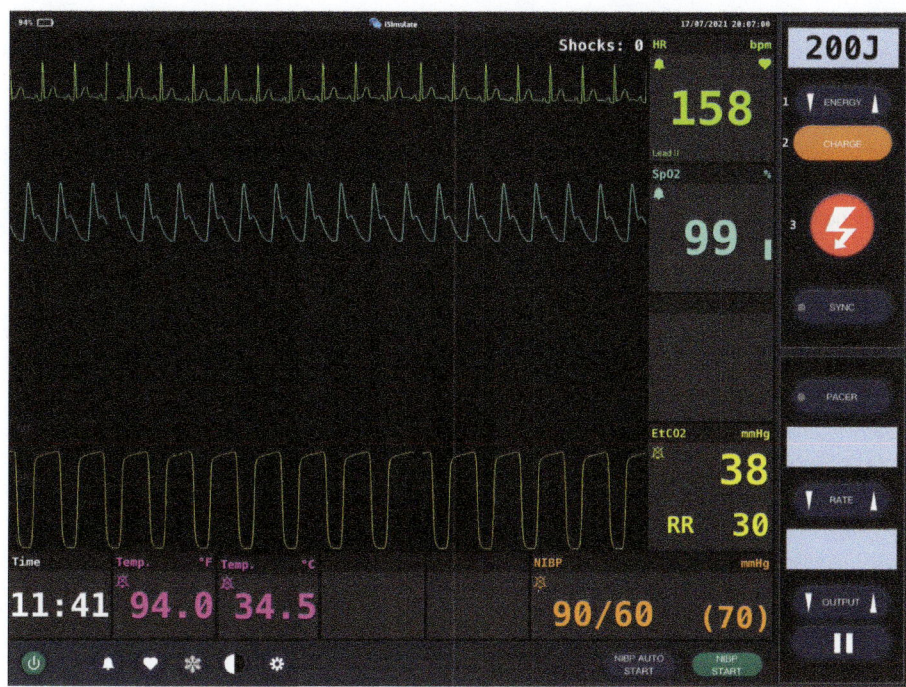

**Figure 8-14** Patient's vital signs while being ventilated.
Courtesy of iSimulate.

**ETCO$_2$:**

- 38 mm Hg
- There is a consistent waveform indicating that the patient is properly intubated.

**Respiratory rate:**

- 30 breaths/min
- The patient is being artificially ventilated at a rate of one breath every 2–3 seconds.

**Blood pressure:**

- 90/60 mm Hg
- This is within the expected range for this patient.

**Temperature:**

- 94°F (34.5°C)
- The temperature in this case indicates that the patient may have been down for longer than described by the aunt and uncle.

**Blood glucose:**

- 178 mg/dL
- This is an elevated glucose, which could be the result of a stress response or due to the administration of epinephrine during resuscitation efforts.

**Weight:**

- Estimated to be 6 kg per the length-based tape

As you are examining the patient, she begins to have a generalized seizure.

## Case Questions

- What treatment would you provide to terminate the seizure activity?
  - Lorazepam 0.1 mg/kg IV was administered to terminate seizure activity.

This patient is a previously healthy 3-month-old female who experienced sudden cardiopulmonary arrest. The patient's aunt and uncle are the legal guardians and report that they found her on the floor outside of her portable playpen after hearing a loud thump. They think she may have climbed out. The patient was briefly responsive immediately after they checked on her following the loud thump, but then had a single episode of emesis after which she became unresponsive. The aunt and uncle contacted EMS at this point.

On EMS arrival, the patient was found in cardiopulmonary arrest with signs of trauma noted on the anterior and posterior chest. Following 10 minutes of resuscitation efforts, the patient experienced ROSC. The patient then experienced generalized seizure activity, which was terminated after a single administration of lorazepam, 0.1 mg/kg IV.

**Detailed Physical Exam**

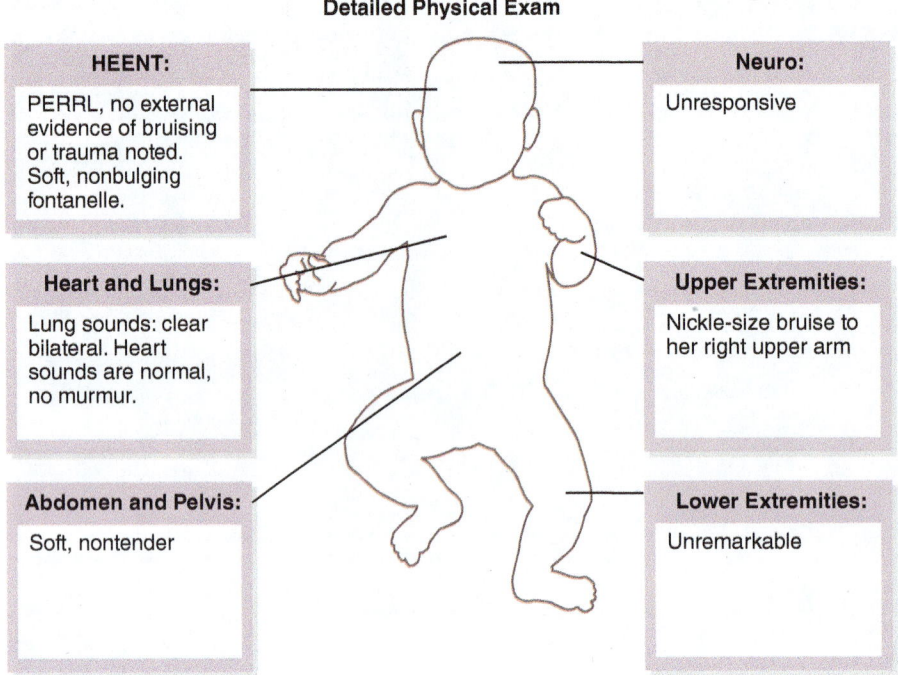

**HEENT:**

PERRL, no external evidence of bruising or trauma noted. Soft, nonbulging fontanelle.

**Neuro:**

Unresponsive

**Heart and Lungs:**

Lung sounds: clear bilateral. Heart sounds are normal, no murmur.

**Upper Extremities:**

Nickle-size bruise to her right upper arm

**Abdomen and Pelvis:**

Soft, nontender

**Lower Extremities:**

Unremarkable

**Figure 8-15** During the secondary survey, a nickel-size bruise is noted on the patient's right upper arm.

© Jones & Bartlett Learning.

The history provided by the guardians does not explain the level of injury noted on physical exam. The patient's level of development is not consistent with ability to climb out of a playpen. The height of the fall which would occur if such an event did happen is unlikely to cause the level of injury seen. The scenario as presented is highly suspicious for nonaccidental trauma. The history, physical exam, and patient presentation are specifically concerning for abusive head trauma.

## Detailed Exam

### HEENT (Figure 8-15):

- **H**ead: No external evidence of trauma. The fontanelle is full and slightly bulging.
- **E**yes: Pupils are dilated and slow to constrict.
- **E**ars: Unremarkable
- **N**ose: Scant mucus present, no rhinorrhea noted
- **T**hroat: Unremarkable

### Chest, heart, and lungs:

- Pulses: Peripheral pulses palpable
- Cardiac auscultation: Regular rate and rhythm with no rub, gallop, or murmur noted
- Lung auscultation: Lungs are clear to auscultation bilaterally; breath sounds are equal.
- Chest exam: No external trauma noted

### Neurologic:

- Unresponsive, with absent tone throughout

### Abdomen and pelvis:

- Soft and nondistended

### Extremities:

- Upper extremities: A nickel-sized bruise is noted on the right upper arm.
- Lower extremities: Unremarkable

### Back:

- Unremarkable

## Treatment

The initial treatment for this patient involves basic life support care with CPR. Vascular access and advanced airway placement should take place as appropriate. Based on the suspicion of trauma, consider c-spine immobilization and precautions if practical.

Attention should be paid to the patient's hypothermia. Warmed fluids can be administered, and the patient should be kept covered as much as possible. Benzodiazepines for the management of seizures are appropriate.

The goal of treatment for this patient is to support cardiopulmonary and hemodynamic status while providing rapid transport to a pediatric tertiary care center. Ongoing management for seizure activity and

## Case Questions

- What conditions are part of your potential differential diagnosis?
  - The differential for this patient includes:
    - Ingestion
    - Trauma
    - Hypothermia
    - Sudden death
    - Abusive head trauma

hypothermia will be critical to prevent further harm while en route to the transport destination. EMS practitioners should be prepared for rapid deterioration and repeat episodes of arrest during transport.

This patient will require advanced neurology and neurosurgical management and should be transported to a destination that is capable of these services when appropriate.

## Ongoing Management

Due to concern for potential deterioration, the patient was closely monitored and continually reassessed during transport. Warmed fluids were administered (20 mL/kg bolus). The patient was kept covered as appropriate with warm blankets, and the head was covered. The patient remained unresponsive and did not require any sedation or paralytic medications. No additional seizures were encountered, however additional doses of lorazepam were kept on hand just in case.

## Case Questions

- Where is the most appropriate treatment destination and why?
  - The child was transported to the pediatric academic hospital located 20 minutes away.
- Can you safely transport this child in your ambulance?
  - Yes, patient was restrained in infant car seat.
- Will you allow the aunt and uncle to ride in the ambulance?
  - The uncle was allowed to ride with EMS personnel, safely seat belted in the front seat.

On arrival to the emergency department, a full report was given to receiving personnel and concerns for possible abuse were passed on to the attending physician.

## CASE WRAP-UP

Diagnosis: Multiple subdural hematomas (nonaccidental trauma)

On arrival to the emergency department the patient remained hypothermic; however, she was hemodynamically stable.

Based on the history, physical exam, and scene report given by EMS personnel, a stat CT scan of the head was performed, revealing multiple subdural hematomas. This information combined with the story that was reported in the EMS patient care report prompted a report to Child Protective Services and local law enforcement.

The patient remained in the hospital for 26 days where emergent subdural hematoma evacuation and neurologic monitoring occurred. Due to the neurologic damage she suffered, her ability to swallow was no longer present and she was not able to safely feed by mouth. A gastronomy tube was placed for her to receive feeds. She began to open her eyes spontaneously on day 8 of admission, however she did not fix or track. Overall, she had some improvement in her neurologic exam and was moving all extremities spontaneously.

The patient was discharged into state care and is currently at a long-term care facility where she continues to receive medical care and developmental therapies in an effort to maximize her potential for regaining function in the future as she recovers.

## CASE TAKEAWAY POINTS

Remember that the parent's or care provider's explanation of a child's injury should be consistent with the child's developmental abilities. A child who is too young to roll over or sit up would not be physically able to climb out a crib or playpen. Always share suspicion for abuse with the staff at the receiving facility.

## LESSON WRAP-UP

Child abuse and maltreatment is a growing problem in the United States despite efforts to intervene and curb this rise. EMS personnel play a critical role in recognizing and breaking the cycle of abuse.

- The U.S. Department of Health and Human Services reports that in 2018 there were nearly 700,000 cases of reported child abuse. The numbers are increasing every year.

- A significant number of permanent disabilities sustained by children are the result of abuse and maltreatment. This includes physical and psychological injuries.

- The youngest victims often suffer the most severe physical abuse.

- The lifetime estimated financial costs associated with child abuse and neglect are estimated to be $124 billion per year.

This is a difficult topic to discuss, and an even more difficult case to encounter in real life. Bear in mind that regardless of what happened prior to your arrival on scene, you are that child's best chance for survival and escape from abuse once you encounter them and begin providing care. The care you provide and documentation you keep will aid in breaking the cycle of abuse.

## REFERENCES

Adamsbaum C, Grabar S, Mejean N, Rey-Salmon C. Abusive head trauma: judicial admissions highlight violent and repetitive shaking. *Pediatrics*. 2010;126(3):546-555.

Altimier L. Shaken baby syndrome. *J Perinat Neonatal Nurs*. 2008 Jan-Mar;22(1):68-76; quiz 77-78. doi:10.1097/01.JPN.0000311877 .32614.69

Barr RG, Treng RB, Cross J. Age-related incidence curve of hospitalized shaken baby syndrome cases: convergent evidence for crying as a trigger to shaking. *Child Abuse Negl*. 2006;30(1):7-16.

Berry J. Recognizing and treating Mongolian blue spots. *Medical News Today*. August 21, 2020. Accessed December 22, 2021. https://www.medicalnewstoday.com/articles/318853

Christianson CW, Block R, Committee on Child Abuse and Neglect. Abusive head trauma in infants and children. *Pediatrics*. 2009;123(5):1409-1411.

Chua RF, Pico J. Dermal melanocytosis. In: StatPearls [Internet]. Treasure Island, FL: StatPearls Publishing. Updated August 3, 2021. https://www.ncbi.nlm.nih.gov/books/NBK557408/

Greenbaum J, Bodrick N, Committee on Child Abuse and Neglect: Section on International Child Health, et al. Global human trafficking and child victimization. *Pediatrics*. 2017;140(6):e20173138.

Hankinson A, Lloyd B, Alweis R. Lime-induced phytophotodermatitis. *J Community Hosp Intern Med Perspect*. 2014;4(4). doi:10.3402 /jchimp.v4.25090

Joyce T, Gossman W, Huecker MR. Pediatric abusive head trauma. In: StatPearls [Internet]. Treasure Island, FL: StatPearls Publishing. Updated August 26, 2021. https://pubmed.ncbi.nlm.nih .gov/29763011/

New York State Department of Health. Shaken baby syndrome: description of the problem. Accessed December 22, 2021. https://www.health.ny.gov/prevention/injury_prevention/shaken_baby _syndrome/description.htm

Ojo P, Palmer J, Garvey R, Atweh N, Fidler P. Pattern of burns in child abuse. *Am Surg*. 2007 Mar;73(3):253-255.

Reijnevelt SA, van der Wal MF, Brugman E, Hira Sing RA, Verloove-Vanhorick SP. Infant crying and abuse. *Lancet*. 2004;364(9442):1340-1342.

U.S. Department of Health & Human Services, Administration for Children and Families, Administration on Children, Youth and Families, Children's Bureau. Child Maltreatment 2018. Published 2020. Accessed December 22, 2021. https://www.acf.hhs.gov/cb /research-data-technology /statistics-research/child-maltreatment

Shmerling RH. What exactly is cupping? *Harvard Health Blog*. June 22, 2020. https://www.health.harvard.edu/blog/what-exactly -is-cupping-2016093010402

Sugar NF, Taylor JA, Feldman KW. Bruises in infants and toddlers: those who don't cruise rarely bruise. Puget Sound Pediatric Research Network. *Arch Pediatr Adolesc Med*. 1999 Apr;153(4):399-403. doi:10.1001/archpedi.153.4.399

Tan A, Mallika P. Coining: an ancient treatment widely practiced among Asians. *Malays Fam Physician*. 2011;6(2-3):97-98.

Zahmani AR. Coining: what you need to know. CCHP Fact Sheets for Families. February 2010. Accessed November 9, 2021. https://cchp.ucsf.edu/sites/g/files/tkssra181/f/Coining_En0210.pdf

# CHAPTER 9

# Obstetric/Newborn Care and Congenital Birth Defects

## LESSON OBJECTIVES

- Review the physiologic changes of the pregnant patient.
- Differentiate between various complications that may occur during pregnancy.
- Discuss management and delivery using XABCDE and the Pediatric Assessment Triangle.
- Identify cardiopulmonary failure and management interventions in a newborn.
- Analyze congenital heart conditions.

## Introduction

The typical human gestational period is approximately 38 weeks, calculated by the first day of the last menstrual cycle. During this period, several physiologic changes occur in multiple organ systems. The pregnant patient's response to illness and trauma may deviate from what medical practitioners expect, due to altered compensatory mechanisms caused by these physiologic changes. In addition, underlying medical disorders may be aggravated during pregnancy. Thus, the typical pattern recognition used to aid prehospital practitioners in rapid diagnosis and treatment may be unreliable.

## Circulatory Changes

As the fetus grows and develops, the volume and content of the circulating blood changes. Red blood cell volume increases by up to 30% to accommodate the growing need to oxygenate rapidly developing tissues. A new circulatory system has been added in parallel with the mother's, and to perfuse this circuit, the maternal cardiac output must increase by up to 50%. This is accomplished by increasing the stroke volume by approximately 30% and by a modest elevation in the resting heart rate. To adequately filter and condition this new blood volume, circulation to the kidneys rises by nearly 80%. During labor, there is a significant rise in cardiac output—nearly 40%. Immediately postpartum it can increase even further.

## Respiratory Changes

As the fetus grows, abdominal pressure is placed on the diaphragm, causing a steady decline in the functional residual capacity (FRC) of the lungs. Despite the decline in FRC, the maternal minute ventilation must increase to facilitate oxygenation of the increased circulating blood volume. This is accomplished by increasing both tidal volume and respiratory rate. During labor, the minute ventilation may double or even triple.

## Renal Changes

The glomerular filtration rate (GFR) increases to 50% more than normal due to the increase in renal blood flow. The increased circulating blood volume and elevated GFR will cause the kidneys to increase in size by up to 30%. The bladder is positioned in such a way that the developing fetus places pressure on it, and pregnant women may experience the need to urinate more frequently (some women experience urinary incontinence).

## Gastrointestinal Changes

Relaxation of certain anatomic sphincters occurs in the pregnant female. Smooth muscle tone in some regions also changes. In the esophagus, these changes lead to increased gastroesophageal reflux and heartburn symptoms. They can also lead to an increased risk of aspiration during airway procedures or when lying flat with a decreased level of consciousness. Increased intra-abdominal pressure further complicates these issues. Intestinal transport time is increased, and constipation often becomes an issue. Pressure on the lower GI tract and decreased venous return can cause varicosities to arise in the form of hemorrhoids around the rectum and vagina.

## Endocrine Changes

The endogenous release of the hormone relaxin increases during pregnancy, causing maternal ligaments to soften. It also influences the vasculature, leading to vasodilation and decreased blood pressure. Thyroid hormone levels increase by approximately 50%. The release of endorphins and enkephalin is also elevated, causing the maternal pain tolerance to be higher. Overall free cortisol levels also rise.

**Table 9-1** summarizes the physiologic changes that occur during pregnancy.

## Fundal Height and Viability

The proper measurement of fundal height is an important skill and can be used to predict possible developmental problems. To properly measure the fundal height, place the patient on her back. Use a flexible tape measure and place the end at the pubic symphysis. Extend the tape to the highest palpable part of the uterus (**Figure 9-1**).

At approximately 20 weeks' gestation, the fundal height measurement correlation with gestational age becomes more accurate in most cases (**Figure 9-2**). The fundal height should have surpassed the maternal belly button by this point. **Table 9-2** describes the measured fundal height correlation with gestational age in weeks.

Deviations between measured fundal height and the reported gestational age could indicate potential pregnancy complications. These could include intrauterine growth restriction, oligo- or polyhydramnios, multiple fetuses, or breech positioning.

## Age of Viability

The consensus among medical practitioners is that 24 weeks of gestation represents the widely accepted age of viability—the age at which survival outside of the womb becomes possible. Survival in this gestational age range is only possible with extensive medical support. Although some neonates born prior to 24 weeks have survived, the survival rates are extremely low, and the medical comorbidities are high.

**Table 9-1** Physiologic Changes of Pregnancy

**Circulatory Changes**
- RBC count and blood volume increase
- Cardiac output increases
  - Stroke volume and heart rate increase
- Renal perfusion increases

**Respiratory Changes**
- FRC decreases
- Tidal volume and respiratory rate increase
  - Overall minute ventilation is increased

**Renal Changes**
- Increased kidney size
- Increased GFR and renal perfusion

**Gastrointestinal Changes**
- Reduced esophageal sphincter tone
- Increased GERD
- Increased risk for aspiration
- Constipation
- Hemorrhoids

**Endocrine Changes**
- Increase in the hormone relaxin
- Ligaments become more lax
- Thyroid hormone increases
- Endorphins and enkephalin are elevated
- Free cortisol rises

*Abbreviations*: FRC, functional residual capacity; GERD, gastroesophageal reflux disease; GFR, glomerular filtration rate; RBC, red blood cell

© Jones & Bartlett Learning.

The overall chances of survival for premature babies ranges from 0% prior to 22 weeks' gestation up to 80% at 27 weeks' gestation.

Past 26 weeks of gestation, premature neonate survival increases substantially. In some areas, the survival rate of neonates born past 26 weeks is as high as 90%. In general, the more access there is to specialized care, the higher the chances of survival. Mothers with access to prenatal care and high-risk medical practitioners tend to fare better than those without these resources.

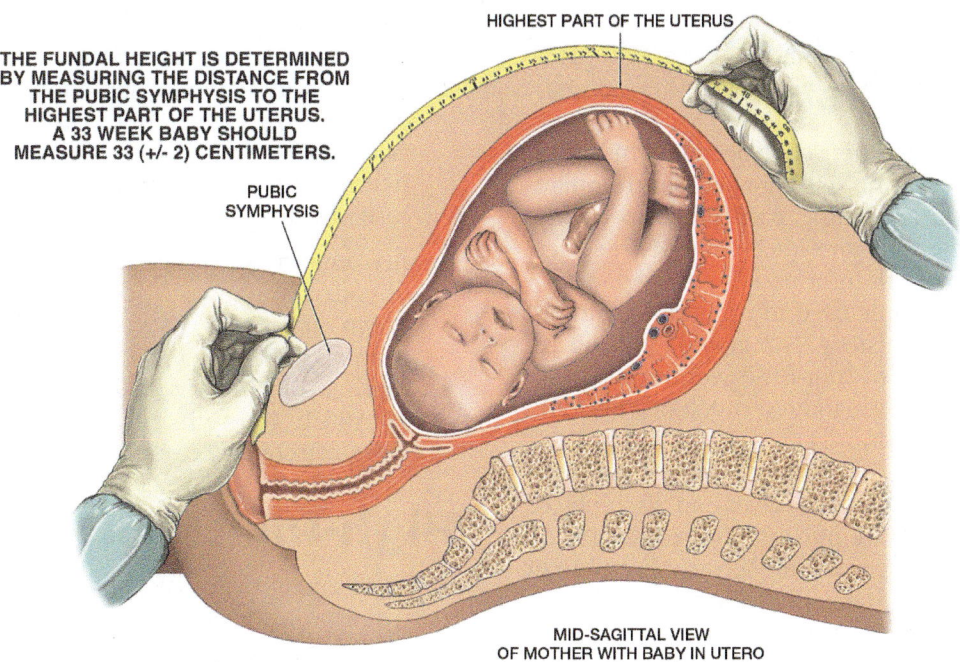

THE FUNDAL HEIGHT IS DETERMINED BY MEASURING THE DISTANCE FROM THE PUBIC SYMPHYSIS TO THE HIGHEST PART OF THE UTERUS. A 33 WEEK BABY SHOULD MEASURE 33 (+/- 2) CENTIMETERS.

HIGHEST PART OF THE UTERUS

PUBIC SYMPHYSIS

MID-SAGITTAL VIEW OF MOTHER WITH BABY IN UTERO

**Figure 9-1** Use a tape measure to measure from the pubic symphysis to the highest part of the uterus to capture fundal height.

© Nucleus Medical Media Inc/Alamy Stock Photo.

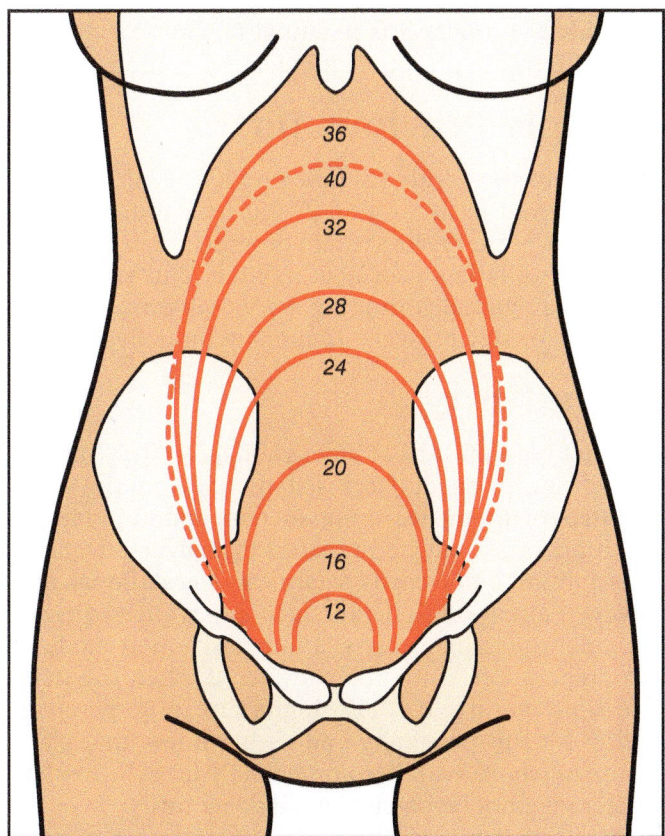

**Figure 9-2** Fundal height measurement should match gestational age. Around 37 to 40 weeks, the fundus moves down about 4 cm as the baby moves down into the pelvic cavity and the body prepares for birthing.

© Jones & Bartlett Learning.

| Table 9-2 Fundal Height and Gestational Age Correlates | |
|---|---|
| 12 weeks | ▪ The fundus rises above the pubic symphysis. |
| 12–20 weeks | ▪ The fundus lies somewhere between the pubic symphysis and the belly button. |
| | ▪ Positioning and height can be variable and difficult to gauge during this time. |
| 20–36 weeks | ▪ Fundal height surpasses 20 cm, and each additional cm in height should correlate with an additional gestational week. |
| | ▪ Viable gestational age is 24 weeks, or a fundal height of 24 cm. |
| | ▪ 26 weeks and beyond are considered extremely viable, with survival rates over 90% in some cases. |
| | ▪ At 36 weeks the fundal height will generally lie just below the xiphoid process. |
| 37–40 weeks | ▪ Fundal height may drop down by up to 4 cm as "lightening" occurs and the fetus drops into the pelvis prior to delivery. |

© Jones & Bartlett Learning.

# Documentation of Pregnancy History

Many prehospital practitioners have been taught how to document pregnancy using G/P (gravida/para) nomenclature. In the healthcare setting, particularly specialized obstetrics environments, more information is required, and documentation of this information is important.

GTPAL is a mnemonic used to properly document a complete pregnancy history. The gravida portion reflects the total number of times the woman has been pregnant, regardless of pregnancy outcome. Episodes of multiple fetuses are counted as one pregnancy. Para, which is a term used to document the number of pregnancies carried past 20 weeks' gestation, is replaced with a more detailed TPAL portion. The TPAL portion represents term births, premature births, abortions or miscarriages, and total living children. **Table 9-3** provides more information.

The following are some examples using the GTPAL charting style:

| Table 9-3 | GTPAL Documentation of Maternal Pregnancy History |
|---|---|
| G—Gravida | <ul><li>Total number of times the woman has been pregnant</li><li>All pregnancies are counted regardless of outcome</li><li>Pregnancies involving multiples are counted as a single pregnancy</li></ul> |
| T—Term | <ul><li>Number of births delivered at term</li><li>Any birth at 37 weeks and 0 days or later is included here</li></ul> |
| P—Preterm | <ul><li>Number of preterm births delivered between 20 weeks and 0 days to 36 weeks and 6 days gestation</li></ul> |
| A—Abortion | <ul><li>All pregnancies ending before 20 weeks and 0 days gestation</li><li>The term "abortion" includes spontaneous (miscarriage) and induced</li></ul> |
| L—Living | <ul><li>The number of currently living children</li></ul> |

- A woman reports she has been pregnant five times. She has had three miscarriages and delivered a set of triplets at 34 weeks' gestation. She is currently pregnant with twins. Her history would be charted as G5 T0 P3 A3 L3. This reflects 5 pregnancies, 0 term births, 3 preterm births, 3 abortions (in this case miscarriages), and 3 living children.

- A woman has just delivered a baby in the back of your ambulance. She reports this is her first pregnancy. She is 39 weeks along. The baby is doing well and currently being held by the mother. Her history would be charted as G1 T1 P0 A0 L1. This reflects 1 pregnancy, 1 term birth, 0 preterm births, 0 abortions, and 1 living child.

# High-Risk Deliveries

Obstetric emergencies can be considered high risk for many reasons. It is helpful to break down high-risk situations into three categories, as follows:

- Maternal factors
- Pregnancy factors
- Delivery factors

**Table 9-4** briefly lists potential factors that can increase the risk in obstetric emergency situations.

## Multiple Previous Births

Pregnant women with multiple previous births (sometimes referred to as "multips," short for multiparous) have an increased risk for rapid progression of delivery. They may only labor for a short time. This should be considered when determining if you will transport immediately or stay on scene to prepare for delivery.

## Prematurity

Neonates born prior to 36 weeks and 6 days have an increased risk for needing resuscitation beyond the standard steps of drying, warming, suction, and stimulation. Practitioners should be prepared to deliver advanced resuscitation to newborns regardless of gestational age; however, attention to details such as advanced airway equipment, vascular access, and resuscitation medication preparation should be considered when the neonate is premature. It is also important to prepare the mother for this possibility and let her know that placing the newborn with her immediately for skin-to-skin contact may not be possible in all situations.

## Multiple Gestation Pregnancies

Pregnancy with multiple gestations (twins, triplets, etc.) is associated with a higher risk of preterm birth,

**Table 9-4** Risk Factors in Obstetric Emergency Calls

| | |
|---|---|
| Maternal | • Multiple previous births<br>• Lack of prenatal care<br>• Substance abuse<br>• Pregnancy-induced medical emergencies:<br>  ◦ Preeclampsia<br>  ◦ Eclampsia<br>  ◦ HELLP syndrome<br>  ◦ Gestational diabetes<br>  ◦ Gestational hypertension<br>• Chronic, preexisting maternal diseases<br>  ◦ Autoimmune diseases<br>    ▫ Lupus<br>    ▫ Crohn disease<br>    ▫ Ulcerative colitis<br>  ◦ Thyroid disease<br>  ◦ Diabetes (nongestational)<br>  ◦ Mental health and psychiatric illness |
| Pregnancy | • Multiple gestation pregnancies<br>• Prematurity<br>• Congenital diseases<br>• Maternal infection or fever<br>• Large or small for gestational age |
| Delivery | • Placenta abruptio<br>• Placenta previa<br>• Breech presentation<br>• Nuchal cord<br>• Prolapsed cord<br>• Meconium |

*Abbreviation*: HELLP, hemolysis, elevated liver enzymes, and low platelets

© Jones & Bartlett Learning.

low birthweight, and need for advanced resuscitation. These neonates will likely require specialized care at a facility with high-level neonatal intensive care unit (NICU) resources.

When field delivery is imminent, additional personnel should be summoned so that adequate attention can be given to mother and babies. The receiving facility should also be notified so that additional NICU teams can be placed on standby for your arrival.

## Meconium

Meconium is the first stool passed by a neonate. This is often thick, green/brown material that is particularly sticky and viscous. When the fetus is stressed or carried past the projected due date, this first stool may be passed in utero. The presence of meconium itself is not an emergency, however it indicates that the fetus is in distress and there is a possibility that the meconium could be aspirated.

Resuscitation for newborns where meconium is noted progresses no differently than resuscitation for other newborns. The only exception is that in cases where there is high suspicion for aspiration of meconium, earlier placement of an advanced airway may be considered.

## Placental Abnormalities

The placenta is vital for fetal health. It helps oxygenate the fetus and process metabolic waste products. Placental abnormalities can arise from several issues, such as the following:

- Positioning
  - Implantation in certain areas may make delivery or cesarean section more difficult or impossible.
  - Positioning over the cervical os can lead to severe hemorrhage.
- Circulation
  - Poor perfusion to the placenta can lead to placental insufficiency, which in turn leads to poor fetal growth and development.
  - Certain illicit substances, such as cocaine and other stimulants, can stunt the growth of the placental vessels and decrease perfusion.
  - Premature separation of the placenta can lead to poor perfusion, bleeding, and fetal demise.

Specific placental emergencies are discussed in more detail next.

### Placenta Previa

The most common location for placental implantation is the uterine fundus. This position allows space for the fetus to transit the birth canal. When the placenta implants in such a manner that it covers the cervical opening, it is called placenta previa (**Figure 9-3**). During the pregnancy, complications from placenta previa are minimal. Once labor starts, and the cervix

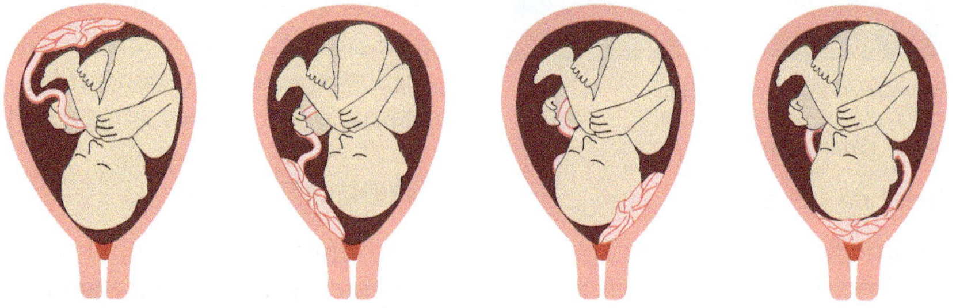

PLACENTA PREVIA

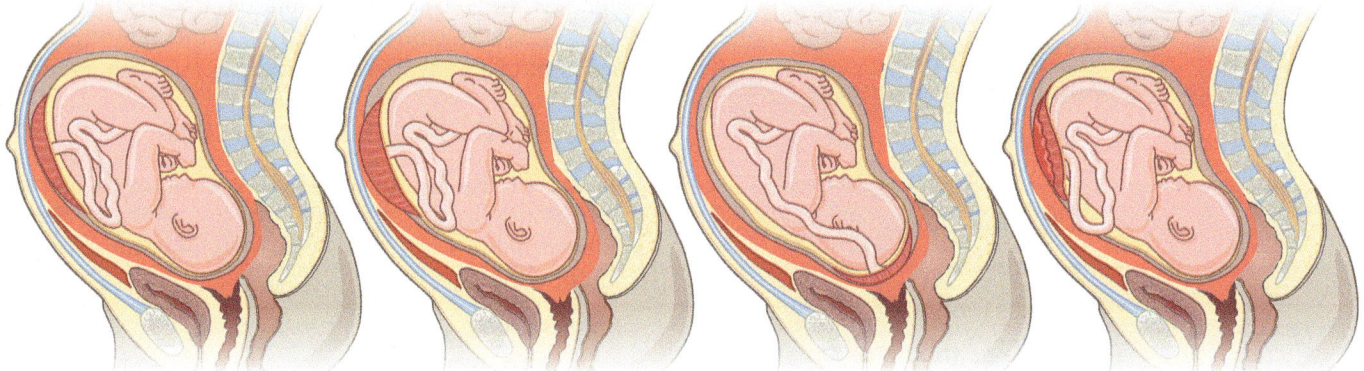

NORMAL          MARGINAL          PARTIAL          TOTAL
PLACENTA

**Figure 9-3** Placenta previa is an abnormal implantation of the placenta on the lower half of the uterine wall, partially or completely covering the cervical opening.
© Betty Ray/Shutterstock.

**Figure 9-4** In placenta abruptio, the placenta separates from the uterus before childbirth. Consider the extent of separation (partial or complete) and the location of separation (marginal or central).
© Jones & Bartlett Learning.

begins to dilate, the vessels that communicate between the placenta and uterus are sheared, and the placental tissue tears. Because of the highly vascular nature of the placenta and the significant amount of blood flow the organ receives, tearing of these tissues is associated with the potential for massive hemorrhage, putting both mother and fetus at risk.

Risk factors for placenta previa include prior occurrences of the condition, multiple gestations, and advanced maternal age, among others.

Placenta previa is usually painless. It will present with moderate to large amounts of bright red blood, usually in the third trimester. Hypotension may be present along with tachycardia. Remember that pregnant women have an elevated heart rate at baseline and their blood pressure response to hypovolemia may be delayed due to increased circulating volume.

Prehospital interventions for placenta previa are limited. The most important step is to recognize the condition and transport rapidly to the closest appropriate facility. A sanitary pad should be placed over the

vagina and attempts should be made to keep track of blood loss. Place the patient in the left lateral recumbent position. Establish large-bore intravenous (IV) access and treat for hypovolemic shock. The patient will likely require a highly skilled obstetrics team and the use of large quantities of blood products, so plan your transport destination appropriately, per local protocols.

## Placenta Abruptio

During normal labor and delivery, the fetus is delivered, and shortly after, the placenta separates and delivers. Ideally, the neonate has been delivered when this separation occurs and there should be no more reliance on the placenta for oxygenation and blood conditioning. In some situations, the placenta separates early, or abruptly, leading to a condition known as placenta abruptio (abruptio placentae; **Figure 9-4**).

Placenta abruptio can be categorized by the location and severity (how much) of the segment that has separated.

- Partial abruptions are described by the location of the segment that has detached.

  - Marginal

    - Separation occurs along the margins of the placenta and bleeding is usually present.

  - Central

    - Separation occurs at the center of the placenta.

    - The margins may stay attached, leading to a buildup of blood under the placenta. Bleeding may not be apparent in these situations.

- Complete abruptions occur when the placenta is completely separated from the uterine wall.

  - Blood loss in these situations can be significant.

  - In some instances, depending on the location of the fetus and the detached placenta, bleeding may be concealed for a period of time.

Bleeding from placenta abruptio is usually darker than from placenta previa. The peak incidence for this condition is around 25 weeks' gestation. Trauma is the most common cause for premature separation.

Signs of placenta abruptio include painful vaginal bleeding around the 25th week of gestation, maternal hypotension, tachycardia, and other signs of distress. In the setting of trauma, bleeding from the vagina of a pregnant women should be considered abruptio placenta until proven otherwise.

Prehospital treatment includes placing sanitary pads on the vagina to estimate blood loss, transport in the left lateral recumbent position, and treatment for hypotension and shock. Fetal distress may be present before maternal distress. Packing of the vagina is contraindicated.

### PLACENTA ABRUPTIO VERSUS PLACENTA PREVIA

Differentiating placenta abruptio from placenta previa can be difficult. It may be helpful to remember:

**Placenta abruptio—painful always**

**Placenta previa—practically painless**

Any bleeding that is painful and associated with trauma or cocaine use should be considered placenta abruptio until proven otherwise. Painless bleeding that is bright red and profuse in the absence of trauma or drug use is suspicious for placenta previa.

When possible, fetal monitoring should be performed. The patient will likely require a highly skilled obstetrics team and the use of large quantities of blood products, so plan your transport destination appropriately.

## Preeclampsia

Preeclampsia is a disorder of pregnancy in which there is hypertension and some form of end-organ dysfunction present in a previously normotensive woman. Hypertension in this case is defined as systolic greater than 140 mm Hg and/or diastolic greater than 90 mm Hg. The blood pressure should be confirmed—usually within about 4 hours. In severe cases (the likely scenario when emergency medical services [EMS] has been called) the confirmatory blood pressure can be taken within a few minutes.

In addition to hypertension, some form of end-organ dysfunction must also be present. The classic example is protein in the urine, representing some element of renal dysfunction. Other examples of end-organ dysfunction that could herald preeclampsia include the following:

- Peripheral edema

- Severe headaches

- Visual disturbance such as floating spots, light sensitivity, blurred vision, or temporary loss of vision

- Nausea and/or vomiting

- Abdominal and/or shoulder pain, usually on the upper right side representing possible liver involvement

- Shortness of breath

- Decreased urination

The precise pathogenesis of preeclampsia is not completely known; however, it is related to a maternal reaction to the placenta. Risk factors include high blood pressure during the patient's most recent pregnancy, obesity, twins/triplets or more, and a chronic history of hypertension or diabetes. Birth and delivery of the placenta is curative, although in some limited cases the condition can persist or recur in the following days to weeks. Although uncommon, preeclampsia can develop within the first 6 weeks following delivery (usually within the first 48 hours postpartum). For this reason it is important to consider preeclampsia in your differential diagnosis when treating a patient who recently delivered a baby.

Prehospital management for preeclampsia is to guard the airway, breathing, and circulation and optimize maternal oxygenation to protect the fetus. Electrocardiogram (ECG) monitoring along with vascular access is important. Mothers will often be volume depleted because of increased proteinuria; however, fluids should be used judiciously as the patient will be hypertensive.

## Eclampsia

Eclampsia can be seen as a progression of untreated, severe preeclampsia. The condition occurs when the criteria for preeclampsia are met and the woman's condition progresses to involve uncontrolled grand mal seizures in the setting of no known seizure disorder. All symptoms of preeclampsia are possible, along with progression to hyperreflexia, oliguria, neurologic deficits, anxiety, and confusion.

The management of eclampsia is the same as for preeclampsia, however the urgency is much higher. Optimal magnesium sulfate dosing for the treatment of preeclampsia and eclampsia has not been identified, so administration should follow local protocols. Magnesium sulfate is thought to trigger cerebral vasodilation, which is why it is used to help prevent seizures in women as well as manage seizure activity. Before administering, ensure the patient has an adequate respiratory rate (usually greater than 16 breaths/min), as effects of magnesium can cause breathing difficulties. The patient should be closely monitored for signs of toxicity, such as hypotension. If toxicity develops, calcium gluconate can be administered per local protocols.

If IV access cannot be obtained, there are recommendations for intramuscular (IM) dosing. A 10-gram IM loading dose of magnesium sulfate can be administered. To accomplish this, the dose should be divided into two syringes, and 5 grams administered into each buttock, to be given every 4 hours as needed.

> Neonates born to mothers who have been on a magnesium infusion will often have poor tone and can have respiratory depression. They may require more assistance breathing and advanced care while the magnesium wears off.

## Abnormal Fetal Presentations

### Bulging Sac

When you check for crowning, there may be instances in which all you can see is a bulging amniotic sac (**Figure 9-5**). In an otherwise uncomplicated pregnancy and birth (full term, adequate prenatal care, etc.), this is not an issue. Medical practitioners may use a gloved

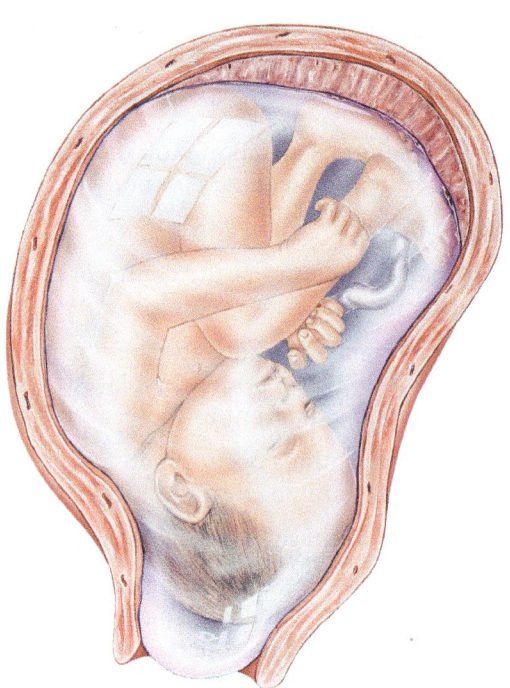

**Figure 9-5** A bulging sac refers to presentation of the amniotic sac on cervical exam.
© Medical Art Inc/Shutterstock.

### HELLP SYNDROME

HELLP syndrome is a rare condition (occurring in 1–2 of 1,000 pregnancies) related to the spectrum of preeclampsia and eclampsia. The hallmark triad symptoms are Hemolysis, Elevated Liver enzymes, and Low Platelets (hence the name).

This is specified as a distinct pathology because the triad of hemolysis, transaminitis, and low platelets are rarely seen in isolation—when one is present, the other two are most likely present or evolving. When severe right upper quadrant pain is present you should consider HELLP syndrome as part of your differential diagnosis. HELLP usually develops in the third trimester of pregnancy but can develop as late as the first week postpartum.

HELLP is a true emergency and requires urgent management by specialized staff in a hospital with advanced maternal–fetal capabilities.

finger to pinch and shear the sac so that it may rupture and delivery can proceed, if allowed by local protocols.

In preterm labor, rupturing the sac is not recommended as it would expose the fetus to the outside environment and bacteria may ascend the birth canal, leading to infection.

## Prolapsed Cord

When a medical practitioner checks for crowning, ideally they should see the top of the fetal head. When the umbilical cord is noted to be the presenting part, this is termed *prolapsed cord* (**Figure 9-6**). Umbilical cord prolapse is an uncommon complication, but it has the potential for severe consequences if not managed appropriately. As the mother continues to push and

the head engages into the pelvis, increasing pressure is placed on the umbilical cord, causing fetal hypoxia and distress.

Multiple births, breech positioning, and shoulder dystocia all increase the risk for prolapsed cord.

When a prolapsed cord is noted, the mother should immediately be placed in a knee-chest position with her hips elevated. Coach the mother not to push as this will increase fetal hypoxia. Rapid transport to a medical facility capable of performing an emergent cesarean section and managing advanced resuscitation of both mother and baby is recommended. The receiving facility should be explicitly notified that there is a prolapsed cord so they can have resources in place to expedite the performance of the emergency c-section.

## Nuchal Cord

A nuchal cord occurs when the umbilical cord loops around the neck of the fetus during birth (**Figure 9-7**). In some cases the cord may even wrap more than once around the neck (double or triple nuchal cord). This presents a risk for tightening and entrapment as the baby progresses down the birth canal.

In most instances of a single nuchal cord, the issue can be resolved by working a finger under the cord and slipping the nuchal segment off the neonate's head. Labor and delivery can progress normally from that point. If the cord is too tight to accomplish this, then clamps should be placed approximately 2 to 4 inches apart and the segment should be cut to facilitate release of the wrapped segment. This is a treatment of last resort as labor will need to progress rapidly after this point, because the baby is no longer receiving placental support.

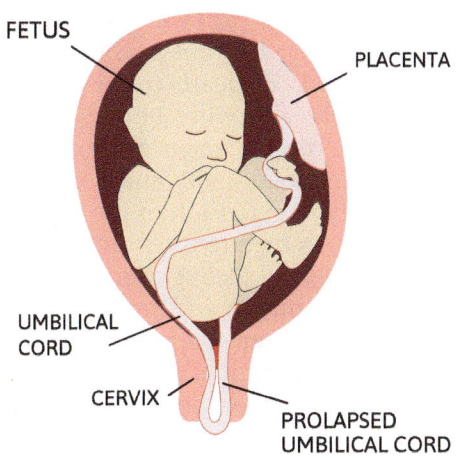

**Figure 9-6** Umbilical cord prolapse is an uncommon but deadly complication.
© Betty Ray/Shutterstock.

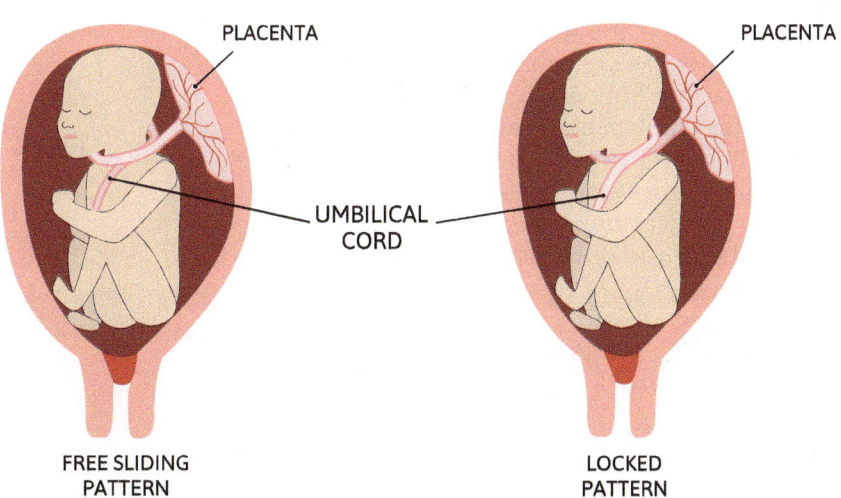

NUCHAL CORDS

**Figure 9-7** A nuchal cord refers to a situation in which the umbilical cord is wrapped around the neck of the fetus during birth.
© Betty Ray/Shutterstock.

## Breech Presentation

Breech presentation is when any part other than the head presents at the cervix (**Figure 9-8**). Breech presentations come in three forms:

- Frank breech
  - The baby's buttocks present first. Both hips are flexed and both knees are extended, resulting in a "folded in half" position with the feet up by the head.
  - This accounts for the majority (66%) of breech presentations.
- Complete breech
  - The baby's hips *and* knees are flexed bilaterally, placing the feet adjacent to the buttocks.
  - In this situation, there may be a limb presentation at the cervix.
- Incomplete breech
  - Both hips are flexed with one knee flexed and one knee extended.
  - This results in one foot by the head and one foot adjacent to the buttocks.
  - In this situation, there may be a limb presentation at the cervix.

The main issue with breech presentation is that the cervix does not open in the same manner that it does in a head-first delivery. This makes successful delivery difficult. Breech presentations also increase the risk for cord prolapse, further complicating matters.

In situations where delivery is not imminent, place the mother in the knee-chest position with the hips elevated and transport rapidly to the closest appropriate facility, providing supportive care along the way.

If delivery is imminent, prepare as you normally would and notify the receiving facility. Support the feet or buttocks as they deliver. As the trunk delivers, allow the feet to dangle while providing support to the delivering torso. The head will typically deliver facedown. If there is difficulty with the head completely passing through the birth canal, this is the only instance when inserting gloved fingers into the vagina is recommended. Place your fingers into a "V" shape and insert them into the vagina, creating a pocket of space to allow for the neonate to breathe. Blow-by oxygen can be administered if necessary.

## Shoulder Dystocia

Shoulder dystocia occurs when the fetal shoulders are too broad or the maternal pelvis is too narrow to facilitate delivery (**Figure 9-9**). Risk factors include maternal diabetes (resulting in large for gestational age neonates), postdate pregnancy, and maternal obesity.

One sign that shoulder dystocia may be present is the "turtle" sign, where there will be some progression of the head, and then it retreats into the birth canal after the contraction finishes and the mother stops pushing.

If delivery is delayed or not possible, fetal distress increases and hypoxia or death could occur. The risk for birth injuries increases with the presence of shoulder dystocia. While clavicle fracture is possible, it is rare due to the increased joint laxity and bone compliance of the newborn. Hyperextension of the shoulder girdle during delivery places high tension on the nerve structures within the brachial plexus. Nerve injuries to the brachial plexus are common due to shearing of the nervous tissues as extreme tension is applied during birth. Palsies of the upper extremities may be seen. These can be extremely life limiting for the newborn as they grow and develop. Erb's palsy is a common form of brachial plexus palsy in which the infant's affected limb hangs from the shoulder and the wrist and hand is in flexion.

Management of shoulder dystocia involves the McRoberts maneuver, in which the mother's hips are

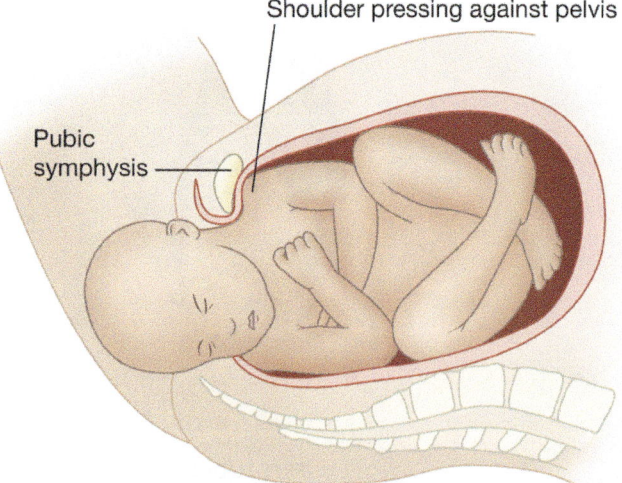

**Figure 9-9** Shoulder dystocia occurs when the fetal shoulders are too broad or the maternal pelvis is too narrow to facilitate unassisted delivery.

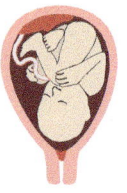 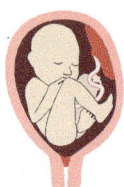 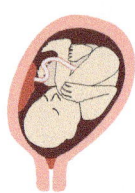 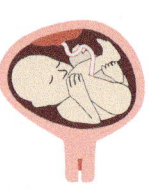

CEPHALIC BREECH OBLIQUE TRANSVERSE

**Figure 9-8** Breech presentation complicates delivery and increases the risk for cord prolapse.

hyperflexed to allow for more room to pass the anterior shoulder. Suprapubic pressure can be applied to the mother to guide the shoulder down and engage the birth canal. With shoulder dystocia and other abnormal fetal presentations, follow local protocols for management. Rapid transport to a facility capable of emergency c-section and advanced neonatal care is recommended.

## CASE STUDY

### Case 1

#### Dispatch

You and your partner respond for an 18-year-old female in labor. It is a mild spring morning with a temperature of 60°F (15.6°C).

#### Case Questions

- What are your initial concerns?
  - This is an 18-year-old in labor. Young mothers are at risk for having inadequate access to prenatal health care. It will be important to determine if her pregnancy has been complicated by any medical conditions or social issues.
- Based on the dispatch information, what is the possible differential diagnosis for this patient?
  - This could be "false labor," or Braxton-Hicks contractions.
  - This could also be true labor and medical practitioners should be prepared for potential complications.
- What equipment should be prepared and brought on scene in cases where imminent delivery might be present?
  - A full obstetric kit should be ready for use on all calls where delivery is possible. This kit should include:
    - Sterile scalpel or scissors
    - Disposable towels and drapes
    - Receiving blanket
    - Bulb suction syringe
    - Umbilical clamps or ties
    - Large plastic bag to contain the delivered placenta
    - Plastic-lined underpads
    - Gown, mask, face shield, and gloves for personal protective equipment (PPE)
    - Oxygen and airway bag for both mother and a newborn
    - Pediatric bag with supplies for newborn resuscitation if needed
- What measures can be taken to prepare the patient compartment in the back of the ambulance for potential delivery and transport?
  - Consider the need for additional equipment and resources if there are complications with the mother or baby, and stage equipment appropriately.
  - Start warming the ambient environment to avoid hypothermia. Turn off air conditioning and turn up the heat. The environment should be borderline uncomfortably warm for prehospital practitioners—this helps decrease the chances that the newborn will be unintentionally cooled to the point of hypothermia.
- If there is family on scene, it may be helpful to give them tasks so that they can help. This will also aid in keeping the delivery environment clear and controlled. What tasks might be appropriate for family members to perform during a home delivery?
  - Consider having someone place towels or linens in a dryer to warm them up so that the baby can be swaddled in a warm blanket.
  - Have family members begin to clear a path so that the mother can be wheeled out on the stretcher when ready for transport.
  - It is important to ask the mother who she wants in the room and who she does not. It is completely appropriate to ask individuals to leave the delivery environment if the mother requests. The mother is entitled to as much privacy as possible during delivery.
  - Allowing the patient's partner or support person to stay in the delivery environment when possible is important if the mother wishes for them to be present. This is a once in a lifetime moment, and normalizing it as much as possible should be the goal.

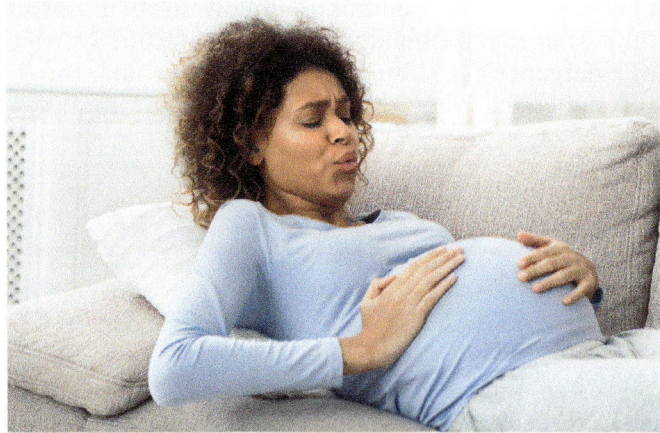

**Figure 9-10** The patient appears to have started labor.
© Prostock-studio/Shutterstock.

## Initial Observations

As you arrive at the front entrance of the residence you are met by the patient's mother, who appears very anxious. She states that the patient's water broke a few hours ago. They tried to wait until the doctor's office was open for the day, but the contractions became so frequent they were concerned that the baby might be about to come. She leads you to the living room where you see the patient lying on the couch, clearly breathing through a contraction (**Figure 9-10**). She is alert and oriented with good signs of circulation and an intact airway and respiratory status.

### Case Questions

- Based on the initial observations, what additional steps might be warranted at this point?

  - If you determine that delivery is imminent, it may be safer to move the mother to a firm flat surface.

  - Delivery of a baby in the back of the ambulance during transport is not ideal and poses a greater risk than delaying transport and delivering on scene in most cases.

  - In cases where delivery has not occurred within 30 minutes, it is reasonable to initiate transport. Contact medical control in these cases for guidance.

  - It may be reasonable to call for a second transport team as there will be two patients on this scene very shortly. Call for backup personnel sooner rather than later.

  - Have a family member gather linens so that fluids and potential incontinence can be contained.

> If contractions are more than 5 minutes apart, delivery is likely not imminent. Once contractions are spaced 5 minutes or less apart, delivery will begin to progress more rapidly.
>
> Any situation in which crowning is visualized or any other fetal part is present at the level of the vagina indicates imminent delivery.

As you are talking with the patient's mother, you are interrupted by the patient screaming, "Help! The baby is coming and I need to push right now!!!"

The decision to transport without delay or to deliver on scene is difficult to make. There are multiple factors that could sway your decision. In most cases, a full-term pregnancy with no prenatal complications can proceed with little risk for resuscitation or complication. If delivery is imminent in these cases, it is reasonable to contact additional resources and attempt delivery on scene prior to transport.

In cases where the patient is preterm or significant prenatal complications have been identified, or if there is a life-threatening condition present in the mother such as placental abnormality or hypertensive emergency (preeclampsia, eclampsia, HELLP) then it is reasonable to initiate transport as rapidly as possible to an appropriate facility. It is likely that significant resources will be needed and there is a high likelihood that mother, baby, or both will require advanced resuscitation. Contact medical control in cases where you are unsure if delivery on scene or rapid transport is necessary.

Make sure you know what facilities around you have advanced resuscitation capabilities and access to advanced neonatal care if necessary. Facilities specializing in high-risk obstetrics and neonatology should are preferred, if available.

## Primary Survey

The primary survey for this patient reveals the following:

**X**—No bleeding is noted.

**A**—The airway is open and patent.

**B**—Respirations are rapid with mild to moderate retractions, but slow in between contractions to an appropriate rate and work of breathing.

**C**—Radial pulses are strong, regular, and rapid. Capillary refill is brisk. The skin is warm and diaphoretic.

**D**—Alert and anxious. Glasgow Coma Scale (GCS) score is 15 (E4, V5, M6).

**E**—The patient is lying on the couch. Her fundus is at the level of the xiphoid. Contractions are coming every 3 minutes or so. A quick visual exam of the vagina reveals crowning is present.

## Case Questions

- Based on your initial impression, is this patient "Quick" or "Not Quick"?

  - This patient qualifies as "Quick," however rapid transport might not be the best decision in this case. Crowning has been noted, and contractions are 3 minutes apart. The mother strongly feels the urge to push. These are all signs that delivery is imminent.

- What questions should be asked that will help you evaluate the risk for complication with the delivery?

  - How far along is she?

    - This patient is at 36 weeks' gestation. Preterm births (36 weeks' gestation or fewer) are more likely to present with complications and/or require resuscitation.

  - Has she been pregnant before? If so, what were the outcomes?

    - This is the patient's first pregnancy. Labor generally progresses more slowly in a woman who has not given birth previously. Also, complications in prior pregnancies suggest an increased risk of similar complications in the current pregnancy.

  - Has the mother received regular prenatal care?

    - Regular prenatal care increases the chances that health issues with mother or baby are identified and treated earlier, before they pose significant risk.

    - Medical conditions such as diabetes, hypertension, and underlying cardiac or pulmonary disease place the mother and baby at increased risk, especially if they are not followed appropriately by a physician.

  - Is the mother on any prescribed medications?

    - Some prescription drugs have associations with fetal birth defects.

    - Knowing what prescription medications the mother is taking may aid in revealing underlying health conditions.

  - Has the mother used any illicit substances during this pregnancy?

    - It is important to ask this question in a nonjudgmental manner. Emphasize that this question is asked for all mothers, and the information is only necessary to make sure you can take care of both her and the baby.

    - Some mothers may be afraid to answer this question honestly as they fear that the baby may be taken away from them by child protective services.

    - The more rapport you can build with the mother, the more likely you are to get an honest answer that facilitates excellent care for both her and the baby.

    - Know what illicit or prescription drugs might cause respiratory depression, hypoglycemia, agitation, or other complications for both mother and baby. In general, it is best to assume that any substance the mother may have taken can cross the placenta and impact the baby's health.

  - Has the patient participated in any high-risk activities during the pregnancy?

    - Alcohol use, tobacco and/or nicotine ingestion, multiple sexual partners, unprotected sex, poor diet, and eating disorders can all negatively impact fetal health.

- What potential complications should you be prepared for?

  - Excessive bleeding is the most common complication during delivery. The expected blood loss with delivery is approximately 500 mL. When blood loss reaches 1,250–1,500 mL, hypotension and hemodynamic collapse can ensue.

- What is your initial treatment for this patient?

  - Treatment should focus on preparation for delivery of the newborn on scene.

  - Call for additional resources to help manage the baby once they have been born.

  - Prepare and stage all obstetric equipment so that it is ready when the baby is born.

  - If time permits, contact online medical direction and inform them that you are preparing for the field delivery of a newborn and will update them if complications arise. This will allow them to mobilize resources and potentially have specialized physicians available for consultation if necessary.

## Stages of Labor

Normal labor and delivery is divided into four stages. Table 9-5 describes these stages in more detail.

## Post-Delivery Care for Mother

After the baby is born and any necessary resuscitation has taken place, it is important to place the baby skin-to-skin with the mother if it is safe to do so. Even though milk may not be being produced and the newborn's suck may be weak, stimulation of the breast and nipple tissue will prompt contraction of the uterus and help with delivery of the placenta and tamponade of uterine bleeding. Massaging of the uterine fundus may also help but avoid aggressive uterine massage as it may disrupt blood clots and lead to uterine atony.

The mother's perineum should be inspected for tears. Direct pressure should be used to stop any external hemorrhage. Never pack any wounds unless instructed to do so by medical control. If packing does take place, it is important to keep a careful count of any pads used, to estimate blood loss and ensure that any sponges used are accounted for and not retained in the vagina.

Vital signs should be continuously monitored and any signs of shock should be treated aggressively. IV access should be obtained if it has not been already and fluids administered if indicated.

| Table 9-5 Stages of Labor | |
|---|---|
| First | ■ Begins with the onset of contractions and ends when the cervix is fully dilated |
| | ■ Contractions last approximately 45 seconds and are spaced 5–30 minutes apart initially |
| | ■ The amniotic sac may rupture and the mucus plug may be expelled (bloody show) |
| | ■ Active labor begins as contractions become more frequent and longer in duration (60 seconds in length, 5 minutes apart) |
| | ■ Cervix dilation begins |
| | ■ Fetus begins to descend into the pelvis and cranial molding takes place |
| | ■ Contractions increase in frequency as the transition phase begins, coming every 2–3 minutes |
| | ■ The cervix becomes fully dilated at 10 cm, ending the first stage of labor and signaling the transition to the second stage |
| Second | ■ Begins with full dilation of the cervix and ends with birth of the neonate |
| | ■ Often referred to as the pushing stage |
| | ■ Contractions lengthen to approximately 90 seconds in duration with 3–5 minutes in between |
| | ■ The baby descends more with each contraction as the abdominal muscles begin to help |
| | ■ The baby will make slow progress, moving forward with contractions, and slightly backward in between, progressing slightly farther with each successive push |
| Third | ■ Begins when the baby is completely delivered and ends with delivery of the placenta |
| | ■ The uterus begins to contract again, separating the placenta from the uterine wall |
| | ■ The uterine contractions also tamponade off any bleeding vessels and slow any remaining hemorrhage |
| | ■ The placenta is ultimately expelled within approximately 5–30 minutes after birth |
| Fourth | ■ May be referred to as the postpartum stage |
| | ■ The first hour after delivery |
| | ■ Mother–baby bonding takes place. Skin-to-skin contact is important |
| | ■ Hormonal changes begin the process of colostrum production |

Do not delay transport to deliver the placenta. It should deliver within 15 to 30 minutes after the delivery of the newborn. Placental delivery usually occurs spontaneously and is rarely an emergency. Once the placenta is delivered it is important to place it in a bag for inspection by a physician trained in pathology at the receiving hospital. Visually examine the placenta to determine if there are any tears or pieces missing. Any portion of the placenta that is retained in the uterus or vagina can cause severe infection and sepsis in the mother.

Postpartum hemorrhage should not exceed 500 mL of blood loss. Once blood loss exceeds this amount the risk for shock increases. Use sponges to absorb blood. These can be weighed at the receiving hospital to estimate blood loss. Visual estimates of blood loss often underestimate severity.

## Detailed Assessment

### History Taking

As your partner prepares the equipment for delivery and you await the arrival of additional resources, you begin to take a detailed history.

**OPQRST:**

- **O**nset: Intermittent with contractions every 2 to 3 minutes lasting approximately 50 seconds
- **P**rovocation/palliation: Pain is contraction induced.
- **Q**uality: Intense achy back pain with pressure felt in the pelvis
- **R**adiation: Back and lower abdomen
- **S**everity: 10/10 during contractions
- **T**iming: 2 hours

**SAMPLER:**

- **S**igns/symptoms: Labor with contractions
- **A**llergies: No known allergies to medications, foods, or the environment
- **M**edications: Prenatal vitamins
- **P**ast medical history: Primigravida, adequate prenatal care, denies any medical problems or prescription medications, denies illicit drug use
- **L**ast oral intake: Dinner yesterday evening
- **E**vents leading up to the emergency: Has gotten considerably worse over the last 2 hours since her water broke
- **R**isk factors: 40 weeks' pregnant

### Vital Signs

As you were discussing the history, the patient was attached to the monitor and the following vital signs were obtained (**Figure 9-11**):

**Heart rate:**

- 101 beats/min
- Expected tachycardia during active labor

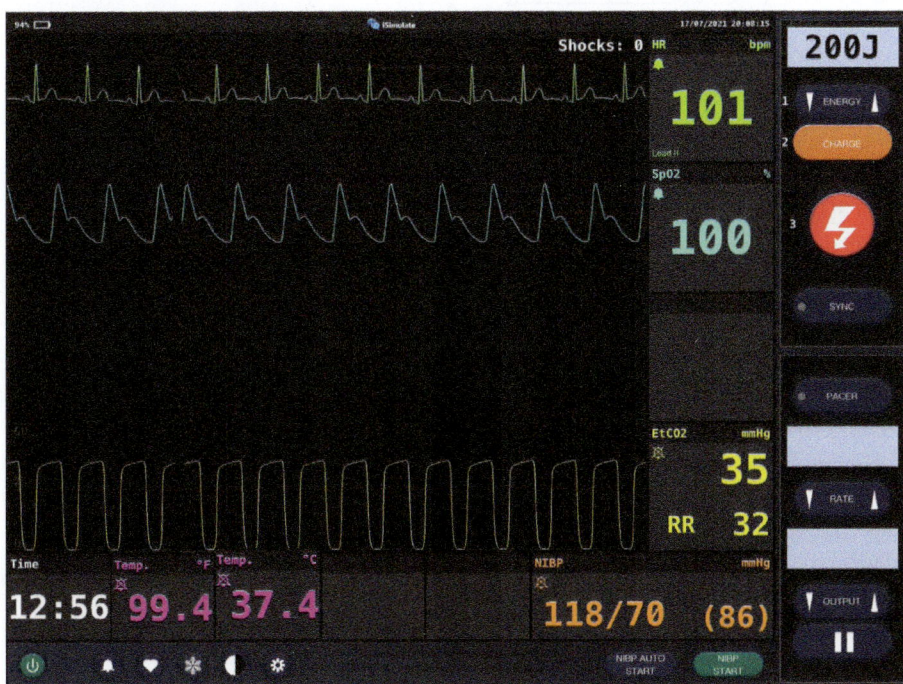

**Figure 9-11** The patient's vital signs are consistent with a patient in labor.
Courtesy of iSimulate.

**SpO$_2$:**

- 100% on room air (RA)

**ETCO$_2$:**

- 35 mm Hg

**Respiratory rate:**

- 32 breaths/min

- Expected tachypnea during active labor

**Blood pressure:**

- 118/70 mm Hg

**Temperature:**

- 99.4°F (37.4°C)

**Blood glucose:**

- 107 mg/dL

You determine that the fetal heart rate is 125 beats/min.

### Case Questions

- What is the expected fetal heart rate during active labor?

  - The expected fetal heart rate in active labor is 140–180 beats/min. Lower or higher heart rates can indicate fetal depression and stress states.

The patient is an 18-year-old female who is G1 T0 P0 A0 L0 at 40 weeks' gestation likely in the second stage of active labor. She is full term and there are no major risk factors for a complicated delivery identified on history or exam. Delivery is imminent based on visualization of crowning and the frequency and duration of contractions (**Figure 9-12**). The EMS crew should prepare for delivery at the scene. Additional resources are en route.

## Detailed Exam

**HEENT:**

- **H**ead: Unremarkable

- **E**yes: PERRL

- **E**ars: Unremarkable

- **N**ose: Unremarkable

- **T**hroat: Unremarkable

**Chest, heart, and lungs:**

- Pulses: Strong peripheral and central pulses palpated

- Cardiac auscultation: Regular rate and rhythm, no rubs, gallops, or murmurs appreciated

- Lung auscultation: Clear in all fields bilaterally

- Chest exam: Unremarkable

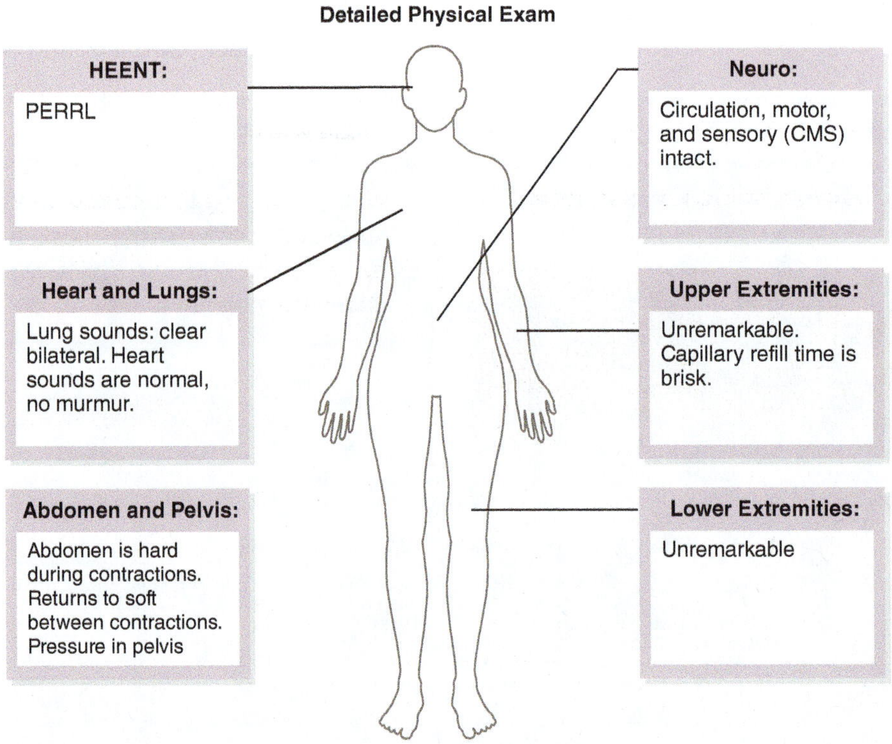

**Detailed Physical Exam**

**HEENT:**

PERRL

**Neuro:**

Circulation, motor, and sensory (CMS) intact.

**Heart and Lungs:**

Lung sounds: clear bilateral. Heart sounds are normal, no murmur.

**Upper Extremities:**

Unremarkable. Capillary refill time is brisk.

**Abdomen and Pelvis:**

Abdomen is hard during contractions. Returns to soft between contractions. Pressure in pelvis

**Lower Extremities:**

Unremarkable

**Figure 9-12** The patient's secondary survey reveals strong pulses and a crowning fetus.

**Neurologic:**

- Neurovascular status intact

**Abdomen and pelvis:**

- Abdomen is hard during contractions. Gravid uterus palpated with fundal height of approximately 39 cm.

**Genitourinary:**

- Crowning is visible. No evidence of frank bleeding. No evidence of prolapsed cord or placenta previa. There is evidence of thick brown/green discharge consistent with meconium present.

**Extremities:**

- Upper extremities: Unremarkable. Capillary refill is brisk.
- Lower extremities: Unremarkable

**Back:**

- Unremarkable

## Case Progression

Given that the baby is crowning and the mother feels the urge to push, the decision to deliver on scene was made (**Figure 9-13**). There is thick, green meconium noted during the delivery.

Given that there is meconium present it is likely this fetus is in distress. This is further backed up by the fact that fetal heart tones were slightly depressed. In addition to the steps taken for a routine delivery, practitioners should be prepared to provide aggressive airway management and resuscitation if the newborn does not respond to the routine steps of newborn care, which include drying, warmth, suction, and stimulation.

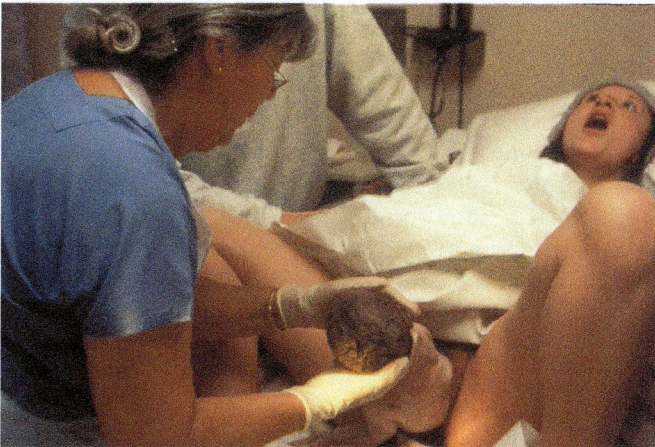

**Figure 9-13** When the baby is crowning and the mother feels the urge to push, the decision to deliver on scene may be made.
© Angela Hampton Picture Library/Alamy Stock Photo.

A meconium aspirator may be useful if thick meconium is noted in the nares or oropharynx.

## Initial Steps for Newborn Care

There is a mnemonic that can be used to remember the initial steps of newborn care: Do What Probably Seems Simple (**Figure 9-14**). This stands for the following:

- Dry
  - Use warm clean linens to dry the infant.
- Warm
  - Maintain a warm environment and provide skin-to-skin contact with mother if appropriate.
- Position
  - Make sure the airway is positioned in such a way that the newborn can breathe.
- Suction
  - If secretions are noted, use a bulb syringe to suction them out. Not all newborns require deep suctioning of the airway.
- Stimulate
  - Stimulate the newborn by flicking the soles of the feet and drying them with clean warm linens.

> **When using bulb suction, always suction the mouth first and then the nose (remember that M—mouth—comes before N—nose). If you suction the nose first, you might stimulate the infant to take a breath, which may cause them to inhale any meconium and fluids into their lungs.**

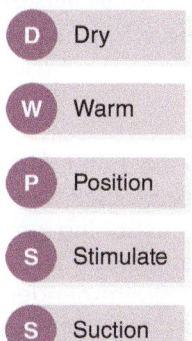

| D | Dry |
| W | Warm |
| P | Position |
| S | Stimulate |
| S | Suction |

**Figure 9-14** Do What Probably Seems Simple is a helpful mnemonic for remembering the initial steps of newborn care.
© Jones & Bartlett Learning.

When drying and warming the newborn, you are taking steps to avoid hypothermia. Hypothermia is a major complicating factor that can lead to further distress and difficulty transitioning after birth. Cool babies often appear as if they are in shock. A hat should be placed on the head to prevent unnecessary heat loss. One of the most important steps in keeping the newborn warm is to dry them and make sure they are not in contact with any damp or moist surfaces. Frequently replace towels and blankets as you use them to dry the neonate. If medical practitioners are not uncomfortably warm in the resuscitation environment, then it is likely too cool for the newborn. Skin-to-skin contact is also important for warmth. If stable enough, place the baby directly against the mother's skin. This will also help reduce postpartum hemorrhage.

Ensure that the baby's head is positioned in such a way that they can maintain an open airway. Also ensure that when they are wrapped, the mouth and nose remain uncovered.

Stimulate the baby by using the linens to dry them and flicking the soles of the feet. Take care to not be overly aggressive—almost any form of stimulation will prompt breathing in an otherwise healthy, term newborn. If the apnea is secondary to medications, toxins, or prolonged hypoxic ischemic event, no amount of stimulation will work and you will need to progress down the airway management protocol. If the newborn remains apneic after 30 seconds of adequate stimulation, positive-pressure ventilation (PPV) will be necessary.

> Although certain methods of aggressive stimulation such as slapping the buttocks, squeezing of the rib cage, flexing of the hips into the abdomen, dilating the anal sphincter, and hot or cold stimuli may have been used historically, these methods are not considered safe or evidence based. They deviate from the standard of care.

Suctioning can be helpful when the airways are occluded by secretions such as amniotic fluid or meconium. However, suctioning provides no protection against fluid aspiration, and routine intrapartum suctioning is no longer recommended.

If secretions are clearly visible, use a bulb syringe to remove them. Suction the mouth first, then the nose. Remember to squeeze the bulb prior to placing it in the mouth, then expel the suctioned materials away from the newborn. If a flexible suction catheter is used, avoid performing deep suctioning or overly vigorous suctioning. This may stimulate the baby's vagal response and cause a precipitous decline in heart rate due to increased vagal tone. Brief, gentle suctioning with a bulb syringe is almost always more than adequate to clear the airway. If bradycardia does occur during suctioning, stop the procedure and provide positive-pressure ventilation if necessary to recover the heart rate.

Practitioners should be aware that light meconium rarely causes significant airway compromise. In the presence of a vigorous, crying infant, no additional steps need to be taken when meconium is present, but be sure to inform the receiving hospital of meconium presence at birth. If the baby is not vigorous and resuscitation is needed, standard algorithms can be followed with no specific steps necessary to treat the meconium aspiration in the field. Severe meconium aspiration will sometimes require aggressive life-sustaining therapies such as high-frequency oscillatory ventilation or extracorporeal membrane oxygenation (ECMO).

## Delayed Cord Clamping

When no complications are present and the newborn does not require resuscitation, it is appropriate to delay cord clamping for 30 to 60 seconds. This has many benefits, including the following:

- Increased hemoglobin and iron stores for the newborn
- Better red blood cell (RBC) volume and less need for RBC transfusion
- Lower incidence of necrotizing enterocolitis and intraventricular hemorrhage

The first clamp should be placed about 10 cm (4 inches) from the baby, with the second clamp placed approximately 5 cm (2 inches) distal to the first. The cord can then be cut with a scalpel or a pair of scissors.

During the cord clamping and cutting process, it is important to keep the baby at the level of the mother to prevent any major transfers of blood to or from the newborn. Holding the baby too high will favor blood flow to the placenta and possibly cause anemia in the neonate. Holding the baby too low will favor blood flow to the newborn and can lead to a condition called polycythemia, where the blood is thickened with too many RBCs.

## Apgar Scoring System

The Apgar scoring system is a quick assessment of appearance, pulse, grimace, activity, and respiratory effort performed at 1 and 5 minutes after birth (**Figure 9-15**). Additional scores can be performed at other intervals if resuscitation is ongoing or there is a change in the newborn's status.

| | Activity (muscle tone) | Pulse | Grimace (reflex irritability) | Appearance (skin color) | Respiration | | | |
|---|---|---|---|---|---|---|---|---|
| 0 points | Absent | Absent | Flaccid | Blue, pale | Absent | Severely depressed | Moderately depressed | Excellent condition |
| 1 point | Arms and legs flexed | Below 100 bpm | Some flexion of extremities | Body pink, extremities blue | Slow, irregular | | | |
| 2 points | Active movement | Over 100 bpm | Active motion (sneeze, cough, pull away) | Completely pink | Vigorous cry | | | |
| Points totaled | | | | | | 0–3 | 4–7 | 8–10 |

**Figure 9-15** The Apgar scoring system.
© Jones & Bartlett Learning.

The 1-minute score is an indicator of how well the baby tolerated the birthing process. The 5-minute score is an indicator of how well the baby is transitioning outside of the womb. The Apgar score does not have prognostic value regarding the possibility of developmental delay or other deficits that may be present as a result of depressed state immediately at birth.

Overall, a scores correlate to the following states:

- Severely depressed: 0–3
- Moderately depressed: 4–7
- Excellent condition: 8–10

The Pediatric Assessment Triangle (PAT) can also be used to quickly evaluate the patient's status. Follow your local guidelines. Some agencies require that Apgar scores be calculated and reported.

## Appearance

Assess the baby's overall tone. If they are moving vigorously, then they likely do not need aggressive resuscitation and simply keeping them dry and warm should suffice. If they are limp and have little or no movement, then quick action is needed. This includes stimulation and other measures to increase the heart and respiratory rates if necessary.

## Work of Breathing

The same indications of respiratory distress of infants can be seen in newborns with difficulty breathing. Nasal flaring, retractions, and sounds such as grunting are all ominous signs. A baby who is crying vigorously has an intact airway and adequate respiratory effort. A baby making no sounds may be apneic or have respiratory failure.

Assess the airway for secretions, and pay close attention for the possibility of meconium. Meconium can stain the baby's face a brown or green color. This may be present in the mouth and airway and can be very irritating if aspirated into the lungs. Meconium ranges from very thin and watery to very thick and soupy. The thicker the meconium, the more likely it is to cause airway complications. Respiratory distress and failure from meconium aspiration may not be apparent immediately. In some cases, lung damage can evolve over the next hours to days. It is important to pass on whether meconium is present or not so that other healthcare practitioners can monitor more closely for signs of respiratory distress.

Any newborn with a weak cry, shallow breathing, poor muscle tone, or poor signs of perfusion requires immediate intervention, including assisted ventilation and chest compressions if the pulse falls below 60 beats/min and does not respond to oxygenation.

Premature infants lack the muscle development and neurologic maturity to tolerate respiratory distress well. They are not capable of extensive use of accessory muscles and can experience respiratory failure even with seemingly small airway complications.

## "Quick" Versus "Not Quick" for Newborns

It may be easy to think that all newborns birthed in the prehospital setting are "Quick." This is not necessarily the case. Although field birth carries some increased risks, most babies are born perfectly healthy with little complication. Table 9-6 lists come general considerations for "Quick" and "Not Quick" newborn situations.

In situations where the infant is determined to be "Not Quick," provide routine newborn care, allow the baby to be skin-to-skin with mother, and transport in a routine fashion. Mother and infant can be safely transported together if policy allows; however, an additional medical practitioner should be taken along in the back of the ambulance to assist with monitoring the additional patient.

In situations where the child is determined to be "Quick," resuscitation and stabilization will need to be provided. Ventilations should be assisted—this will resolve nearly all instances of newborn bradycardia. If the neonate does not respond to assisted ventilations, then the EMS practitioner should search for an underlying cause. These causes may include the following:

- Maternal drug use
- Congenital heart defects
- Hypoglycemia
- Aspiration
- Physical lung or airway malformations

**Table 9-6** Characteristics of "Quick" Versus "Not Quick" in Newborns

| Not Quick | Quick |
|---|---|
| Term gestation | Premature |
| Clear amniotic fluid | Poor muscle tone |
| Good muscle tone | Meconium present |
| No respiratory distress | Apneic or signs of respiratory distress |
| Actively crying | Weak or absent cry |
| Tolerating skin-to-skin with mother | Gasping respirations |
| Initial Apgar of 8 or above | Apgar of 7 or less that does not respond to initial interventions |

© Jones & Bartlett Learning.

In cases where maternal drug use is the suspected cause, note that treatment with naloxone (Narcan) or other medications is no longer indicated because of the risk of withdrawal symptoms, such as seizures.

## Newborn Resuscitation

When a newborn does not respond to the routine steps of newborn care (dry, warm, position, suction, stimulate) or they are clearly apneic and pulseless immediately after birth, the prehospital practitioner must proceed with resuscitation. Resuscitation for a newborn involves several components: warm, dry, stimulate, suction, PPV, chest compressions, and medications. Other resuscitation steps include establishment of IV access and advanced airway placement. Resuscitation is worked through systematically, and not all newborns will need all components. Determining which patients need what components of resuscitation can be difficult when EMS practitioners are under pressure. However, most newborns delivered in the prehospital environment do not require treatment beyond the warm, dry, stimulate steps (or possibly suction).

### Ventilations

Prehospital practitioners should begin ventilations immediately for newborns who are apneic or those who have a pulse less then 100 beats/min after the initial DWPSS (dry, warm, position, suction, stimulate) steps have been taken. Central cyanosis not responsive to blow-by oxygen within 30 seconds of birth is also an indication for PPV. If there is any question as to the appearance of the newborn or if the respiratory effort appears inadequate, PPV is likely indicated.

Positive-pressure ventilation can help the newborn transition to life outside of the womb by providing opening pressure to the lower airways. This opening pressure may be difficult for stunned, weak, or stressed newborns to generate.

Great care should be used when providing PPV to the newborn. The lungs are tiny and only require approximately 20 to 25 mL of air for a term newborn. Practitioners should give only enough air to cause the chest to subtly rise. Common issues with ventilation include poor mask seal and hyperextension of the airway. Practitioners must remember that the newborn airway is flexible, and hyperextension will generally result in narrowing of the airway, leading to greater resistance to ventilation.

The initial ventilatory rate for newborns is 40 to 60 breaths/min. Ensure adequate time for exhalation. The goal is to keep the heart rate above 100 beats/min.

If practitioners are using a self-inflating bag with peak end-expiratory pressure (PEEP) valve, a PEEP of 5 cm $H_2O$ should be used to prevent alveolar collapse at the end of exhalation. The seal must be kept in place

> **Heart rate is the key indicator that newborn resuscitation efforts are effective.**

for PEEP to work. Additionally, peak inspiratory pressure (PIP) of 20 to 25 cm $H_2O$ may be required initially to inflate the lungs. As you continue with breaths, the peak pressures may gradually come down while lung compliance increases.

As the heart rate increases above 100 beats/min, overall color improves, and the newborn begins to display signs of increasing activity and respiratory effort, trial a discontinuation of PPV and provide stimulation to the newborn to see if they can maintain their own respiratory effort. If they remain vigorous and the heart rate holds, consider placing them skin-to-skin with mother and monitoring closely.

Always be prepared for deterioration and resume PPV if necessary. When deterioration occurs during PPV, evaluate for technical issues such as oxygen disconnection, kinked or obstructed endotracheal (ET) tubes, poor mask seal, or other faulty equipment. Auscultate breath sounds and evaluate for asymmetry which might indicate dislodged or displaced ET tubes or pneumothorax. Take corrective action as necessary—check the mask and adjust if needed, reposition the head to open the airway, suction the mouth first followed by the nose, increase pressure if there is no chest rise, and consider an advanced airway.

## Chest Compressions

It is important to remember that the vast majority (over 90%) of newborns respond to routine steps of newborn care (DWPSS). Of those who do not respond to routine care, most will respond to simple ventilatory assistance. Only a small subset of newborns will require chest compressions or medications when the routine steps of newborn care and proper ventilatory assistance have been provided. In these cases, there is likely some outlying factor which has complicated the status of the newborn during the pregnancy or delivery.

Any newborn with a heart rate less than 60 beats/min that has not responded within 30 seconds of administering adequate respiratory assistance should receive chest compressions. Application of a cardiac monitor or additional signs of cardiac collapse are not necessary. It should be muscle memory for practitioners to act upon heart rate less than 60 beats/min not responding to 30 seconds of ventilatory assistance (PPV); initiate chest compressions without delay.

Oxygenation and ventilation are the most effective newborn resuscitation steps. For this reason, the coordination for cardiopulmonary resuscitation (CPR)

is different than the standard 30:2 or 15:2 provided to children. Compressions must be paused to allow for adequate oxygen delivery and exhalation time, and the rate of compressions and breaths per minute is higher overall. This is necessary to meet the high metabolic demands of newborns.

The compression-to-ventilation ratio for newborns is 3 to 1, resulting in 120 actions per minute, each action lasting approximately 0.5 seconds. The cadence to call out is, "push, push, push, breathe." This sequence of three rapid compressions (allowing for full recoil each time) and one breath is repeated throughout the entire resuscitation. Reassess every 30 to 60 seconds or when the patient shows signs of life or clinical status change.

When the newborn can sustain a heart rate over 60 beats/min with good peripheral perfusion, compressions can be stopped. The patient will often still require ventilatory assistance for a period following chest compressions.

## Medications

The only medication routinely used in neonatal resuscitation is epinephrine. The standard dose is 0.01 mg/kg of a 1:10,000 solution. Epinephrine is indicated when a newborn's heart rate remains less than 60 beats/min despite adequate ventilation, oxygenation, and chest compressions for at least 30 seconds.

Epinephrine may be administered via the ET tube, however this is the least reliable route of administration and should be avoided whenever possible. If the endotracheal route is used while vascular access is obtained the dose is substantially higher: 0.05–0.1 mg/kg. Epinephrine administration can be repeated every 3–5 minutes while resuscitation proceeds.

Volume resuscitation using normal saline may be considered when significant maternal hemorrhage is present and there is concern for neonatal hypovolemia. The initial starting bolus is 10 mL/kg. This generally should not exceed 40 mL total volume per bolus. In cases where there is a known cardiac defect, volume resuscitation should be cautiously considered, as cardiac overload can easily occur. Smaller bolus amounts of 5 mL/kg should be used in these situations, and only when absolutely necessary.

## Initial Observations

- Pediatric Assessment Triangle (**Figure 9-16**)
  - Appearance
    - Weak cry, brownish-green tint around the face and mouth
  - Work of breathing
    - Flaring present

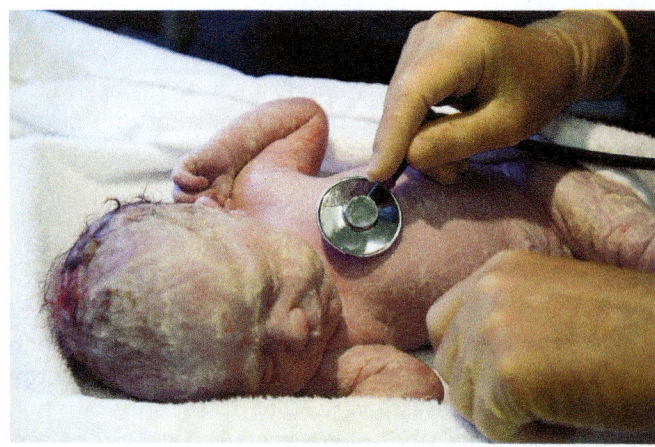

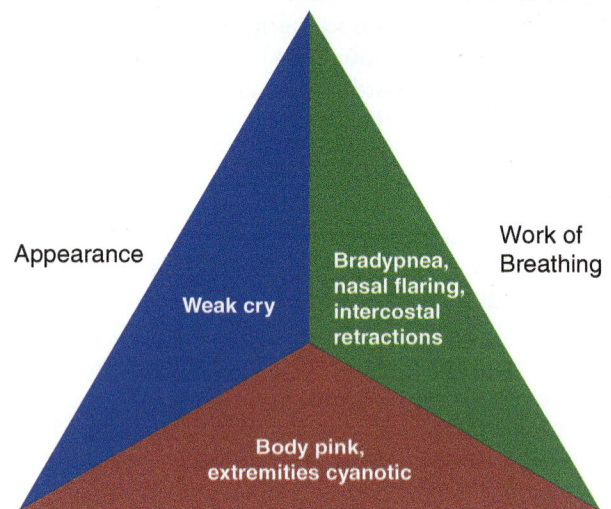

Appearance

Work of Breathing

Weak cry

Bradypnea, nasal flaring, intercostal retractions

Body pink, extremities cyanotic

Circulation to Skin

**Figure 9-16** The infant is now also a patient.

A. © RapidEye/E+/Getty Images; B. Used with permission of the American Academy of Pediatrics, Pediatric Education for Prehospital Professionals, © American Academy of Pediatrics, 2000.

- **R**etractions present with slow respiratory rate
- **A**udible airway sounds present, gurgling
- **P**ositioning—head positioned appropriately
- Circulation
  - Good perfusion centrally, acrocyanosis present

## Case Questions

- Is this patient "Quick" or "Not Quick"?
  - Based on the slow respiratory rate and obvious increase in work of breathing, this patient requires quick initial interventions to support respiratory effort and maintain circulation.

Acrocyanosis, or cyanosis of the peripheral extremities such as the hands and feet, is a common finding in newborns. In the setting of normal respiratory effort, vigorous activity, and good signs of central perfusion, it is considered benign and usually resolves within 24 to 48 hours.

## Primary Survey

The primary survey for this patient reveals the following:

**X**—No bleeding noted

**A**—Open and patent

**B**—Poor respiratory effort with nasal flaring and intercostal retractions. Adventitious lung sounds bilaterally with referred upper airway sounds indicating nasal congestion.

**C**—Palpable brachial pulses with a rate less than 100 beats/min. Capillary refill time approximately 4 seconds. Peripheral cyanosis present, but good perfusion centrally.

**D**—Overall depressed. Apgar = 6 (A1, P1, G1, A1, R2)

**E**—Yellow-green tint on the skin

## Case Questions

- Based on the findings noted in the primary survey, what would your initial interventions and treatment include?
  - The initial treatment for this newborn should include the routine steps of DWPSS and rapid transition to ventilatory support if there is no improvement in respiratory effort within 30 seconds. Additional suctioning of the nose and mouth may be necessary if there are visible secretions.
  - When time permits and protocols allow, check the blood glucose level of the newborn. Hypoglycemia is an easily reversible cause of newborn respiratory depression.

Practitioners should be aware that acceptable blood glucose levels in the newborn are generally lower than in adults. Any value greater than 45 mg/dL is acceptable in a newborn.

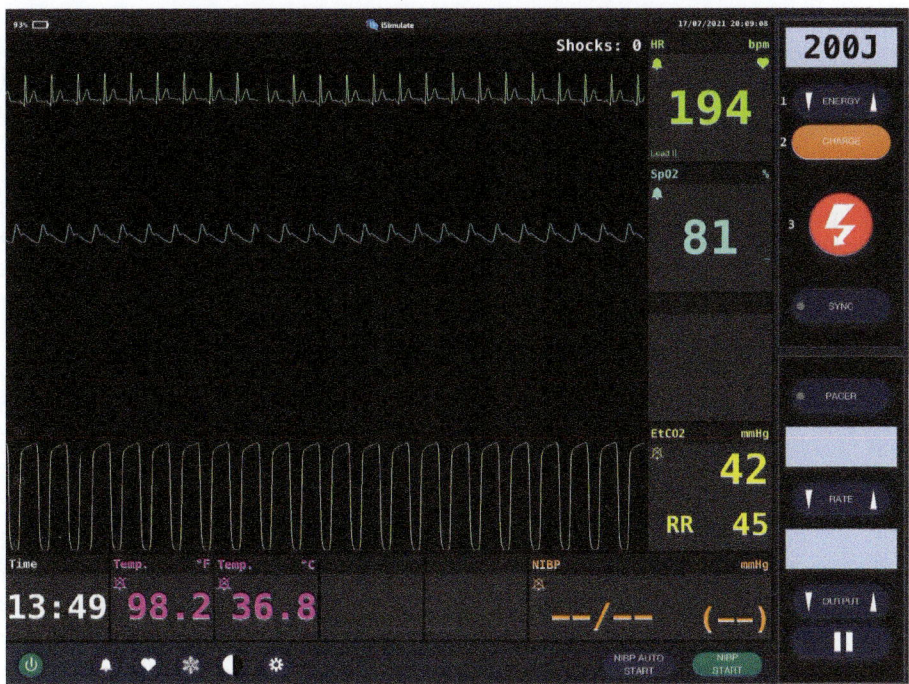

**Figure 9-17** Heart rate and respiratory effort are the key indicators to guide neonatal resuscitative efforts.

Courtesy of iSimulate.

## Detailed Assessment

### Vital Signs

As you are performing DWPSS and assisting ventilations, the patient was attached to the monitor and the following vital signs were obtained (**Figure 9-17**):

**Heart rate:**

- 194 beats/min
- This is improved over the pulse of less than 100 beats/min initially encountered during the initial assessment.
- This is tachycardic for a newborn, however tachycardia is preferred over bradycardia in general. The newborn is stressed, but based on the PAT initially, central perfusion appears adequate.

**SpO$_2$:**

- 81% RA
- This improves with positive-pressure ventilation.
- While SpO$_2$ is a data point that can be trended, it should not be used as the sole determinant of resuscitation.
- Heart rate, respiratory effort, and overall activity should be used as key indicators of resuscitation success.

- It generally takes infants at least 10 minutes to be in the mid 90s for oxygen saturation.

**ETCO$_2$:**

- 42 mm Hg

**Respiratory rate:**

- Initially the patient was given PPV at a rate of approximately 40 breaths/min.
- After 1 minute of PPV, the newborn now has a respiratory rate of 45 breaths/min with adequate effort, and improved work of breathing.

**Blood pressure:**

- Not obtained
- Central capillary refill is now 2 to 3 seconds after DWPSS and ventilatory assistance.

**Temperature:**

- 98.2°F (36.8°C)

**Blood glucose:**

- 64 mg/dL

## Newborn Pulse Oximetry

Immediately after birth, there is a transition from fetal to neonatal circulation. This involves the resolution of cardiac shunts that were required for life inside the womb.

These shunts do not resolve immediately, however, and the decrease in pulmonary vascular resistance is gradual over the first few hours of life. As shunts such as the ductus arteriosus and foramen ovale resolve, the mixing of oxygenated and deoxygenated blood gradually decreases. This is reflected in the preductal oxygen saturation that is obtained on the right upper extremity of the newborn.

**Table 9-7** shows expected preductal oxygen saturations based on the newborn's age in minutes.

| Table 9-7 Expected Preductal Oxygen Saturation for Term Newborns | |
| --- | --- |
| 1 minute | 60–65% |
| 2 minutes | 65–70% |
| 3 minutes | 70–75% |
| 4 minutes | 75–80% |
| 5 minutes | 80–85% |
| 10 minutes | 85–95% |

© Jones & Bartlett Learning.

## Meconium Delivery

The presence of meconium alone is not itself an emergency. Most patients with meconium-stained fluid do not get meconium aspiration syndrome and have a normal transition to newborn life (**Figure 9-18**). When there is persistent respiratory distress or poor circulation, neonatal resuscitation can proceed per the normal algorithm, with special attention paid to the airway and potential need for invasive ventilation with an ET tube.

## Treatment

In this scenario practitioners cannot lose track of the fact that there are still two patients to consider.

### Newborn Management

Overall management for the newborn in this case includes basic life support (BLS) management of the airway. Positive-pressure ventilation and oxygen as necessary to target expected preductal oxygen saturation values should be adequate. Suctioning of the nose and airway as necessary to keep the passages clear and reduce work of breathing will also be helpful.

ALS practitioners should be aware that routine intubation solely for the purposes of deep tracheal and

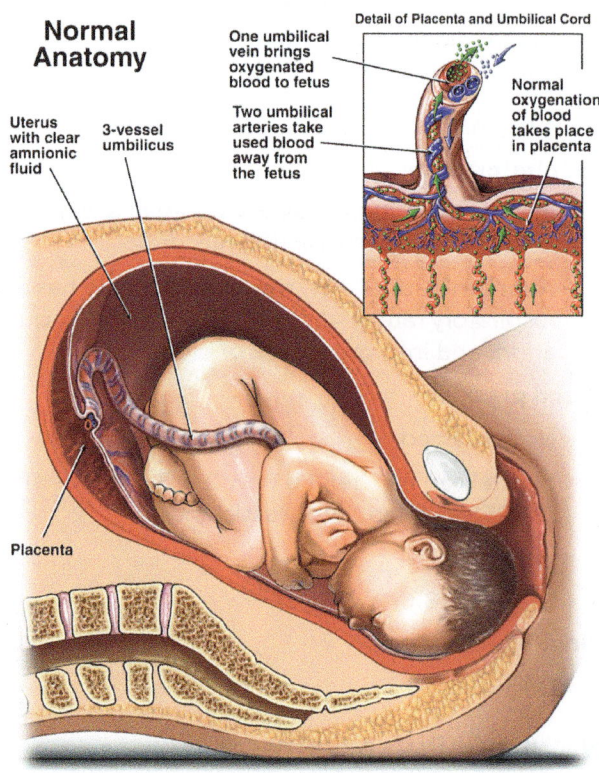

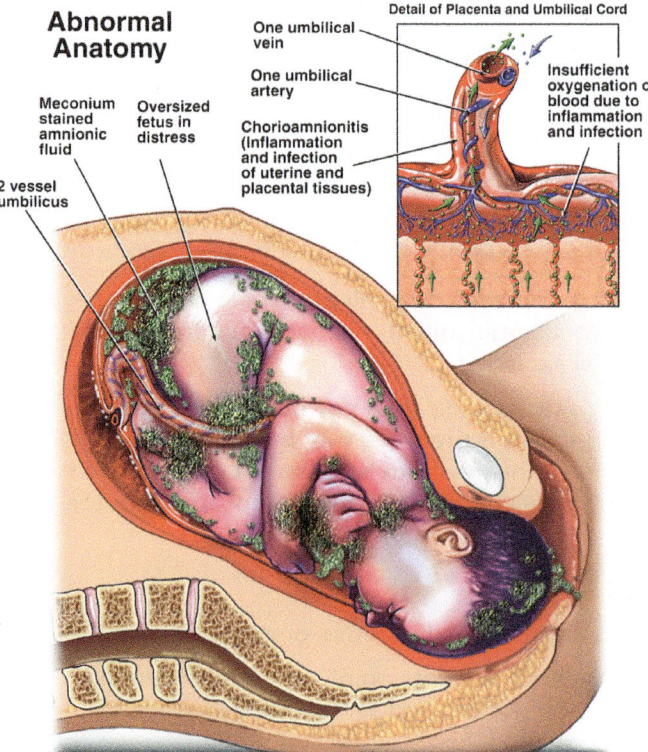

**Figure 9-18** Meconium aspirated into the lungs causes inflammation of the lungs (pneumonitis) and increases the risk of lung infection.

© Nucleus Medical Media Inc/Alamy Stock Photo.

airway suctioning is not recommended. If PPV fails to perk up respiratory effort, then intubation and suctioning may be necessary, however this is only needed in a select few cases.

There is no specific critical care management for this patient in the immediate postpartum period. If the patient requires transport to a higher level of care, a neonatal specialty care transport team may utilize other forms of ventilatory assistance, such as oscillatory ventilation. Inhaled nitric oxide for the treatment of pulmonary hypertension may also be used. In some severe cases of meconium aspiration syndrome, ECMO may be necessary. This is only available at pediatric specialty care centers.

## Maternal Management

In the immediate postpartum period, special attention should be paid to signs of excessive hemorrhage. Sanitary pads should be used to estimate the blood loss. Amounts up to 500 mL are generally considered normal. As this amount approaches 1,000 mL or more, significant concern for hypovolemic shock exists. Vascular access should be obtained and fluids administered for hypovolemia if it is suspected. Provide fundal massage if necessary.

Overall care should focus on mother—baby bonding if both patients are stable enough to tolerate this.

## Ongoing Management

During transport, the mother and baby are continually reassessed for deterioration. There is no sign of maternal hemorrhage, and the newborn's 5- and 10-minute Apgar scores increased to 9 (A2, P2, G1, A2, R2).

### Case Questions

- What is the most appropriate treatment destination and why?
  - Generally, if both mother and baby have good general appearance and are stable, they can be transported together to the closest appropriate facility. Where possible, transport to the

hospital where the mother had planned to deliver the baby.

- Can you safely transport this child in your ambulance?
  - There are few commercially available devices that can safely transport a patient the size of a newborn. Consult local protocols for guidance when initiating transport. The ideal transport method for unstable newborns would be in a purpose-built neonatal isolette that has been approved for emergency transport and has temperature regulation and patient monitoring capabilities. These units cost tens of thousands of dollars and are utilized by pediatric/neonatal specialty care transport teams. They are not practical for use in general emergency services systems.
  - In cases in which both mother and baby are stable, you must balance the benefit of mother–baby bonding through skin-to-skin contact with the risk of transporting the newborn unsecured on the mother's chest. When transporting a stable mother and newborn, consider transporting using kangaroo care. This is a method of holding the baby against the mother to provide skin-to-skin contact.
- Will you allow grandmother to ride in the ambulance?
  - If protocols allow, permit a family member to ride in the ambulance safely secured in a seat. In this case, the patient's mother decided to follow in her personal vehicle so she could have transportation while at the hospital.

**Evidence shows that skin-to-skin contact between newborn and mother stabilizes the newborn's heart rate and breathing and aids in thermoregulation, among other benefits.**

### CASE WRAP-UP

Diagnosis: Mother, vaginal delivery with no complications; Newborn, meconium aspiration.

The mother and patient were admitted to the local hospital. The mother was admitted to the postpartum ward and the newborn went to the NICU as a precaution. Empiric antibiotics were started while the physicians waited for blood cultures to see if blood

cultures produced any growth. The baby also had some grunting and mild retractions which required approximately 36 hours of high-flow nasal cannula treatment prior to being weaned to room air. Mother was fine post birth; infant was transferred to NICU from ED and released to stepdown unit after 3 days of treatment.

## CASE TAKEAWAY POINTS

Meconium-stained fluid and possible meconium aspiration is common, occurring in up to 15% of deliveries. Very few of these patients go on to develop the more serious meconium aspiration syndrome which requires advanced life support care.

Practitioners should be ready to deal with meconium-stained fluid in any birth situation; however, babies who are born postterm, involved in a stressful protracted labor situation, or are full-term and small for gestational age are at higher risk for passage of and possible aspiration of meconium.

Field care for these babies involves routine delivery and resuscitation, preparation for advanced airway placement, and transport to a hospital with the capabilities to provide advanced care to newborns.

# Congenital Heart Defects

Congenital heart defects (CHDs) are the result of malformation in the structure of the heart, valves, or circulatory anatomy in utero. Congenital means present at birth, and as such, these defects are not acquired, but rather present during development. The terms *defect*, *disease*, and *lesion* are often used interchangeably when discussing CHDs.

CHDs are often classified by the presence or absence of cyanosis. They may also be further classified as causing obstruction to systemic blood flow. Table 9-8 classifies some of the major congenital heart defects.

A convenient shorthand to help practitioners differentiate among the major types of congenital defects is to consider the infant's skin tone; infants with a heart defect typically present as either pink (or well-perfused in darker-skinned children), blue, or gray:

- "Pink baby": Acyanotic heart defect
- "Blue baby": Cyanotic heart defect
- "Gray baby": Obstructive heart defect

Table 9-9 provides more information on the pink/blue/gray baby presentations.

The following sections describe some of the most common defects. This information is meant to provide an introduction and is not comprehensive. A full description of defects, palliation, and critical care management is beyond the scope of this course.

# Cyanotic Heart Defects

Cyanotic CHD lesions occur when there is mixing of deoxygenated blood from the right side of the heart with oxygenated blood from the right side of the heart, leading to a lower arterial oxygen content in the blood that is perfusing the systemic circulation.

### Table 9-8 Major Congenital Heart Defects

| Cyanotic | Acyanotic | Obstructive |
| --- | --- | --- |
| Tetralogy of Fallot | Septal defects<br>- Atrial septal defect (ASD)<br>- Ventricular septal defect (VSD) | Coarctation of the aorta |
| Transposition of the great arteries (TGA)* | Patent ductus arteriosus (PDA) | |
| Total anomalous pulmonary venous return (TAPVR)** | | |
| Truncus arteriosus | | |
| Tricuspid atresia | | |

*May be referred to as transposition of the great vessels, or TGV, in some texts.
**May be referred to as total anomalous pulmonary venous connection, or TAPVC, in some texts.

**Table 9-9** Congenital Heart Defects: Infant Presentation

| Baby Presentation | Blue | Gray | Pink | Blue |
|---|---|---|---|---|
| **Age** | <2 weeks | <2 weeks | 1–6 months | 1–6 months |
| **Pulmonary vs. systemic congestion** | Poor lung circulation | Poor lung circulation and perfusion | Respiratory congestion | Blood return in the lungs is obstructed |
| **Class** | Right obstruction condition | Left obstruction condition | Left to right shunt | Mixing right to left shunt |
| **Presentation** | Central cyanosis | Cardiogenic shock | Heart failure | Cyanosis and heart failure |
| **Findings** | $SpO_2$ <80%; Chest X-ray: black lungs ECG: RVH | Differential $SpO_2$, BP, and pulse in right upper extremity vs. lower extremities Slow capillary refill; Chest X-ray: white lungs ECG: LVH; in >7 days of life RVH in newborn | Hepatomegaly; murmur; Chest X-ray: white lungs ECG: Possible extreme tight axis deviation or AV block | $SpO_2$ <80%; Hepatomegaly; Chest X-ray: white lungs |
| **Treatments** | Prostaglandin E1; intubate; oxygen and inhaled nitric oxide | Prostaglandin E1; intubate; minimal oxygen with PPV and inhaled nitric oxide; antibiotics; IV fluid therapy; epinephrine and dopamine; milrinone or dobutamine | Minimal oxygen with PPV or intubate; careful IV fluid therapy; diuretics; milrinone or dobutamine | Minimal oxygen with PPV; antibiotics; restrict IV fluid therapy; diuretics |
| **Conditions** | Tricuspid atresia; pulmonary atresia; pulmonary stenosis; Ebstein's anomaly | Hypoplastic left heart syndrome; coarctation of aorta; interrupted aortic arch; aortic stenosis or atresia | Patent ductus arteriosus; ventricular septal defect; arteriovenous malformation; arteriovenous canal defect | Total anomalous pulmonary venous return; truncus arteriosus; double outlet right ventricle; transposition of the great arteries with ventricular septal defect or patent ductus arteriosus |

*Abbreviations*: LVH, left ventricular hypertrophy; RVH, right ventricular hypertrophy

Data from Strobel AM, Lu Le N. The critically ill infant with congenital heart disease. *Emerg Med Clin North Am*. 2015;33(3):501-518.

Cyanotic heart lesions are sometimes classified as the "terrible Ts":

- Tetralogy of Fallot
- Transposition of the great arteries
- Total anomalous pulmonary venous connection
- Truncus arteriosus
- Tricuspid atresia

## Tetralogy of Fallot

Tetralogy of Fallot (ToF) accounts for approximately 10% of congenital heart disease cases (4–5 births per 10,000) and is one of the most common CHDs to require surgery early in life (**Figure 9-19**). While ToF is often referred to as four defects, it really is a single defect leading to four manifestations. In patients with ToF, the infundibular septum fails to fuse and divide the ventricles, leading to the following:

- Large ventricular septal defect (VSD)
- Overriding aorta
- Pulmonary valve stenosis (referred to as right ventricular outflow tract obstruction in some texts)
- Right ventricular hypertrophy

The severity of ToF is largely dictated by the degree of pulmonary valve stenosis and how obstructed the right ventricular outflow tract is. Patients with relatively unobstructed flow may grow into their toddler years and only become affected when significant cardiac output is required. In patients with severely stenotic pulmonary valves, simply feeding from a bottle or at the breast as a newborn can be enough to cause them to have a cyanotic spell.

The cause for cyanotic spells in ToF ("tet spells") is multifactorial, and there is still much debate regarding the exact etiology. When a patient with ToF is acyanotic and not in distress, the flow of blood through the VSD is left to right, and pulmonary blood flow is largely unobstructed. In conditions where the pulmonary vascular resistance is increased, the blood flow gradient across the VSD favors right to left flow, which leads to an increased amount of deoxygenated blood flowing into the left heart and subsequently entering the systemic circulation. This occurs when the infant cries, feeds, or is otherwise distressed. In a toddler this can occur during periods of heavy play.

To rapidly correct this, the gradient must be switched to favor left to right flow again. This means that systemic vascular resistance must be increased to the point that the left ventricle pumps more blood across the VSD than it does through the aortic valve. The simplest form of correction involves the patient

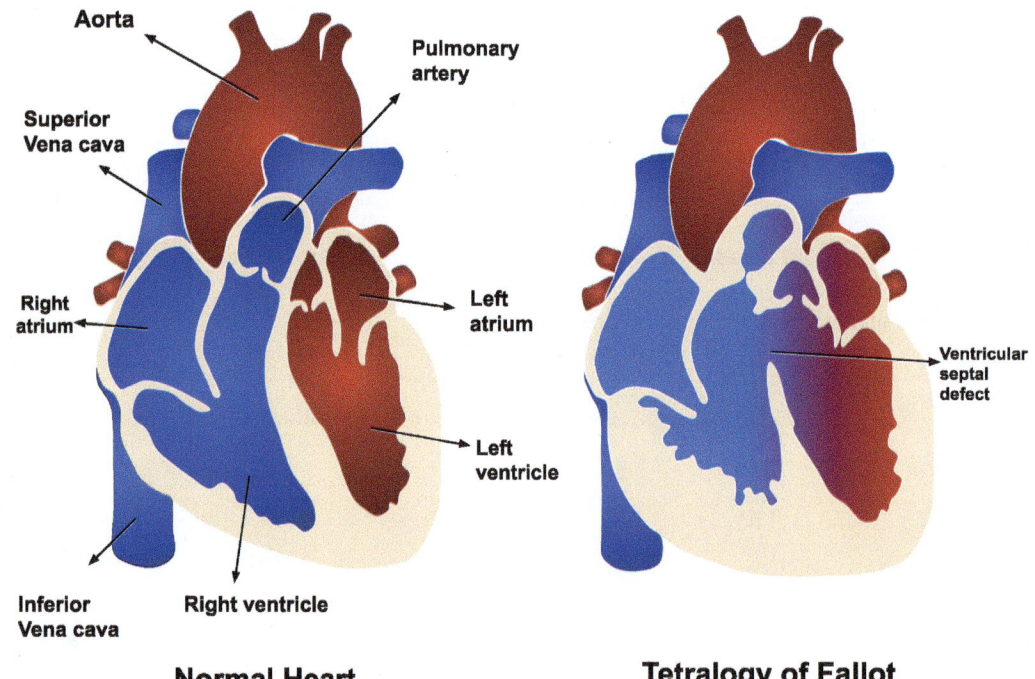

**Normal Heart**                **Tetralogy of Fallot**

**Figure 9-19** Tetralogy of Fallot is a single defect that leads to four manifestations.

squatting or pushing the knees up to the chest in supine or nonambulatory children. Medications or interventions that reduce pulmonary vascular resistance can also achieve this same effect.

The definitive management for children with ToF is surgical correction. Timing of surgery is based on severity, and ideally takes place after the patient has had adequate time to grow and gain weight. Timing is also based on symptom burden. Patients who are failing to thrive and have significant symptomatic burden will require surgical palliation sooner than those who are thriving and have low symptom burden.

## Transposition of the Great Arteries

Transposition of the great arteries (TGA) occurs in approximately 5 out of 10,000 births in the United States. The association of the pulmonary valve and right ventricular outflow tract (RVOT) with the right heart, and the aortic valve and left ventricular outflow tract (LVOT) occurs early in embryologic development. There is a complex set of events that occurs which leads to a septation and division of the great vessels, along with a twisting within these vessels that causes them to deliver blood as intended. In TGA this septation and twisting does not occur appropriately.

The definitive management is surgical and requires significant pre- and postoperative follow-up care.

## Truncus Arteriosus

In truncus arteriosus there is a single dysmorphic valve present for both the pulmonary and systemic arterial circulations. This single "trunk" valve provides blood flow for the entire pulmonary, systemic, and coronary circuits. The blood flow provided comes from both the left and right ventricles. This trunk is positioned above the ventricular septum and allows for significant mixing of oxygenated and deoxygenated blood.

Management is surgical and requires an advanced pediatric hospital with these capabilities.

## Tricuspid Atresia

Tricuspid atresia involves absence or severe dysmorphology of the tricuspid valve. Because the tricuspid valve is essentially absent in tricuspid atresia, the right atrium must shunt blood through an atrial septal defect. The blood then flows through the left atrium and then to the left ventricle. For oxygenation to occur, there must be a VSD present for blood to flow into the diminished right ventricle, where it then flows into the pulmonary circulation for oxygenation. A large left to right shunt must be favored

or else pulmonary blood flow is absent. The left ventricle performs the work for both the pulmonary and systemic circulation.

Prostaglandin to maintain a PDA will be necessary early in life to manage the blood flow between the pulmonary and systemic circuits. A three-stage surgical palliation is required to definitively manage this condition.

# Acyanotic Heart Defects

## Septal Defects

Defects in the septation of both the atria and ventricles are fairly common and often go undiagnosed, because they rarely cause symptoms. However, when septal defects are large, or there is a functional change in the pressure gradient such that the blood flow favors right to left shunting, hypoxia and cyanosis can occur.

Atrial septal defects (ASDs) are almost universally asymptomatic unless they are large. They rarely have a murmur, as the atria do not generate enough force to cause turbulent flow across the septal defect. One of the main risks that is present when ASDs are left intact is stroke as the result of a thrombus traveling from the venous circulation (often the lower legs) through the ASD and into the cerebral vasculature. In the normal heart, this thrombus would generally traverse the lungs where it would lead to a pulmonary embolism. In the setting of an ASD, the thrombus may pass from the right to the left atrium and subsequently be sent to the brain by way of the carotid arteries. This is a known risk and correction of ASD solely for this reason is often determined on a case-by-case basis, depending on the size and other risk factors.

Ventricular septal defects (VSDs) are common as well. These defects may have a murmur depending on size. Although it is counterintuitive, large VSDs often have soft or absent murmurs. Flow becomes more turbulent as the radius of the defect decreases, meaning that small defects often have the most turbulent flow, leading to more severe murmurs.

VSDs may close on their own (as is the case in most muscular VSDs), may be left uncorrected and require watchful waiting, or in some cases correction is pursued. This is determined on a case-by-case basis in consultation with a pediatric cardiologist and cardiothoracic surgeon.

Atrial and ventriculoseptal defects do not typically lead to cyanosis as the pressure gradient favors left to right shunting of blood, and the amount of blood shunted is not enough to cause symptomology.

# Obstructive Heart Defects

## Coarctation of the Aorta

Coarctation of the aorta (CoA) occurs when there is a stricture in the aorta, typically near the area where the ductus arteriosus connects the pulmonary artery to the aortic arch. This leads to restricted blood flow into the distal circulation.

Clinical manifestations of CoA include differential cyanosis (dusky or cyanotic lower extremities with well perfused upper extremities), palpable upper extremity pulses with weak or absent lower extremity pulses, and blood pressure differentials between the upper and lower extremities.

The degree of symptoms is dictated by the amount of stricture. Some patients have very few symptoms, whereas others may be severely affected in the first week of life.

# Sign and Symptoms of Congenital Heart Defects

Congenital heart defects or critical lesions should be on the differential diagnosis for any newborn or infant with respiratory distress that does not respond well to adequate ventilation and oxygenation. Nearly all respiratory issues should respond to effective oxygenation and ventilation, and persistent cyanosis with the application of supplemental oxygen or assisted ventilation typically indicates that the pathology is not inherent to the lungs. The heart is the next most likely culprit.

Age can also be a clue regarding what type of congenital heart lesion may be present. Table 9-10 describes the age of onset associated with some congenital heart defects. This information is just a guide, and you should be aware that every patient will present differently based on the degree of their defect and other circumstances.

**Table 9-10** Congenital Heart Defects Causing Congestive Heart Failure at Different Times During Infancy

| Age | Type of Congenital Heart Disease |
|---|---|
| Newborn | Hypoplastic left heart |
| | Severe pulmonic insufficiency |
| | Tetralogy of Fallot (te-'tral-ə-jē of fä-'lō) |
| | Severe tricuspid insufficiency |
| | Third-degree atrioventricular block |
| | Supraventricular tachycardia (SVT) |
| | Total anomalous pulmonary venous return |
| | Transposition of the great vessels |
| First month | Aortic coarctation with patent ductus arteriosus |
| | Ventricular septal defect (VSD) |
| | Tricuspid atresia |
| | Truncus arteriosus |
| First 6 months | Ventricular septal defect (VSD) |
| | Patent ductus arteriosus |
| 6–12 months | Ventricular septal defect (VSD) |
| | Endocardial fibrolastosis |

© Jones & Bartlett Learning.

---

## CASE STUDY

## Case 2

### Dispatch

You and your partner are dispatched to an apartment building for a 10-month-old male turning blue and currently crying. It is a cool summer evening. The air temperature is 76°F (24.4°C; Figure 9-20).

### Case Questions

- What are your initial concerns?
  - A child reported as turning blue is always concerning. This means that there is something causing hypoxia and cyanosis.

- Based on the dispatch information, what is the possible differential diagnosis for this patient?

  - Based on this dispatch information, the most likely differential diagnosis is a respiratory issue. A viral upper respiratory infection, bacterial infection, asthma, or other pulmonary issue might be causing cyanosis. Choking should also be considered. The possibility of a congenital heart defect cannot be excluded.

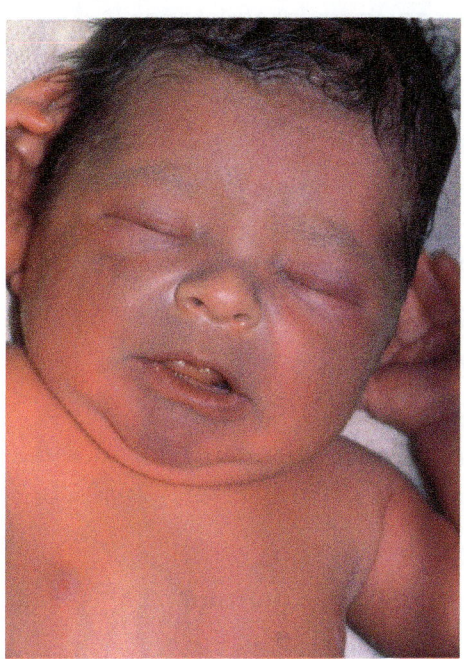

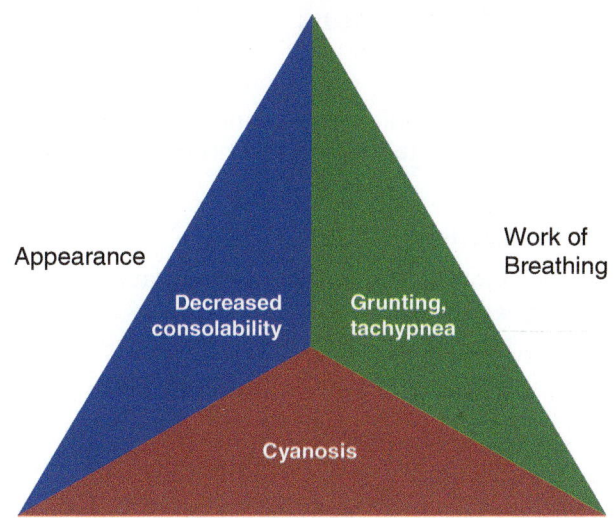

Appearance

Decreased consolability

Work of Breathing

Grunting, tachypnea

Cyanosis

Circulation to Skin

**Figure 9-20** This patient has a history of cyanosis beginning at age 6 weeks.

A. © St Bartholomew's Hospital, London/Science Source B. Used with permission of the American Academy of Pediatrics, Pediatric Education for Prehospital Professionals, © American Academy of Pediatrics, 2000.

## Initial Observations

As you arrive on scene, you are met by the father at the door. He escorts you to a bedroom in the house where the mother is holding the baby, desperately trying to console him. The father informs you that the patient has had intermittent cyanosis when he gets agitated since he was 6 weeks old. He has been diagnosed with tetralogy of Fallot; however, he has not yet had surgical repair, as his symptoms have been controlled and he is growing well. They have an appointment with their cardiologist next month to discuss surgical correction as the cyanotic episodes have been getting more frequent.

- Pediatric Assessment Triangle

  - Appearance

    - Inconsolable, crying loudly and persistently. You note that the patient is severely tachypneic.

  - Work of breathing

    - **F**laring not present

    - **R**etractions not present

    - **A**udible airway sounds include persistent grunting

    - **P**ositioning not present

  - Circulation

    - Cyanosis present

**Many patients with ToF will have symptoms that remain controlled until they reach an age where cardiac output demand exceeds their ability to compensate. As infants grow older and begin to crawl or walk more, the frequency of tet spells may increase, necessitating surgical correction.**

## Case Questions

- Based on your initial impression, is this patient "Quick" or "Not Quick"?

  - This patient is "Quick." Any patient with cyanosis and a known cardiac defect should be transported without delay to a pediatric specialty center. Your ability to manage this patient's oxygenation in the field will be limited because this is not a respiratory issue.

## Primary Survey

The primary survey for this patient reveals the following:

**X**—No bleeding found

**A**—Patent

**B**—Rapid respirations with audible grunting

**C**—Brachial pulses are palpable and rapid. Capillary refill time is 3 seconds. Skin is cyanotic.

**D**—Pediatric GCS is 12 (E4, V2, M6).

**E**—No rashes or bruising noted. Mother is holding baby.

### Case Questions

- Based on the findings noted in the primary survey, what would your initial interventions and treatment include?

  - Knowing that this patient has ToF and they are encountering a tet spell, initial treatment should include immediate placement into a knee-chest position, as shown in **Figure 9-21**.

  - To promote blood flow back across the VSD in left to right fashion, placing the knees to the chest will increase systemic vascular resistance, increasing left ventricular pressure, causing blood to follow the path of least resistance—into the right ventricle. This will increase right ventricular pressure and lead to increased blood flow through the pulmonic valve into the lungs for oxygenation.

  - Calming the patient will also help reduce pulmonary pressures and increase pulmonary blood flow.

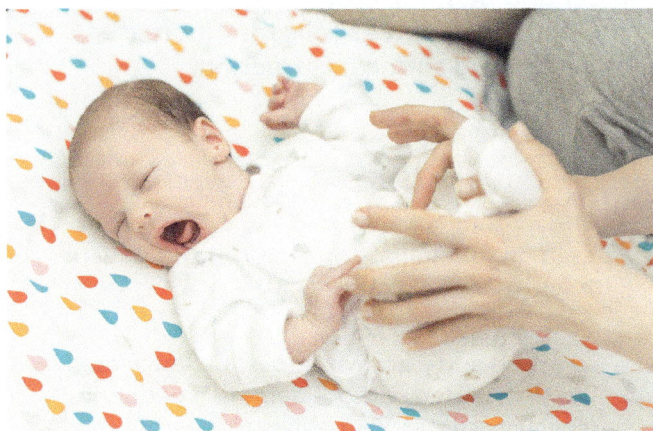

**Figure 9-21** Initial treatment for a tet spell is to place the patient in the knees-to-chest position.
© DeymosHR/Shutterstock.

Hypercyanotic tet spells occur when the pulmonary vascular resistance increases and right to left blood flow across the large VSD occurs. Older children may feel these spells occurring and instinctively squat to increase systemic vascular resistance. Younger children may require assistance doing this.

EMS treatment involves immediate knee-chest positioning, calming the child, and providing oxygen to decrease pulmonary vascular resistance (**Figure 9-21**).

### ADDITIONAL SIGNS AND SYMPTOMS OF TOF

- Bluish color of skin due to low concentration of $O_2$ in blood (cyanosis)
- Shortness of breath
- Syncopal episodes
- Poor weight gain, failure to thrive
- Tiring easily
- Irritability
- Prolonged crying
- Possible heart murmur

## Detailed Assessment

### History Taking

As your partner applies the monitor and takes vital signs, you begin to take a detailed history.

**OPQRST:**

- **O**nset: Sudden
- **P**rovocation/palliation: Increased agitation and crying lead to cyanosis
- **Q**uality: No discomfort
- **R**adiation: None
- **S**everity: Unable to obtain
- **T**iming: 20 minutes

**SAMPLER:**

- **S**igns/symptoms: Tachypnea, cyanosis, grunting
- **A**llergies: No known allergies to medications, foods, or the environment
- **M**edications: None

- **P**ast medical history: Tetralogy of Fallot, uncorrected
- **L**ast oral intake: Formula bottle approximately 2 hours ago
- **E**vents leading up to the emergency: Has gotten worse over the last 20 minutes
- **R**isk factors: History of uncorrected ToF and history of cyanosis

## Vital Signs

As you were discussing the history, the patient was attached to the monitor and the following vital signs were obtained (**Figure 9-22**):

**Heart rate:**

- 177 beats/min
- The patient is tachycardic, likely from the agitation and hypoxia.

**SpO$_2$:**

- 70% RA
- While this patient is hypoxic and cyanotic, it may not be as bad as it seems. Uncorrected congenital heart defect patients often have lower baseline oxygen saturations than the general population.
- It is important to ask the parents about the patient's baseline SpO$_2$.

- In this case the parents inform you that his baseline SpO$_2$ is normally 82% and above.

**ETCO$_2$:**

- 32 mm Hg

**Respiratory rate:**

- 63 breaths/min
- The patient is increasing his minute ventilation in an effort to correct systemic hypoxia.

**Blood pressure:**

- 110/78 mm Hg

**Temperature:**

- 98.6°F (37°C)
- The absence of fever reduces the concern for infectious etiology or complication.

**Blood glucose:**

- 94 mg/dL

The patient is a 10-month-old male with history of uncorrected tetralogy of Fallot presenting with 20 minutes of agitation, crying, and cyanosis. There are no signs or symptoms of infectious etiology at this time and the patient's clinical history, presentation, and exam are consistent with reversal of shunt flow across the VSD leading to symptomatic tet spell (**Figure 9-23**).

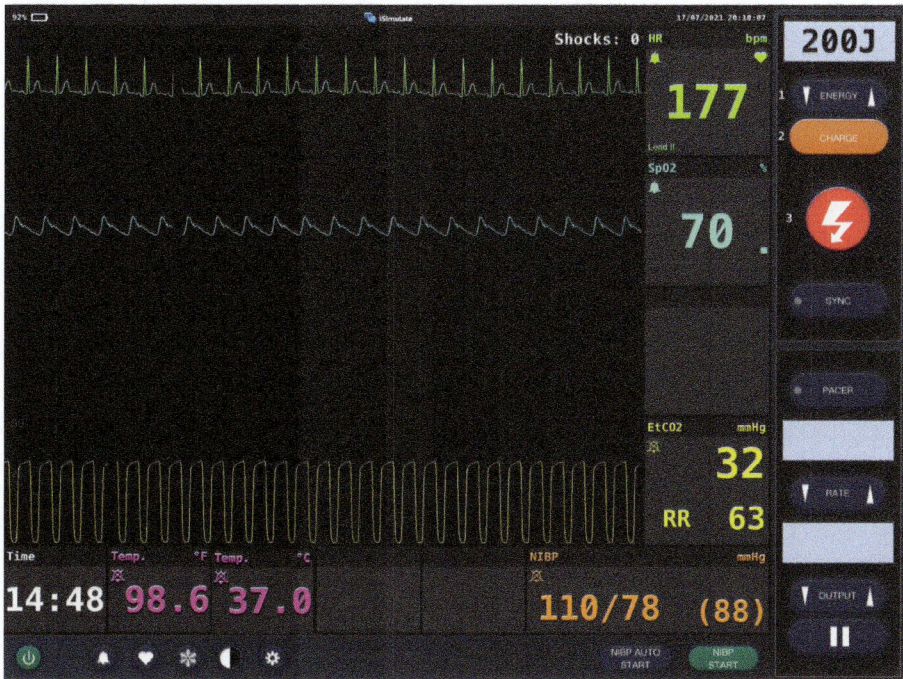

**Figure 9-22** It is important to determine this patient's baseline oxygen saturation level.

Courtesy of iSimulate.

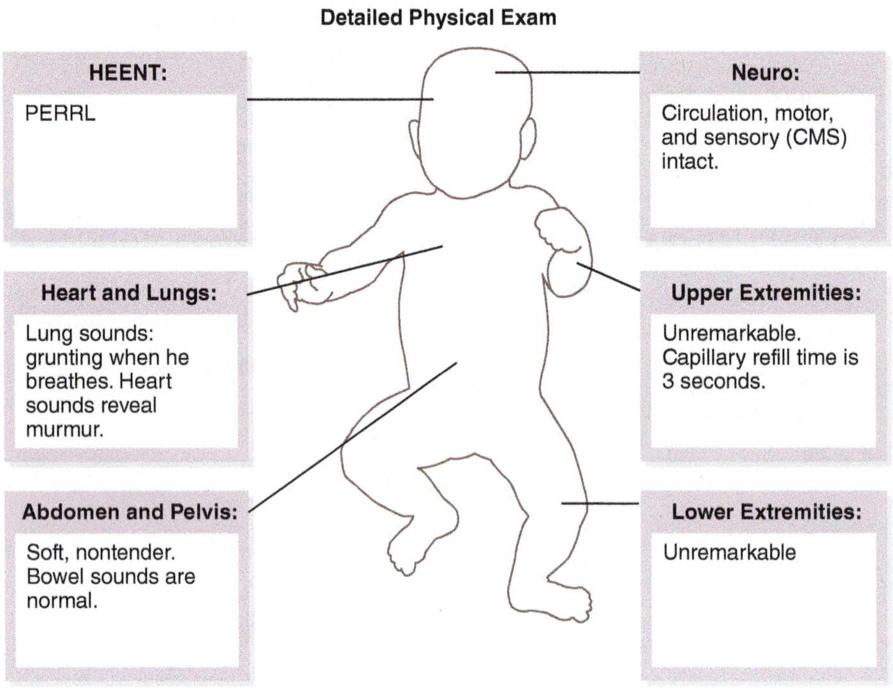

**Detailed Physical Exam**

**HEENT:**
PERRL

**Neuro:**
Circulation, motor, and sensory (CMS) intact.

**Heart and Lungs:**
Lung sounds: grunting when he breathes. Heart sounds reveal murmur.

**Upper Extremities:**
Unremarkable. Capillary refill time is 3 seconds.

**Abdomen and Pelvis:**
Soft, nontender. Bowel sounds are normal.

**Lower Extremities:**
Unremarkable

**Figure 9-23** Results of the patient's secondary survey.
© Jones & Bartlett Learning.

## Detailed Exam

**HEENT:**

- **H**ead: Unremarkable
- **E**yes: PERRL
- **E**ars: Unremarkable
- **N**ose: Unremarkable
- **T**hroat: Unremarkable

**Chest, heart, and lungs:**

- Pulses: Palpable and strong
- Cardiac auscultation: Harsh systolic murmur present
- Lung auscultation: Audible grunting, otherwise clear
- Chest exam: Symmetric movement and no trauma visible, diffuse cyanosis present

**Neurologic:**

- Neurovascular status intact
- Patient is agitated and crying.

**Abdomen and pelvis:**

- Unremarkable

## Case Questions

- Can you safely transport this child in your ambulance?
  - You ask the father to get the patient's car seat from his vehicle, and you secure it to the cot for transport.
- Will you allow the parents to ride in the ambulance?
  - The mother rides up front and the father follows behind in his vehicle.
- What is the most appropriate treatment destination and why?
  - You choose to transport this patient to the tertiary pediatric hospital approximately 35 minutes from the scene. Although there are multiple hospitals that are closer, this patient has stabilized and the parents have clustered care with their cardiologist and cardiothoracic surgeon at that hospital. You discuss with your partner that if the patient decompensates, you will divert to a closer hospital where they can provide emergency treatment and arrange for critical care transport.

**Extremities:**

- Upper extremities: Diffuse cyanosis present. Capillary refill time is 3 seconds.
- Lower extremities: Diffuse cyanosis present.

**Back:**

- Unremarkable

## Treatment

Prehospital management for this patient is limited; however, there are some initial therapies that can promote increased pulmonary circulation and oxygenation.

Immediately place the patient in a knee-chest position. Calm the patient and make sure there is a low-stimulation environment. Establish IV access as medication therapy may be necessary if the patient continues to decompensate. Make sure a cardiac monitor is applied and the patient is assessed frequently.

Supplemental oxygen is beneficial to reduce pulmonary vascular resistance. Target the patient's baseline saturation and be careful not to overshoot. In this case a baseline saturation of 82% should be targeted.

Establish an IV saline lock en route. In some cases, IV morphine may be helpful. The exact mechanism is unclear; however, the reduction of pulmonary vascular resistance is likely to play a role. The initial dose is 0.05–0.2 mg/kg IV, with a maximum single dose of 2–4 mg.

## Ongoing Management

You and your partner take the child to the ambulance immediately for transport. In the back you place the patient in a knee-chest position as your partner places him on oxygen and obtains IV access. You ask one of the parents to help calm the child and hold them in a knee-chest position as you draw up a dose of morphine to administer.

After morphine is administered, the patient calms significantly.

### CASE WRAP-UP

Diagnosis: Tetralogy of Fallot with tet spell

On arrival to the hospital the patient was in stable condition. He was admitted to the pediatric cardiac intensive care unit where his condition was optimized, and he was boarded for an initial palliative surgery that would provide additional blood flow to the lungs. His full corrective surgery was scheduled for a few months later, at which time the surgeon repaired the VSD and pulmonary stenosis. The other two defects were corrected by virtue of the first two defects being repaired.

This patient made a full recovery within approximately 6 weeks of surgery.

### CASE TAKEAWAY POINTS

Tetralogy of Fallot is the most common heart condition in children who have survived untreated beyond the neonatal period. It affects males and females equally, at a rate of 3 to 5 per 10,000 live births, and accounts for 7% to 10% of congenital defects. Surgery is usually required to fix the defect within the first year of life, with predicted 30-day survivorship after repair at 90% to 99%.

### LESSON WRAP-UP

It is important to be familiar with the contents of your obstetric kit. This will require you to review it from time to time, as utilization of this kit is a high-risk, low-frequency event. Recognition of obstetric and neonatal complications can be difficult, but EMS practitioners must be prepared for this.

Do not neglect to care for the mother after delivery. It can be easy to become focused on the newborn, however maternal hemorrhage and other postpartum complications require immediate attention to prevent mortality.

Familiarity with congenital heart defects is necessary to maintain a high index of suspicion and recognize these issues in the prehospital environment. Prehospital management for these defects is limited, however there are some interventions that are important to know. They can be lifesaving.

## REFERENCES

American College of Obstetricians and Gynecologists. Delayed umbilical cord clamping after birth. ACOG Committee Opinion No. 814. *Obstet Gynecol*. 2020;136:e100-106.

American College of Obstetricians and Gynecologists. Quantitative blood loss in obstetric hemorrhage. ACOG Committee Opinion No. 794. *Obstet Gynecol*. 2019;134:e150-156.

Aziz K, Lee HC, Escobedo MB, et al. Part 5: neonatal resuscitation 2020 American Heart Association guidelines for cardiopulmonary resuscitation and emergency cardiovascular care. *Pediatrics*. 2021;147(Suppl 1):e2020038505E.

Beaird DT, Kahwaji CI. EMS, prehospital deliveries. In: StatPearls [Internet]. Treasure Island, FL: StatPearls Publishing. Updated February 25, 2019. https://www.ncbi.nlm.nih.gov/books/NBK525996/

Centers for Disease Control and Prevention. Improved national prevalence estimates for 18 selected major birth defects—United States, 1999–2001. *Morb Mortal Wkly Rep*. 2006;54(51):1301-1305.

Dayan PS, Starc TJ, Berezow J, Vitberg YM, Tsze DS. Treatment of tetralogy of Fallot hypoxic spell with intranasal fentanyl. *Pediatrics*. 2014;134(1):E266-E269.

Diaz-Frias J, Guillaume M. Tetralogy of Fallot. In: StatPearls [Internet]. Treasure Island, FL: StatPearls Publishing. Updated October 14, 2019. https://www.ncbi.nlm.nih.gov/books/NBK513288/

Kanter KR, Kogon BE, Kirshbom PM, Carlock PR. Symptomatic neonatal tetralogy of Fallot: repair or shunt? *Ann Thorac Surg*. 2010;89(3):858-863. doi:10.1016/j.athoracsur.2009.12.060

Mayo Clinic. Tetralogy of Fallot. Accessed December 23, 2021. https://www.mayoclinic.org/diseases-conditions/tetralogy-of-fallot/symptoms-causes/syc-20353477

Mazurek P. Prehospital recognition and care of neonatal congenital heart defects. EMS1. Updated May 2017. Accessed December 23, 2021. https://www.ems1.com/ems-products/neonatal-pediatric/articles/prehospital-recognition-and-care-of-neonatal-congenital-heart-defects-C0SLoetllXO4CULD/

McCowan LM, Figueras F, Anderson NH. Evidence-based national guidelines for the management of suspected fetal growth restriction: comparison, consensus, and controversy. *Am J Obstet Gynecol*. 2018 Feb;218(2):S855-S868.

Myrhaug HT, Brurberg KG, Hov L, Markestad T. Survival and impairment of extremely premature infants: a meta-analysis. *Pediatrics*. 2019;143(2):e20180933.

O'Brien C, Marshall AC. Tetralogy of Fallot. *Circulation*. 2014;130(4):e26-e29. doi:10.1161/CIRCULATIONAHA.113.005547

Papageorghiou AT, Ohuma EO, Gravett MG, et al. International standards for symphysis-fundal height based on serial measurements from the Fetal Growth Longitudinal Study of the INTERGROWTH-21st Project: prospective cohort study in eight countries. *BMJ*. 2016;355:i5662. doi:10.1136/bmj.i5662

Sayed Ahmed WA, Hamdy MA. Optimal management of umbilical cord prolapse. *Int J Womens Health*. 2018;10:459-465. doi:10.2147/IJWH.S130879

Snyder SR. Prehospital childbirth part 2: fetal complications. *EMS World Online*. Published November 2013. Accessed December 23, 2021. https://www.hmpgloballearningnetwork.com/site/emsworld/article/11192112/prehospital-childbirth-part-2-fetal-complications

Touati GD, Vouhé PR, Amodeo A, et al. Primary repair of tetralogy of Fallot in infancy. *J Thorac Cardiovasc Surg*. 1990 Mar;99(3):396-403.

# CHAPTER 10

# Children With Special Healthcare Needs

## LESSON OBJECTIVES

- Describe specific concerns when working with children with special healthcare needs.
- Identify modifications to assessment techniques for children with special healthcare needs.
- Differentiate between the various types of complications experienced by children with special healthcare needs.
- Discuss management of special needs pediatric patients.

## Introduction

In the United States, 1 out of every 5 children has some sort of special healthcare need. In some cases, this need is a single issue, whereas in others the child may have a complex medical condition that involves multiple organ systems. The spectrum of special healthcare needs includes medical, developmental, physical, and emotional issues beyond what is routinely required for well childcare.

Special needs children have a diverse array of needs. In some cases, these needs include subspecialty physician care, frequent hospitalization, mental healthcare services, in-home health services, and prescription medications. The wide variety of needs that these children encounter can place a significant emotional and financial strain on the entire family.

As medical care and technology have advanced, children who would have died in early infancy are now living well into their adult years. In the 1970s, individuals with conditions such as cystic fibrosis rarely lived past their teenage years due to complications from their illness. These children are now living well into their 40s. That represents an almost tripling of life expectancy in only five decades. The fact that these children are living longer increases the need for awareness from prehospital practitioners.

## Cognitive Versus Physical Disabilities

In decades past, the term *mental retardation* was broadly used to describe any individual with a cognitive handicap. That term has fallen out of favor, and the preferred terminology of *intellectually disabled* is now more widely used and accepted.

*Cognitive impairment* is another term that can be used to describe intellectual disability. Examples of cognitive impairment include autism spectrum disorder (ASD) and attention deficit/hyperactivity disorder (ADHD). Both of these conditions are covered in Chapter 11, *Pediatric Behavioral Health*.

Physical disabilities are those that impact the child's ability to independently complete their activities of daily living. It is important to note that certain intellectual disabilities can also impact a child's ability to perform age-appropriate activities of daily living. While in some cases physical and cognitive disabilities coexist in the same patient, one should never assume that a physically disabled individual has cognitive impairment, or that a physically able individual possesses full cognitive abilities.

Chronic conditions that lead to physical disability include asthma, cerebral palsy, trisomy 21, cystic fibrosis, muscular dystrophy, spina bifida, hemophilia, bronchopulmonary dysplasia, and congenital heart defects.

## Assessment

Caregivers are the best resource to aid prehospital personnel in the assessment of a child with special healthcare needs. They will know the child's baseline status and be able to assist in assessing whether the child is altered compared to their baseline. They will also be able to assist prehospital practitioners with the use of specialty equipment or other assistive technology that the child uses. It is important for prehospital practitioners to not get distracted by the child's equipment. It is completely appropriate to ask for help from the caregiver—you are not expected to know how to operate every piece of specialty equipment you encounter in the field.

Modifications in the way you conduct your assessment will likely have to be made in many cases. Minor illnesses can be devastating and even life threatening for children with special needs. It is important to assess the child compared to their own baseline, not the baseline of other children of that same age. Even among children with similar special needs, there can be a wide range of abilities and presentations. It is critical that you determine exactly what is deviating from the child's baseline health status. For example, a child with a tracheostomy may always have secretions at baseline, however a caregiver might call 911 because the secretions have changed color and are more copious.

Caregivers also know what interventions will help and which ones might exacerbate the condition. They also know how to move and mobilize a child to facilitate a full exam. Some children with conditions such as cerebral palsy or muscular dystrophy may have contractures that make moving them in certain ways dangerous or painful. The caregiver will know how to position them in such a way that they may be safely and completely examined.

Communicate with the child using a developmentally appropriate approach.

## Tracheostomy Tubes

In children who have chronic respiratory failure that requires mechanical ventilation or those who have trouble clearing their oral secretions, which leads to recurrent aspiration or pulmonary infections, a tracheostomy tube may be necessary to keep the airway open and free of oral secretions (**Figure 10-1**).

Tracheostomy tubes, like endotracheal (ET) tubes, come in both cuffed and uncuffed varieties. Like an ET tube, the cuff is inflated with air, foam, or sterile water.

There are single- and dual-lumen tracheostomy tubes. A double-lumen style has a hollow outer cannula that remains in place, with a removable inner

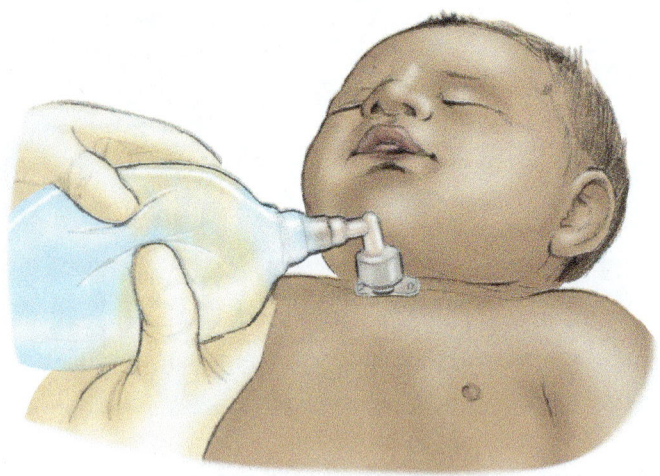

**Figure 10-1** Oxygen and ventilatory assistance can be delivered through a tracheostomy tube.

© Jones & Bartlett Learning.

cannula that can be easily removed for suctioning and cleaning. Many patients with a tracheostomy produce copious secretions, which can adhere to the cannula and reduce the diameter, leading to increased airway resistance and increasing the work of breathing for the patient. The double-lumen style offers the benefit of being able to easily remove and clean the inner cannula, which in some cases is disposable. In smaller patients, having an internal cannula inside of an outer cannula would reduce the diameter too much for practical use. These patients will utilize a single-lumen cannula. Cannulas may also come with fenestration in the superior end to allow for air to go up through the tube into the oropharynx. This aids the patient by allowing them to speak more easily. Oxygen and ventilatory assistance can be provided through a tracheostomy tube if necessary. Blow-by oxygen, a special tracheostomy mask, or a bag-valve mask (BVM) attached to the tracheostomy tube may be used for therapy.

One of the most common complications of tracheostomy tubes is obstructions due to mucus plugging. This can lead to significant respiratory distress and even respiratory failure. To clear an obstructed tracheostomy tube, perform the following steps:

- Place padding underneath the child's shoulders to optimize airway positioning.

- Ensure that the tube is not displaced by confirming that the wings of the tube are against the neck and verify that the obturator (rigid piece of plastic used to keep the shape of the tube during insertion) is not inside the tube.

- If the child has a fenestrated tube, remove the decannulation plug.

- If the child has a dual-lumen tube, remove the inner lumen.

- If the previous steps do not work, then a flexible suction catheter can be inserted to suction out the mucus. Use caution to not insert the suction catheter too far as it can cause irritation of the carina and lead to bradycardia.

- If the obturator is available, it can be passed through the tube to clear plugs that are present within the device itself. Plugs located below the device will not be dislodged by the obturator, however.

# Cerebrospinal Fluid Shunts

Some children have conditions that lead to excessive cerebrospinal fluid (CSF) in the brain (**Figure 10-2**). This can be due to poor drainage, poor absorption, or excessive production. In these cases, a shunt can be inserted to aid in preventing elevated intracranial pressure due to CSF buildup. These shunts work by draining excess fluid from the ventricles of the brain. The most common locations for this drainage to go is into the peritoneum where it can be reabsorbed—this is known as a ventriculoperitoneal shunt (VP shunt). In some cases, the fluid is drained from the ventricles into the right atrium of the heart—this is known as a ventriculoatrial shunt (VA shunt). Either type of shunt is susceptible to obstruction, infection, or other malfunctions.

When a shunt becomes obstructed, the most common initial complaint will be headache. In nonverbal children this may manifest as increased irritability or inconsolability. This can progress to ataxia, altered level of consciousness, Cushing triad, herniation, and ultimately death if the obstruction is not relieved emergently. Some shunts have a bulb that allows for the device to be accessed and CSF to be removed. This is a procedure that should be done in sterile fashion in a hospital setting. If the patient is showing signs of herniation (increased blood pressure, bradycardia, and altered respiratory pattern) you should treat it as you would any other head injury with elevated intracranial pressure. Maintain an open airway and optimize breathing. Elevate the head to 30 to 45 degrees. Assist ventilation and consider hyperventilation if the child is demonstrating signs of Cushing triad.

When fever is present in a patient with a shunt, it should be considered a shunt infection until proven otherwise. These children must be transported to a hospital where CSF samples can be taken for culture and antibiotics initiated.

# Central Venous Catheters

Children who require long-term vascular access for the administration of medications such as chemotherapy, immunosuppressants, or other pharmacotherapies may have a central venous catheter placed (**Figure 10-3**). These catheters are sometimes called ports or "porta-caths." These devices can be tunneled under the skin, positioned directly through the chest, or placed in the arm. They may be single or double lumen.

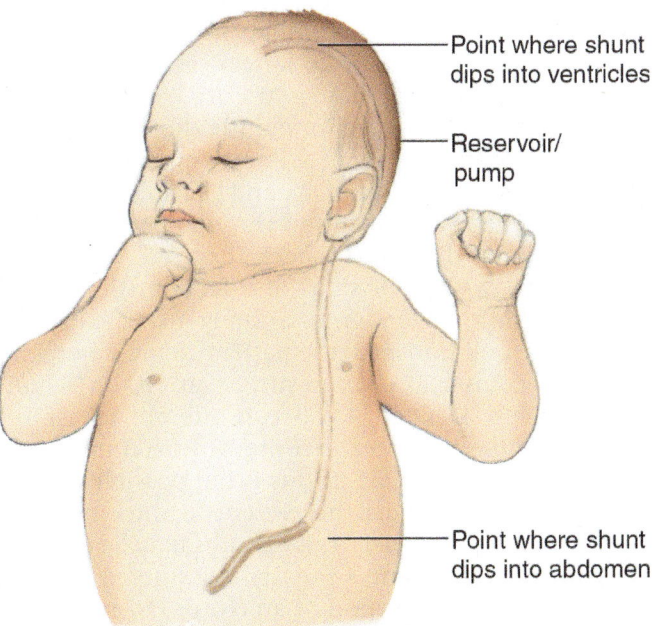

Point where shunt dips into ventricles

Reservoir/pump

Point where shunt dips into abdomen

**Figure 10-2** A cerebrospinal fluid shunt aids in maintaining normal brain pressure in a child with hydrocephalus.

© Jones & Bartlett Learning.

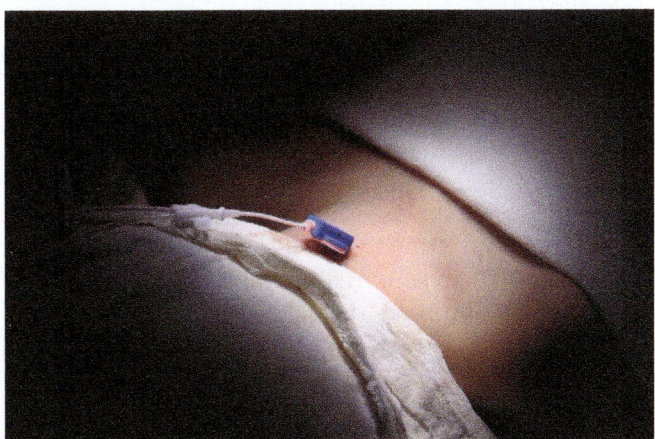

**Figure 10-3** Central venous catheters provide a route to administer nutritional support or medications such as chemotherapy and antibiotic therapy.

© Johner Images/Getty Images.

One of the most serious complications of these catheters is infection. Children with infected catheters will often present with fever, although in some cases, such as children with cancer who are on immunosuppressants, typical signs of infection may not be seen. The area around the catheter may be red, inflamed, and painful to the touch. Do not expect to see purulent buildup or abscess formation in neutropenic individuals, as they lack sufficient immune response to form an abscess. The most common sign in these patients is pain and redness in the area around the catheter.

These catheters can also become dislodged while coughing or if they are pulled on with too much force. This becomes particularly relevant when dealing with children, who are often unaware that they need to be gentle with these devices. Air embolism is a less common complication.

Children who receive total parenteral nutrition (TPN) through these devices may become hypoglycemic if the device becomes obstructed during their nutrition infusion. It may be necessary to obtain intravenous (IV) access and infuse dextrose-containing fluids for patients in these situations.

Most agencies do not allow prehospital practitioners to access central catheters due to infection risk. If you encounter a catheter that appears to be malfunctioning there are a few steps you can take to gain control of the situation. If a central venous catheter is leaking, clamp the exposed end (if possible) to stop the flow of blood. Utilize a clean hemostat with the jaws wrapped in gauze to prevent further damage to the catheter. If you are unable to clamp the device for any reason, apply direct pressure with clean, sterile gauze. If you suspect an air embolism has occurred (coughing, chest pain, shortness of breath) the catheter should be clamped and oxygen should be administered. Place the patient on their left side in a head-down position to prevent the embolism from traveling to the brain. As mentioned, patients receiving nutrition through these devices may require a glucose infusion through a peripheral IV if their catheter becomes obstructed or otherwise nonfunctional. If the patient experiences a reaction to the fluids or medications being administered through the catheter, immediately stop the infusion and transport the patient to the hospital. Bring the fluid for analysis. Use caution when handling chemotherapy medications as they can be toxic and absorbed through the skin.

# Feeding Tubes

Some children do not possess the oral motor skills needed to safely feed themselves by mouth. In these cases, when they feed by mouth, there is a significant risk for aspiration and lung infection. Feeding tubes may be used to

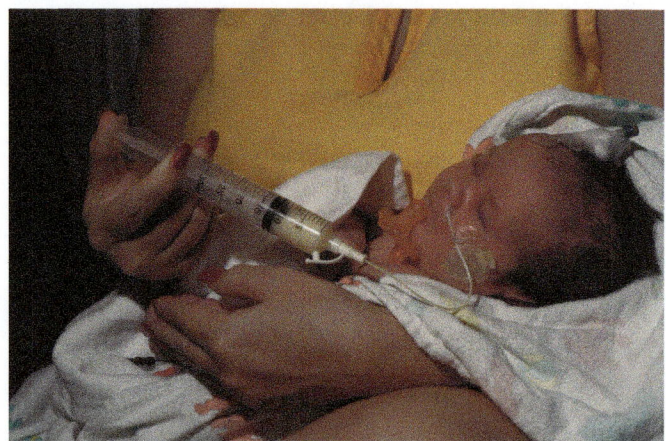

**Figure 10-4** Feeding tubes may be used to provide nutrition safely to patients who do not possess the oral motor skills to safely feed themselves by mouth.
© Rick's Photography/Shutterstock.

provide nutrition safely to these patients without the risk of aspiration (**Figure 10-4**). Feeding tubes may also be used in situations where there is an anatomic obstruction or esophageal disruption preventing oral feeding.

Feeding tubes come in many different varieties. The name of the tube generally tells the practitioner how the tube is positioned. **Table 10-1** lists various feeding tube types and their positioning.

The most common complication encountered with feeding tubes is dislodgement. In many cases the tube may simply fall out of place. This can happen when the cuff or balloon that retains any of the percutaneous tubes (ones that go through the abdominal wall) ruptures and the tube is no longer secure. In the case of orogastric (OG) or nasogastric (NG) tubes that are inserted through the nose or mouth, the most common symptom of dislodgement will be aspiration of feeds, leading to coughing, choking, and gagging.

If a tube that is inserted through the abdominal wall becomes dislodged, check the area for bleeding or leakage. Assess for signs of infection such as redness, warmth, or tenderness. Apply a sterile dressing to the site and transport the patient to the emergency room for reinsertion. If you suspect an NG or OG tube has become dislodged, you can attempt to aspirate from the tube and test the contents with litmus paper to see if they are acidic. If this is not possible or practical, simply transport the patient to the emergency department (ED) where radiographs may be obtained to confirm placement. In many cases parents will be trained in the reinsertion of an NG or OG tube.

If you transport a patient with a dislodged feeding tube to the ED, make sure to bring the original device with you. It can help the ED staff determine the replacement size needed.

### Table 10-1 Types of Feeding Tubes

| | |
|---|---|
| Nasogastric | Inserted through the nostril with the distal tip resting in the stomach |
| Nasojejunal | Inserted through the nostril with the distal tip located transpylorically in the jejunal area of the small intestine |
| Orogastric | Inserted through the mouth with the distal tip resting in the stomach |
| Orojejunal | Inserted through the mouth with the distal tip located transpylorically in the jejunal area of the small intestine |
| Gastrostomy | This tube is surgically placed through the abdominal wall with the distal tip in the stomach. This will sometimes be referred to as a G tube or G button. |
| Gastrojejunal | This tube is surgically placed through the abdominal wall and has two lumens. One lumen is in the stomach (the gastric lumen) and the other lumen is in the jejunum (the jejunal lumen). These will sometimes be referred to as GJ tubes. |
| Percutaneous endoscopic gastrostomy (PEG) | This is a subset of gastrostomy tubes that is placed endoscopically through the abdominal wall with the distal tip in the stomach. |

© Jones & Bartlett Learning.

# Vagal Nerve Stimulator

Vagal nerve stimulators (VNS) are devices that are surgically placed under the skin on the left chest in a manner similar to a pacemaker (**Figure 10-5**). These devices are programmed to provide stimulation to the vagus nerve when activated by a magnet. They are most commonly used for the treatment of seizures but may also be used for the treatment of depression.

If you encounter a seizing patient with a VNS, you may assist the parent in activating the device.

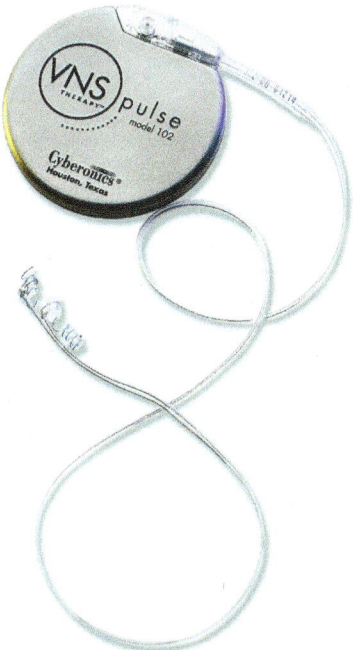

**Figure 10-5** A vagal nerve stimulator is programmed to provide intermittent stimulation to the left vagus nerve leading to the brain.

© Cyberonics, Inc./Getty Images News/Getty Images.

When EMS has been called, it is likely that the device has failed to terminate the seizure, and you should proceed as you normally would for a seizing patient. Focus on the airway, breathing, and circulation. Use caution when defibrillating or performing procedures such a needle decompression. Additionally, practitioners need to be cognizant that they may need to alter their landmarks when performing defibrillation or needle decompression to avoid the VNS device.

# Additional Forms of Assistive Technology

There is a wide variety of assistive technology to help medically complex children perform their activities of daily living (**Figure 10-6**). These devices perform all sorts of tasks. **Table 10-2** provides a small listing of assistive technology devices that EMS professionals may encounter in the field.

EMS should make every effort to provide reasonable accommodations and to transport these devices with the patient when able to safely do so. Coordinate with the caregiver to transport devices that are too large to safely fit in the ambulance, such as specialty wheelchairs.

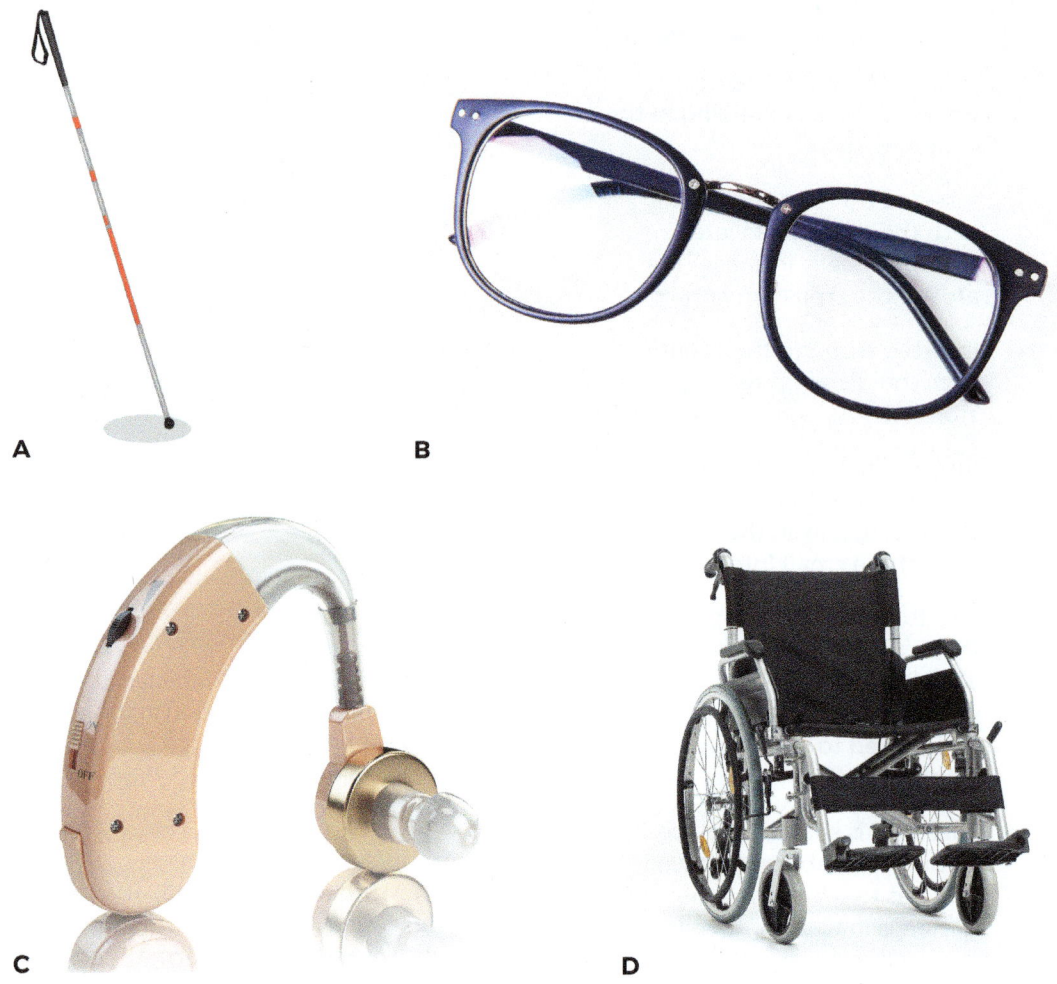

**Figure 10-6** Types of assistive devices. **A.** Walking cane. **B.** Eyeglasses. **C.** Hearing aid. **D.** Wheelchair.

**A.** © Selda Can/Shutterstock; **B.** © Vulp/Shutterstock; **C.** © Maxx-Studio/Shutterstock; **D.** © xiaorui/Shutterstock.

## Table 10-2 Types of Assistive Technology Devices

| Mobility | | Communication | |
|---|---|---|---|
| Mobility | ■ Wheelchairs<br>■ Walkers<br>■ Prosthetic limbs<br>■ Braces<br>■ Seating devices | Communication | ■ Communication card<br>■ Communication tablet<br>■ Text-to-speech device<br>■ Word or picture board |
| Vision | ■ Eyeglasses<br>■ Magnifiers<br>■ Walking canes | Cognition | ■ Task list<br>■ Picture-based instruction book<br>■ Timers |
| Hearing | ■ Headphones<br>■ Hearing aids<br>■ Cochlear implants | Calming | ■ Weighted compression vest<br>■ Weighted blanket<br>■ Noise cancelling or muffling headphones |

# CASE STUDY

## Case 1

### Dispatch

You and your partner respond to a residence for a 2-year-old female with a tracheostomy who is having difficulty breathing (**Figure 10-7**). It is a cold spring evening. The outside temperature is 45°F (7.2°C).

#### Case Questions

- What are your initial concerns?
  - The initial concerns for this call include a child with a history of respiratory issues having trouble with her tracheostomy tube. This is a situation with the potential for a "can't ventilate, can't oxygenate" scenario if the tracheostomy is failing.
- Based on the dispatch information, what is the possible differential diagnosis for this patient?
  - The differential diagnosis for this case includes tracheostomy plugging, dislodgement, or failure. In addition to issues with the tracheostomy, the patient could be having respiratory trouble not related to the tracheostomy itself. This could include viral or bacterial respiratory infections, asthma, or bronchiectasis.

### Initial Observations

As you arrive at the front entrance of the home, you are met by the patient's parents. The patient is being held by her mother, and she appears to be in respiratory distress. The father informs you that she has cystic fibrosis.

- Pediatric Assessment Triangle
  - Appearance
    - Restless
  - Work of breathing
    - **F**laring present
    - **R**etractions present
    - **A**udible airway sounds are present. There are copious secretions and audible rhonchi.
    - **P**ositioning not present
  - Circulation
    - Skin warm and clammy

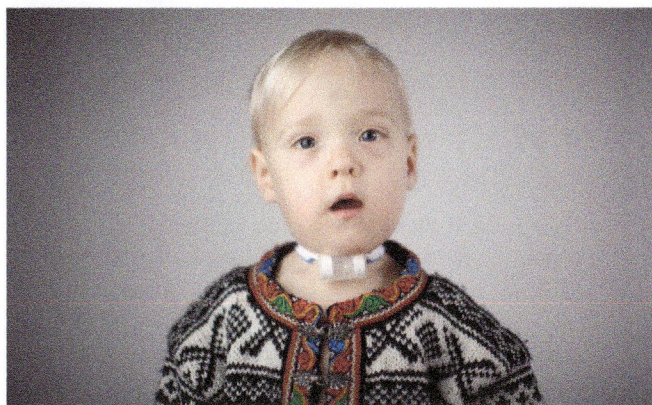

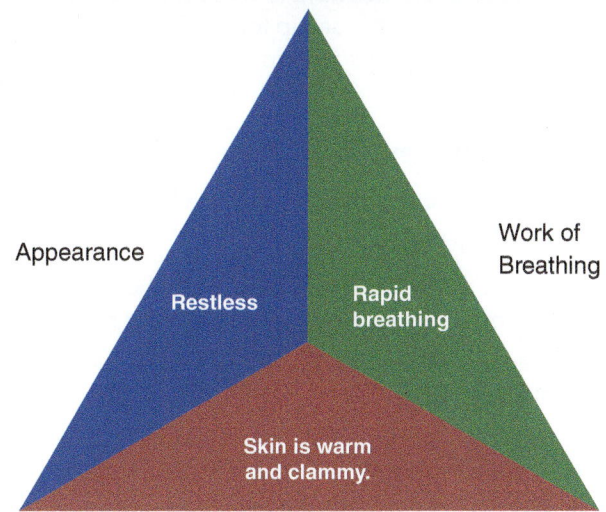

**Figure 10-7** Your patient is a 2-year-old child with a tracheostomy tube who is having trouble breathing.

A. PVstock.com/Alamy Stock Photo; B. Used with permission of the American Academy of Pediatrics, Pediatric Education for Prehospital Professionals, © American Academy of Pediatrics, 2000.

The parents advise you that the patient had a new tracheostomy tube placed about a week ago for recurrent pulmonary infections secondary to her underlying cystic fibrosis.

Cystic fibrosis is a genetic defect in the chloride ion transporter, which results in thick mucus secretions. Cystic fibrosis is discussed further in Chapter 2, *Respiratory Emergencies*. These secretions are difficult to produce, which leads to recurrent respiratory infections and diminished respiratory function. This condition also affects the exocrine pancreas and leads to difficulty with digestion of certain nutrients.

Because this patient has a new tracheostomy tube, the parents may not be fully comfortable with it. Even though most hospitals have an extensive support and training program for patients with new tracheostomy tubes to provide parents with the resources to care for these medically fragile children, nothing can truly prepare caregivers for a situation where their child is actively decompensating.

## Case Questions

- Based on your initial impression, is this patient "Quick" or "Not Quick"?

  - This patient likely has a plugged tracheostomy. Her underlying medical condition makes it difficult to assess how far from her baseline her current level of respiratory distress is. This patient is "Quick" because her only available airway is currently plugged and if EMS personnel are not able to clear the blockage, there is a possible setup for a "can't ventilate, can't oxygenate" scenario.

## Primary Survey

The primary survey for this patient reveals the following:

**X**—No bleeding found

**A**—There is an open tracheostomy tube with bubbling mucinous secretions pouring from it.

**B**—Rapid and regular. There are audible rhonchi bilaterally.

**C**—Brachial pulses are strong and rapid. Capillary refill time is brisk. The skin is warm and clammy.

**D**—Glasgow Coma Scale (GCS) score is 15 (E4, V5, M6). The patient is alert and restless.

**E**—Lying in the mother's arms

## Case Questions

- Based on the findings noted in the primary survey, what would your initial interventions and treatment include?

  - The initial treatment for this patient should include aggressive suctioning of the tracheostomy tube in an effort to clear the mucus plug. Humidified oxygen should be used if available to loosen the plug. Avoid

the use of nonhumidified oxygen as it can make secretions thicker by drying them out. Although saline lavage is sometimes used in the hospital setting, the use of lavage should be limited to experienced practitioners who are able to perform saline lavage in such a manner that saline does not drift into the lungs where it will collect and further impair gas exchange.

- What are your differential diagnoses for this patient?

  - Although mucus plug is the most likely cause of this patient's respiratory distress, other differential diagnoses should be considered. This patient could also be choking on a foreign body, or she could have a respiratory infection.

## Suctioning a Tracheostomy

Suctioning is used when there is mucus or other debris clogging the tracheostomy tube. It can help prevent or alleviate tube obstructions. If you can see or hear secretions, the patient is in respiratory distress, the patient is desaturated, and they are unable to clear the tube with their own cough, suctioning is indicated.

To perform suctioning, you will need a suction device, an appropriately sized flexible suction catheter, sterile water, some 4 × 4 gauze, and proper personal protective equipment (PPE; including eye and face protection). See **Table 10-3** for recommended suction catheter sizes.

Most families will have their own suction equipment in the home. It is appropriate to use this when available if it is functional. It will likely already be sized and ready for use. If not available you will need to use your own equipment from the ambulance.

Prior to suctioning make sure to preoxygenate the patient with a BVM. Place 1 to 2 mL of normal saline or sterile water into the tube to help loosen any thick secretions. Select an appropriately sized suction catheter and insert the catheter no further than the length of the tracheostomy tube, approximately 2 inches (5 cm) in most cases. A spare tracheostomy tube can be used to estimate the distance of insertion. If the patient begins to cough and gag, you have likely inserted the suction catheter too far. Never force the suction catheter against resistance.

Suction pressure should be 80 to 120 mm Hg. Never exceed 120 mm Hg of suction pressure as it could cause

**Table 10-3** Recommended Suction Catheter Sizes

| Tube Size | 3.0 mm | 3.5 mm | 4.0 mm | 4.5 mm | 5.0 mm | 6.0 mm | 7.0 mm and > |
|-----------|--------|--------|--------|--------|--------|--------|--------------|
| Fr size | 7 | 8 | 8 | 10 | 10 | 10–12 | 12 |

trauma to tissues that are pulled into the catheter or collapse the lower airways. Cover the suction port and suction for 3 to 5 seconds while withdrawing the catheter. Use a basin full of saline or sterile water to clear the suction catheter and allow the patient to recover their oxygen saturation before making another suction pass. If the patient becomes cyanotic or bradycardic, immediately terminate the suction attempt and provide assisted ventilations.

Continue suctioning passes until the airway is clear. Reoxygenate the patient with blow-by oxygen or a BVM between attempts.

## Detailed Assessment

### History Taking

As your partner sets up to suction and applies the patient monitor, you begin to take a patient history.

**OPQRST:**

- **O**nset: Gradual
- **P**rovocation/palliation: None
- **Q**uality: None
- **R**adiation: None
- **S**everity: Unknown
- **T**iming: 60 minutes

**SAMPLER:**

- **S**igns/symptoms: Respiratory distress

- **A**llergies: No known allergies to medications, foods, or the environment
- **M**edications: Pancrelipase, multivitamins, Pulmozyme, ivacaftor, albuterol, inhaled Tobramycin
- **P**ast medical history: Cystic fibrosis diagnosed at age 8 months, steatorrhea, pancreatic insufficiency, chronic recurrent respiratory infections. Tracheostomy tube insertion approximately 1 week ago.
- **L**ast oral intake: Dinner 2 hours prior to parents calling 911
- **E**vents leading up to the emergency: Respiratory distress shortly after eating dinner
- **R**isk factors: Cystic fibrosis, new tracheostomy

### Vital Signs

As you were discussing the history, the patient was attached to the monitor and the following vital signs were obtained (**Figure 10-8**):

**Heart rate:**

- 153 beats/min
- This patient is tachycardic, likely related to agitation and hypoxia.

**SpO₂:**

- 92% RA
- The obstructed tracheostomy tube has led to decreased $SpO_2$.

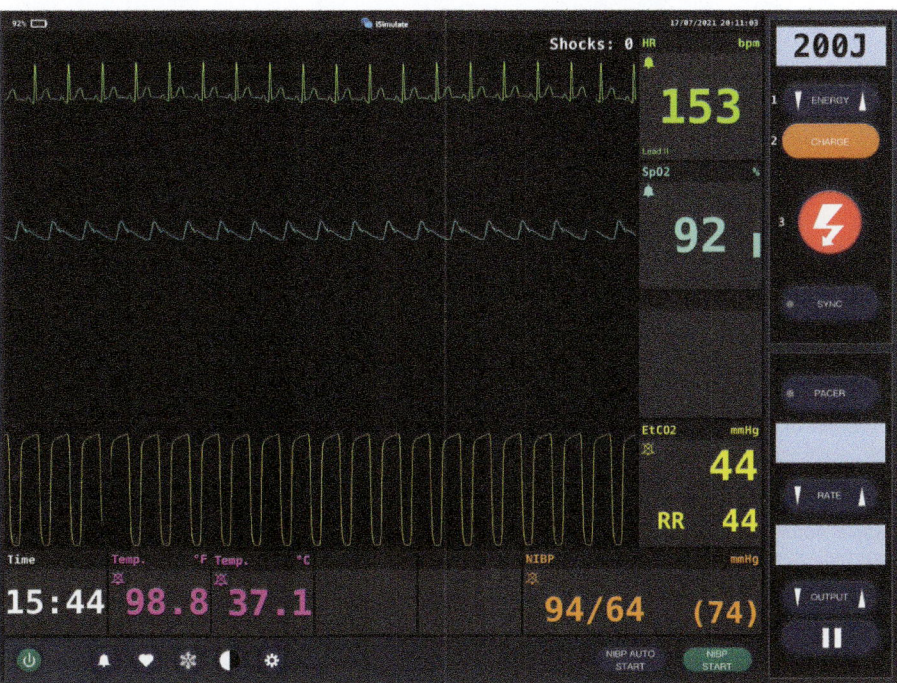

**Figure 10-8** Patient's vital signs indicate tachypnea and tachycardia.

Courtesy of iSimulate.

**ETCO₂:**

- 44 mm Hg

**Respiratory rate:**

- 44 breaths/min
- The patient is tachypneic.

**Blood pressure:**

- 94/64 mm Hg
- This is an adequate blood pressure for this patient.

**Temperature:**

- 98.8°F (37.1°C)

**Blood glucose:**

- 102 mg/dL

Along with the rhonchi and secretions, the vital signs indicate that the patient has intact perfusion with respiratory distress and mild hypoxia.

The patient is a 2-year-old female with history of cystic fibrosis and recent tracheostomy tube placement presenting with sudden-onset respiratory distress likely related to mucus plugging. She is currently hemodynamically stable with signs of mild hypoxia.

## Detailed Exam

**HEENT (Figure 10-9):**

- **H**ead: Unremarkable

- **E**yes: PERRL, unremarkable
- **E**ars: Unremarkable
- **N**ose: Some secretions
- **T**hroat: There is a new tracheostomy in place. No leaking or bleeding is noted around the insertion site. There are copious secretions inside the tube.

**Chest, heart, and lungs:**

- Pulses: Present and palpable peripherally
- Cardiac auscultation: Regular rate and rhythm with no rubs, gallops, or murmurs auscultated.
- Lung auscultation: Rhonchi are heard bilaterally with significant referred upper airway congestion suggestive of mucus plugging.
- Chest exam: There is symmetric chest rise bilaterally.

**Neurologic:**

- Neurovascular status intact. The patient is restless and easily agitated.

**Abdomen and pelvis:**

- Unremarkable

**Extremities:**

- Upper extremities: Unremarkable
- Lower extremities: Unremarkable

**Back:**

- Unremarkable

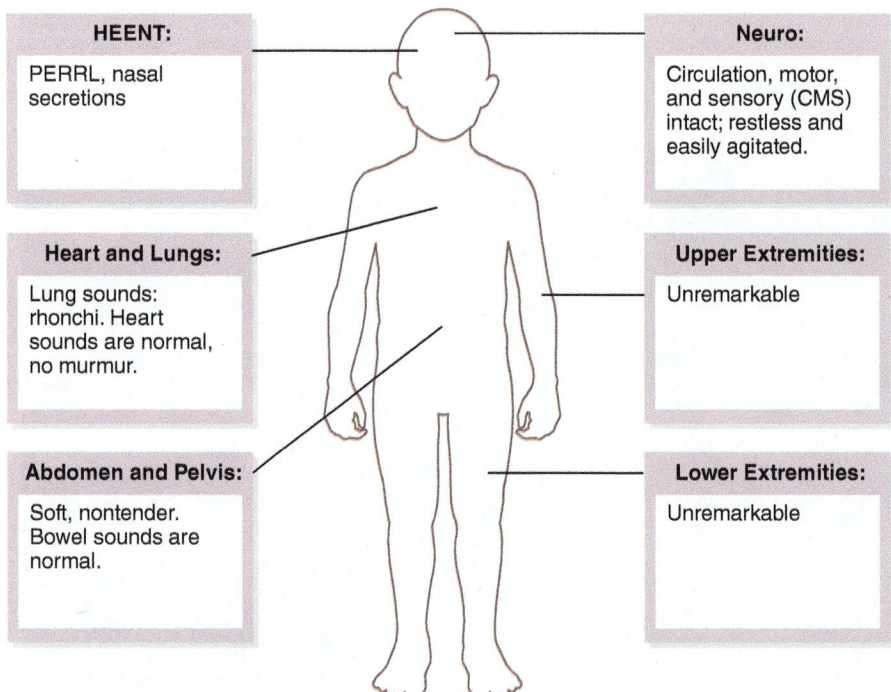

**Detailed Physical Exam**

**HEENT:**
PERRL, nasal secretions

**Neuro:**
Circulation, motor, and sensory (CMS) intact; restless and easily agitated.

**Heart and Lungs:**
Lung sounds: rhonchi. Heart sounds are normal, no murmur.

**Upper Extremities:**
Unremarkable

**Abdomen and Pelvis:**
Soft, nontender. Bowel sounds are normal.

**Lower Extremities:**
Unremarkable

**Figure 10-9** Details of the patient's secondary survey.

## Treatment

This patient should be treated with aggressive respiratory support aimed at clearing the upper airway obstruction. Practitioners should be prepared for rapid deterioration.

Practitioners should set up to suction the airway. Administer humidified oxygen if available. ALS practitioners can prepare to replace the tracheostomy tube if a spare is available and suctioning is unsuccessful.

There is little role for bronchodilators and inhaled or systemic steroids in this case. The primary issue is related to upper airway obstruction from secretions, not inflammation. However, if there was wheezing or signs of lower airway obstruction present, inhaled beta agonists and corticosteroids may be beneficial.

Critical care practitioners may set up for and anticipate the need for advanced airway insertion. Pharmacologically assisted intubation (PAI) may be necessary if the patient is in a "can't ventilate, can't oxygenate" scenario. When the decision to intubate a patient with a tracheostomy is made, the most experienced practitioner should be the one to attempt intubation. The patient's anatomy will likely be abnormal, and practitioners should anticipate a difficult airway insertion. This should be a last resort and only attempted when ventilation via BVM is unsuccessful and with medical control approval.

## Ongoing Management

After suctioning the patient, the oxygen saturation rose to 95% with blow-by humidified oxygen. The patient was loaded for transport and the parents requested that you take the patient's chest physiotherapy vest with her to the hospital. The patient remained stable throughout the remainder of the transport.

### Case Questions

- What is the most appropriate treatment destination and why?
  - The child was taken to the academic children's hospital, bypassing less specialized adult EDs in favor of a hospital where the patient's multiple subspecialists (pulmonology and endocrinology) are located.
- Can you safely transport this child in your ambulance?
  - You utilized the patient's car seat from her parents' vehicle to safely secure her to the patient stretcher.
- Will you allow the parents to ride in the ambulance?
  - The mother rode in the patient compartment safely secured to the bench seat, while the father followed behind, bringing the patient's other in-home equipment.

### CASE WRAP-UP

Diagnosis: Tracheostomy blockage and bronchiectasis

At the hospital this patient received a chest x-ray and computed tomography (CT) scan due to history of possible aspiration. These imaging studies revealed bilateral tram track opacities and hyperinflation, suggestive of bronchiectasis, and widening of the upper airway with excessive mucus buildup. She was continued on humidified oxygen and an aggressive pulmonary toilet regimen including inhaled hypertonic saline and bag suctioning, and chest physiotherapy was initiated. Her respiratory status improved significantly over the next 24 hours and she was discharged home. The family was provided with additional education and resources for dealing with tracheostomy emergencies in the future.

### CASE TAKEAWAY POINTS

Obstruction is the most common respiratory emergency in children with a tracheostomy tube (**Figure 10-10**). EMS practitioners should be capable of dealing with this emergency should they be called to assist.

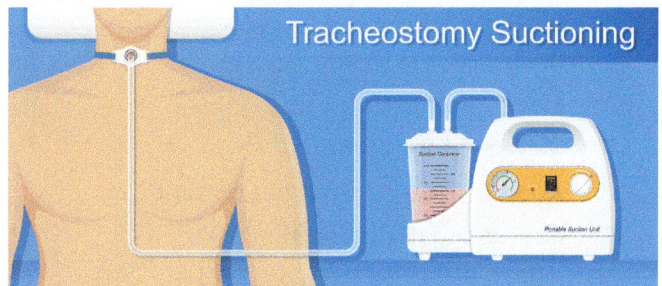

**Figure 10-10** Obstruction is the most common cause of severe respiratory distress in pediatric patients with a tracheostomy.
© rumruay/Shutterstock.

# CASE STUDY

## Case 2

### Dispatch

You and your partner respond to a home for a 5-year-old male who is actively seizing (**Figure 10-11**). It is a hot summer afternoon. The outside temperature is 88°F (31.1°C).

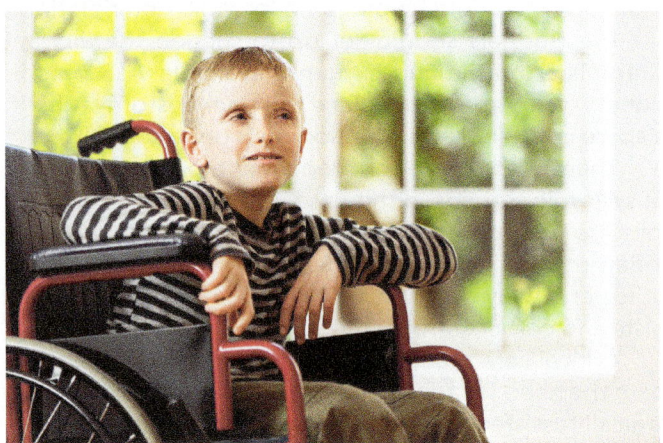

### Case Questions

- What are your initial concerns?
  - The initial concern in this call is that a 5-year-old is having an uncontrolled seizure. This could lead to respiratory and possibly cardiac arrest if it goes untreated.
- Based on the dispatch information, what are the possible differential diagnoses for this patient?
  - The differential diagnosis for seizure activity is broad. Seizures may be due to epilepsy or febrile in nature. Toxic exposure or ingestion and hypoglycemia can also lead to seizure activity. Nonaccidental trauma leading to traumatic brain injury should also be included.

### Initial Observations

As you arrive on scene you are met at the front door of the house by a preteen child telling you that everyone is around in the back of the house on the patio. As you go around the back you see two parents crouched down by a school-age child lying on the patio, who you assume to be the patient, with a specialty wheelchair nearby. The patient is no longer seizing, and the parents tell you they administered rectal diazepam.

- Pediatric Assessment Triangle
  - Appearance
    - Lethargic
  - Work of breathing
    - Breathing is slow and regular
    - **F**laring not present
    - **R**etractions not present
    - **A**udible airway sounds not present
    - **P**ositioning not present
  - Circulation
    - Skin is flushed.

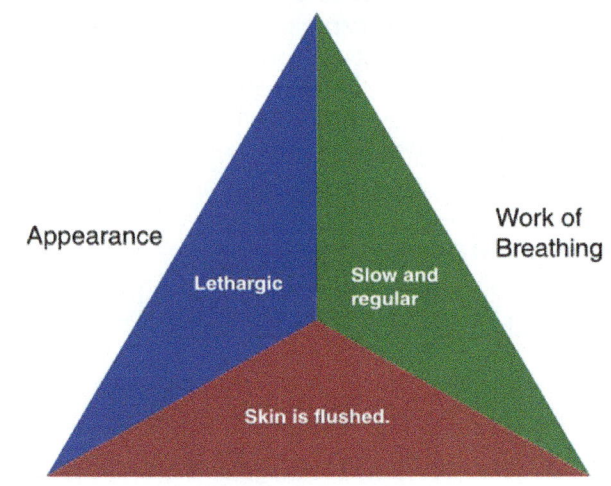

**Figure 10-11** The patient is a 5-year-old boy who is reported to be having an uncontrolled seizure.
© RapidEye/iStock/Getty Images Plus/Getty Images.

### Case Questions

- Based on your initial impression, is this patient "Quick" or "Not Quick"?
  - This patient is "Quick." He has an altered level of consciousness and recent seizure activity. Even though you have not yet obtained a history, the presence of a medical-grade wheelchair suggests that he may have a complex underlying illness.

## Primary Survey

The primary survey for this patient reveals the following:

**X**—No bleeding found

**A**—Patent

**B**—Slow and regular

**C**—Radial pulses are strong and regular, capillary refill time is brisk. The skin is flushed.

**D**—GCS is 9 (E2, V2, M5).

**E**—Lying on the floor; postictal state

You ask the parents about the patient's typical baseline neurologic status. They inform you that he is normally alert and oriented. Sometimes he has mild drooling, but he is able to communicate verbally. He has mild strabismus. They inform you very clearly that he is not at his neurologic baseline.

### Case Questions

- Based on the findings noted in the primary survey, what would your initial interventions and treatment include?

  - The initial treatment for this patient should include measures to protect the airway and optimize breathing. The patient does not appear to be actively seizing any longer, so medication administration is not immediately necessary. You may consider examining the airway to ensure there is no vomitus or secretions that could be aspirated, and suction if necessary. Consider obtaining IV access in case the seizure activity starts again.

## Detailed Assessment

### History Taking

As your partner applies the monitor and sets up for IV access, you begin to take a more detailed history.

**OPQRST:**

- **O**nset: Sudden
- **P**rovocation/palliation: None
- **Q**uality: None
- **R**adiation: None
- **S**everity: None
- **T**iming: 10 minutes

**SAMPLER:**

- **S**igns/symptoms: Seizure activity lasting approximately 5 minutes
- **A**llergies: No known allergies to medications, foods, or the environment
- **M**edications: Rectal diazepam
- **P**ast medical history: Low birthweight, maternal insulin-dependent diabetes mellitus and preeclampsia, seizure activity on day 2 of life
- **L**ast oral intake: Lunch 1 hour prior to the seizure
- **E**vents leading up to the emergency: Outside playing with his family
- **R**isk factors: Cerebral palsy, past medical history of seizures

## Types of Cerebral Palsy

Cerebral palsy is the most common motor disorder among pediatric patients. It is an umbrella term for a group of disorders that affect an individual's capability to move and maintain balance. In some cases the condition is accompanied by intellectual disability; however, many patients are cognitively intact.

Cerebral palsy is usually classified by the type of movement disorder involved. The movement disorder is dictated by the area of the brain that is affected. **Table 10-4** describes the classification, prevalence, etiology, and clinical description of some of the most common forms of cerebral palsy.

Cerebral palsy is a spectrum, and the signs and symptoms range from subtle to quite obvious. Children who have delayed motor or coordination milestones should be evaluated for cerebral palsy by their pediatrician, especially if risk factors are present.

### Vital Signs

As you were discussing the history, the patient was attached to the monitor and the following vital signs were obtained (**Figure 10-12**):

**Heart rate:**

- 81 beats/min
- This is within the expected range for this patient.

**SpO$_2$:**

- 93% RA

**ETCO$_2$:**

- 39 mm Hg

**Respiratory rate:**

- 20 breaths/min

**Table 10-4** Types of Cerebral Palsy

| Classification | Percentage Affected | Common Etiologies | Clinical Description |
|---|---|---|---|
| Spastic diplegia | 13–25% | Periventricular leukomalacia | Both legs > arms |
| Spastic hemiplegia | 21–40% | Neonatal stroke<br>Cortical malformations | One side of the body<br>Arm > leg<br>Sensory deficits |
| Spastic quadriplegia | 20–43% | CNS infection<br>Cerebral dysgenesis<br>Perinatal/postnatal events | All limbs<br>Arms ≥ legs |
| Dyskinetic | 12—14% | Severe perinatal asphyxia | Involuntary movements exacerbated by stress, excitement, or fever |
| Ataxic | 4–13% | Early prenatal events<br>Genetic | Uncoordinated, unsteady movements<br>Slow, jerky, and/or explosive speech |

© Jones & Bartlett Learning.

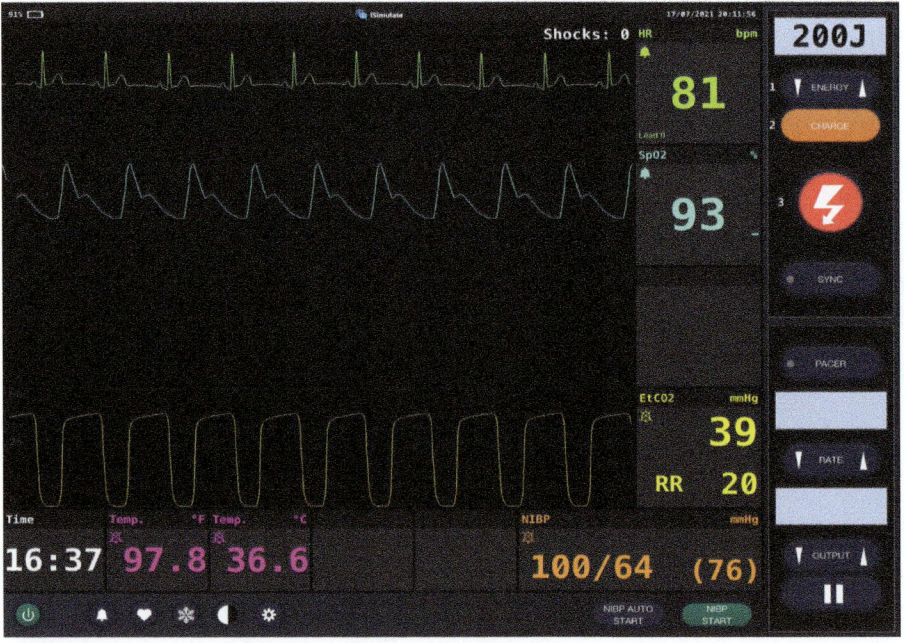

**Figure 10-12** This patient's vital signs are reassuring.
Courtesy of iSimulate.

**Blood pressure:**

- 100/64 mm Hg

**Temperature:**

- 97.8°F (36.5°C)

**Blood glucose:**

- 100 mg/dL

The vital signs for this patient are reassuring. He has an intact circulatory and respiratory status. He does not

**Detailed Physical Exam**

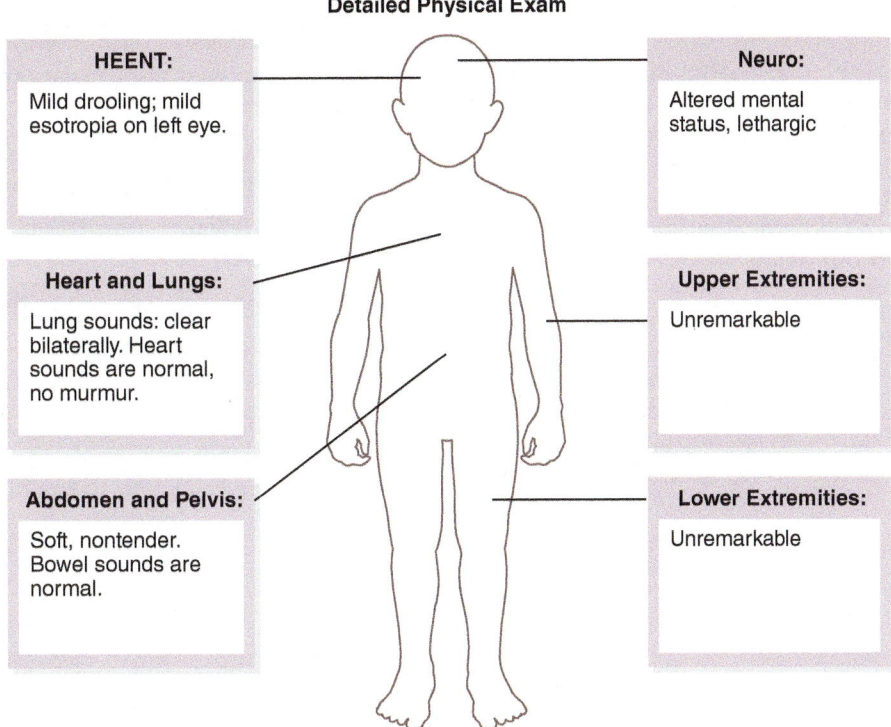

**HEENT:**
Mild drooling; mild esotropia on left eye.

**Neuro:**
Altered mental status, lethargic

**Heart and Lungs:**
Lung sounds: clear bilaterally. Heart sounds are normal, no murmur.

**Upper Extremities:**
Unremarkable

**Abdomen and Pelvis:**
Soft, nontender. Bowel sounds are normal.

**Lower Extremities:**
Unremarkable

**Figure 10-13** Detailed assessment reveals that the patient is not yet back to his baseline.

© Jones & Bartlett Learning.

have fever or other signs of infection, which would support possible febrile seizure. He does not appear to be at risk of imminent decompensation.

The patient is a 2-year-old male with history of seizures and cerebral palsy presenting with seizure activity lasting approximately 5 minutes. He is currently hemodynamically stable with no signs of respiratory compromise. He is not yet back to his neurologic baseline.

## Detailed Exam

**HEENT (Figure 10-13):**

- **H**ead: Unremarkable
- **E**yes: PERRL, sluggish to react, left esotropia noted
- **E**ars: Unremarkable
- **N**ose: Unremarkable
- **T**hroat: Unremarkable
- **M**outh: Mild drooling present

**Chest, heart, and lungs:**

- Pulses: Peripheral pulses palpable throughout
- Cardiac auscultation: Regular rate and rhythm with no rubs, gallops, or murmurs

- Lung auscultation: Clear bilateral breath sounds with good air entry and aeration
- Chest exam: Symmetric chest expansion

**Neurologic:**

- Altered mental status; lethargic and difficult to arouse

**Abdomen and pelvis:**

- Soft and nontender. Bowel sounds are present and normal.

**Extremities:**

- Upper extremities: Unremarkable
- Lower extremities: Unremarkable

**Back:**

- Unremarkable

## Treatment

The initial treatment for this patient should include diligent attention to maintaining an open and patent airway with aggressive ventilatory support as needed to maintain adequate oxygenation and ventilation.

Supplemental oxygen should be provided to maintain $SpO_2 > 94\%$.

Advanced life support crews should establish IV access in case another seizure occurs. Drawing up the appropriate dose of medication in anticipation of additional seizure activity is advisable so there is no delay in providing the medication.

Rapid transport to a pediatric specialty care center should be initiated without delay.

## Ongoing Management

The patient is loaded into the ambulance and secured to the stretcher using an appropriately sized pediatric transport device. He remains lethargic throughout the transport, and no additional seizure activity occurs.

### Case Questions

- What is the most appropriate treatment destination and why?
  - You transport him to the academic pediatric hospital where his subspecialists practice.
- Can you safely transport this child in your ambulance?
  - The patient was secured to the stretcher safely.
- Will you allow the parents to ride in the ambulance?
  - His mother rides in the front of the ambulance and his father follows along, transporting the patient's wheelchair to the hospital.

## CASE WRAP-UP

Diagnosis: Seizure due to underlying cerebral palsy

At the hospital the patient is monitored closely in the ED for additional seizure activity. He returns to his neurologic baseline within a few hours of arrival. His labs are normal and there is no concern for any other underlying pathology. His parents are comfortable transporting him home and continuing to observe him. He is discharged home to follow-up with his pediatrician and neurologist.

## CASE TAKEAWAY POINTS

Cerebral palsy is a leading cause of motor movement disorders in children. It is generally acquired during pregnancy or at birth. It occurs in 2 out of 1,000 live births in the United States. Seizure activity is often present in cerebral palsy, occurring in up to 30% of patients. The age of onset is generally in the first 2 years of life.

## LESSON WRAP-UP

*Children with special healthcare needs* is an umbrella term that covers a wide range of pediatric patients with chronic health conditions and disabilities. EMS practitioners should attempt to expand their knowledge base regarding pediatric chronic medical conditions. This will help improve prehospital treatment and overall outcomes.

For children with chronic medical conditions, the caregiver is often the most important source of information for assessing the patient's baseline mental status. The caregiver can also help operate the patient's medical equipment and assist in providing medical treatment when appropriate. They are often an expert in their child's condition.

Do not be intimidated by the technology. The caregiver is a valuable resource in helping utilize this equipment. You are not expected to know how to operate it, and it is completely appropriate to ask for help when attempting to operate it.

## REFERENCES

American Academy of Pediatric Dentistry. Special health care needs [definition]. In: *The Reference Manual of Pediatric Dentistry*. Chicago, IL: AAPD; 2020:19.

American Thoracic Society. Care of the child with a chronic tracheostomy. *Am J Resp Crit Care Med*. 1999;161(1). doi:10.1164 /ajrccm.161.1.ats1-00

Blumenstein I, Shastri YM, Stein J. Gastroenteric tube feeding: techniques, problems and solutions. *World J Gastroenterol*. 2014;20(26):8505-8524. doi:10.3748/wjg.v20.i26.8505

Centers for Disease Control and Prevention. Children and youth with special healthcare needs in emergencies. Reviewed January 6, 2021. Accessed December 23, 2021. https://www.cdc.gov/childrenindisasters/children-with-special-healthcare-needs.html

Cystic-fibrosis.com. How long do patients with cystic fibrosis live? Published July 30, 2019. Accessed November 10, 2021. https://cystic-fibrosis.com/life-expectancy

Harris CA, McAllister JP. Obstruction of cerebrospinal fluid drainage systems. In: *The Cerebrospinal Fluid Shunts*. Nova Science Publishers; 2016:273-291.

Jones S, Nursing Clinical Effectiveness Committee. Tracheostomy management. The Royal Children's Hospital Melbourne. Updated April 2018. Accessed December 23, 2021. https://www.rch.org.au/rchcpg/hospital_clinical_guideline_index /Tracheostomy_management/

Mehta AK, Chamyal PC. Tracheostomy complications and their management. *Med J Armed Forces India*. 1999;55(3):197-200. doi: 10.1016/S0377-1237(17)30440-9

Ross KR, Chmiel JF, Konstan MW. The role of inhaled corticosteroids in the management of cystic fibrosis. *Paediatr Drugs*. 2009;11(2):101-113. https://doi.org/10.2165/00148581-200911020-00002

Trieschmann U, Cate UT, Sreeram N. Central venous catheters in children and neonates: what is important? *Images Paediatr Cardiol*. 2007;9(4):1-8.

World Health Organization. Assistive technology for children with disabilities, creating opportunities for education, inclusion, and participation: a discussion paper. 2015. Accessed December 23, 2021. https://sites.unicef.org/disabilities/files/Assistive-Tech-Web.pdf

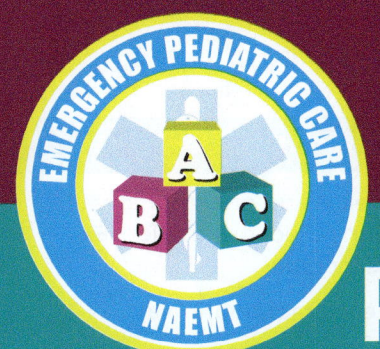

# CHAPTER 11

# Pediatric Behavioral Health

## LESSON OBJECTIVES

- Identify types of pediatric behavioral health disorders.
- Recognize signs and symptoms of behavioral health disorders.
- Discuss the management of pediatric behavioral health disorders.
- Use the most appropriate pediatric behavioral health management intervention based on the patient's assessment findings.

## Introduction

The term *behavioral health disorder* covers an extensive range of conditions affecting the mood, thinking, and behavior of individuals. As children grow and develop throughout their early years, they reach certain developmental milestones. These milestones include learning how to properly socialize and integrate among their peers. This involves learning how to respond to social situations, regulate emotions, and develop coping strategies for everyday fears and concerns.

Although all children may experience brief periods during which they become dysregulated and find themselves unable to cope with stressful situations, occasionally exhibiting disruptive behavior in and of itself does not constitute a behavioral health disorder. When children consistently find themselves unable to cope and their dysregulation affects their daily life, social interactions, and peer relationships on a consistent basis, they may have developed a behavioral health disorder. Parents and healthcare practitioners should take note when a child exhibits serious, persistent changes in the way they act or cope with their emotions and whether these changes interfere with daily life.

## Attention Deficit/ Hyperactivity Disorder (ADD/ADHD)

ADHD is the most common behavioral health disorder in pediatrics patients. This disorder is characterized as a group of symptoms present for a minimum of 6 months, in multiple environments, with an onset prior to age 12 years. The median age of onset is age 6 years.

ADHD is divided into three subtypes: inattentive, hyperactive/impulsive, and combined. The classification is based upon which symptoms predominate in the child's condition. Symptoms can be further classified as mild, moderate, or severe. A standardized screening tool, such as the Vanderbilt ADHD Diagnostic Rating Scale (VADRS) is utilized to screen for the condition. It is important to note that these standardized tools screen for ADHD, but they do not diagnose the condition. The diagnosis is based on the clinical judgment of a trained clinician, considering the results from the screening tools, history reported by the parents, and in many cases reports from teachers at the patient's school.

The most common symptoms of ADHD include hyperactivity, inattention, impulsivity, and forgetfulness. When these symptoms begin to affect the child's ability to maintain peer relationships, perform academically, or impact the safety of themselves or those around them, an ADHD diagnosis may be considered in the appropriate clinical context.

The first-line pharmacologic treatment in children 6 years and older is stimulant medication such as d-amphetamine. Additional medications, such as guanfacine, may be considered.

Early recognition of ADHD is critical as it is commonly associated with other behavioral health disorders, and early treatment and control can impact the patient academically and socially. ADHD has been categorized in some texts as a learning disorder, as the impaired attention and impulsivity may impact academic performance, which in turn can lead to difficulty forming peer relationships. Medication and cognitive behavioral therapy can aid in helping these patients both socially and academically.

# Anxiety

When a child does not outgrow their fears or worries, or when they become so serious that they begin to affect the child's everyday life, they may be considered to have an anxiety disorder. Specific anxiety disorders are listed in **Table 11-1**.

Patients with anxiety will manifest the condition in three symptoms groups: behaviors, thoughts, and somatic symptoms.

Behaviors and thoughts are somewhat self-explanatory. Somatic symptoms are more complex, however. Somatic symptoms include actual vital sign changes, along with other symptoms that are clinically present on examination. These symptoms can include tachycardia, diaphoresis, dizziness, shortness of breath, tingling hands, and syncopal episodes or altered levels of consciousness.

When considering anxiety as the potential cause of a patient's symptoms, it should be noted that the catecholamine "dump" that occurs with anxiety, leading to the somatic symptoms, also occurs in other medical conditions, such as shock. Medical causes for anxiety symptomology should be evaluated and ruled out before considering anxiety as the sole cause of the patient's behavioral symptoms. Anxiety is a diagnosis of exclusion.

When assessing anxiety and the patient's response to medical therapy, certain scales have been developed to assess the patient's condition. One such scale, the Richmond Agitation-Sedation Scale, allows the practitioner to monitor the patient's anxiety and sedation

| Table 11-1 Types of Anxiety Disorders | |
|---|---|
| Phobias | An extreme and often irrational fear of an object or situation. Examples include:<br>■ Spiders (arachnophobia)<br>■ Dogs (cynophobia)<br>■ Tight spaces (claustrophobia) |
| General anxiety | Excessive and uncontrollable worry about things in general, including:<br>■ Life<br>■ The future<br>■ Friendships<br>■ Academic performance<br>■ Feelings of impending doom |
| Social anxiety | A fear of unfamiliar people (particularly adults) or social situations. Being in public may cause severe distress. |
| Separation anxiety | Being irrationally afraid of anticipated or actual separation from a caregiver or loved one. |
| Panic disorder | Sudden, unexpected attacks that consist of dyspnea, shaking, tachycardia, and a sudden intense fear of something intangible.<br>■ The typical onset of panic attacks begins in puberty.<br>■ Emergency medical services (EMS) is often called for panic attacks as the patient can appear severely dyspneic, complain of chest pain or tightness, and seem very ill. |

© Jones & Bartlett Learning.

levels. It is a 10-point scale with four levels of agitation/anxiety and five levels of sedation. Practitioners should be familiar with the tools that their institution uses to monitor anxiety and sedation.

Treatment for anxiety starts with ensuring the safety of yourself and your partner. Approach the child slowly and try to get on their level. Use a calm voice and avoid the tendency to increase your tone or volume, as the child may increase their tone and volume in response. Assess for previous history of anxiety, and try to determine if there are any known triggers present. Remove any triggers if you can. Attempt to determine if the patient has any preexisting strategies they use for dealing with their anxiety, whether these are behavioral strategies or pharmacologic therapies.

In most cases anxiety can be managed with behavioral coaching, such as having the patient go through deep breathing or redirection to discussion of a topic that helps to reduce their anxiety. Monitor the patient's end-tidal $CO_2$ ($ETCO_2$) and attempt to coach their breathing to maintain a normal level between 35 and 45 mm Hg. Pharmacotherapy should be a last resort; do not use sedative medications if this is the patient's first episode of acute anxiety. Using medications can alter their mental status and make assessment difficult for the emergency department clinician. When medications must be used to protect yourself or the patient, benzodiazepines are a good first-line choice. Ketamine may also be used in certain situations if allowed by protocol, but caution should be used any time a medication is administered.

# Depression

Depression may be considered as a diagnosis if a child exhibits persistent, severe sadness or hopelessness for a period of 2 weeks or longer. Symptoms include the loss of joy from activities from which the child previous gained pleasure, persistent sadness, hopelessness, sleep–wake cycle disturbance, or even self-destructive behavior or increased risk taking.

Depression can be difficult to identify in younger children, as they may present with anger, irritability, or aggression. Changes in eating and energy patterns should also be considered red flags.

Recognizing signs of depression is important, as this paves the way for intervention and treatment. Although this condition is relatively uncommon, it still affects 3.2% of children between ages 3 and 17 years.

Treatment for depression includes taking steps to ensure the safety of yourself, your partner, and the patient. Establish trust by using appropriate eye contact and speaking calmly and clearly. Allow the patient time to talk—this is not the time to be perceived as "rushing" the patient. Use reflective listening and try to repeat back a summary of what the patient has told you to demonstrate that you are listening to them. Take steps to be empathetic and demonstrate that empathy to the patient. Do not force the patient to talk if they wish to remain silent. In suicidal or homicidal patients, law enforcement should be contacted if the patient is refusing care, and the patient should be taken into protective custody.

Patients with undiagnosed or inadequately treated depression are at significant risk for suicidal ideation and suicide attempts.

# Bipolar Disorder

Bipolar disorder is relatively uncommon in the pediatric population and generally not diagnosed until late adolescence at the earliest, although there have been breakthrough cases in which the condition was diagnosed in younger children. Bipolar disorder was previously known as manic depressive disorder. It is characterized by dramatic swings in mood from manic episodes to depression.

Manic episodes are characterized by an increased level of activity and energy. These patients may be seen as "the life of the party" and may have intense silliness or happiness. They can also be short tempered, have episodes of insomnia, experience difficulty with focus, and in some cases become hypersexual.

Depressive episodes are characterized by much less activity than normal. Frequent sadness, difficulty concentrating, increased anger and irritability, and altered eating or sleeping habits may be present. These changes in mood are often unprovoked and unpredictable.

Treatment for bipolar disorder includes medications and psychotherapy. Personal safety must be the top priority. Include the caregiver in the patient's care when able to do so in a safe manner. Limit the number of personnel on scene and have a single individual directly engage with the patient when possible to avoid sensory overload and decrease the potential audience for outbursts. Speak clearly and calmly, avoiding the tendency to match the patient's cadence, tone, and volume. Move slowly when approaching the patient so as not to startle them. Even though the child may start off silly, happy, and engaging, be prepared for their mood to change quickly. They can easily deteriorate into anger and violence. Have a plan, and discuss with your partner whether and when to use physical restraints or pharmaceutical management, per local protocols, if patient, bystander, or practitioner safety is a concern.

Pharmacologic agents such as benzodiazepines are the mainstay first-line treatment for acute episodes of mania and agitation. Always ensure that you are monitoring the patient's respiratory and circulatory status any time you use physical restraint or pharmaceutical management of a patient. Never transport a patient with a behavioral health emergency, particularly bipolar disorder, alone in the back of the ambulance without a chaperone.

When suicidal or homicidal ideation is present, law enforcement should be on hand to escort the patient to the hospital along with EMS personnel.

# Schizophrenia

Similar to bipolar disorder, schizophrenia is rare in children and is typically seen in late adolescence at the earliest. Schizophrenia is a complex disorder affecting how a person feels, thinks, and behaves. Psychosis related to schizophrenia may be a slow spiral or a rapid deterioration. Early onset schizophrenia often presents insidiously and evolves over time, usually manifesting its earliest signs at times of significant transition, such as going off to college, the death of a loved one, or other major life changes.

The diagnosis of schizophrenia prior to age 12 years is almost unheard of. The late 20s is the peak age of onset for schizophrenia; however, a small subset of patients is diagnosed with early onset schizophrenia younger than 18 years.

The diagnosis is often made after the patient experiences their first psychotic episode. Symptoms typically fall into three categories as follows:

- **Psychotic symptoms.** Delusions, hallucinations, and thought disorders (e.g., thought insertion, thought broadcasting)

- **Negative symptoms.** No emotional or facial expressions (blunt affect), lack of motivation, decreased feeling of pleasure, poverty of speech (not talking very much)

- **Cognitive symptoms.** Difficulty paying attention or processing information to make rational decisions

As mentioned earlier, schizophrenia is often an insidious process in children and adolescents; however, it can also occur suddenly, with a psychotic break occurring out of nowhere with little warning.

Treatment for patients with schizophrenic episodes starts with ensuring the safety of yourself, your partner, and the patient. Include the caregiver if it does not escalate the patient's anger or mood. Establish trust, and limit the number of personnel directly engaging with the patient. Having personnel back off when appropriate can help relieve feelings of paranoia and persecution. Speak clearly and calmly, avoiding the tendency to match the patient's cadence, tone, and volume. Do not attempt to alter, correct, or advise the patient's hallucinations. These hallucinations are real to the patient. Be prepared to take appropriate action to maintain the safety of yourself, your partner, and the patient if the patient should become aggressive. Have a plan established regarding whether, when, and how you will use physical restraints or pharmaceutical management. Benzodiazepines are the most common first-line acute treatment for psychosis in the field. Contact law enforcement for assistance with patients who have active suicidal or homicidal ideations.

# Posttraumatic Stress Disorder (PTSD)

Posttraumatic stress disorder (PTSD) develops in some pediatric patients who have witnessed or experienced significant traumatic events. The trauma does not have to be directed at the child. Seeing a parent be the victim of physical harm or abuse, witnessing a car accident, or other events can lead to PTSD in a child. Patterns of physical, emotional, and sexual abuse also can lead to PTSD. Children who have been victims of kidnapping, witnessed the death of a family member, or suffered from neglect or abandonment are susceptible to developing PTSD.

The duration and intensity of the trauma, along with the patient's age at the time of exposure tie together to inform the diagnosis of PTSD. Symptoms of PTSD include reliving of the trauma, nightmares, intense fear, outbursts of anger or physical violence, hopelessness, anxiety, and sleep disturbance.

PTSD is often associated with ongoing psychological issues into adulthood, including anxiety and conduct disorder. It is important to identify the any triggers that the patient has from their past trauma and avoid them if possible. For example, children who have a history of sexual abuse may be triggered by physical restraints. It may be easier to manage the patient's symptoms without the use of restraints, and they should be avoided in patients who are not combative.

Treatment for PTSD involves ensuring personal safety first and foremost. Use a calm voice and avoid the tendency to match the cadence, tone, and volume of the patient. Monitor $ETCO_2$ when able. This can provide information regarding whether the patient is hypo- or hyperventilating and can guide the coaching of breathing exercises. Benzodiazepines and ketamine can be used as a last resort if pharmaceutical management is necessary.

# Suicide Attempts and Suicidal Ideation

Suicide is the second leading cause of death in children ages 10 to 17 years. Common causes of suicide include firearms, overdose, and strangulation or hanging. Boys and men are more likely to use firearms and have a successful suicide attempt than girls and women. Girls and women are more likely to ingest pills or other toxins.

Suicide is reaching epidemic proportions in the United States. The Centers for Disease Control and Prevention (CDC) reports that suicide rates for individuals between the ages of 10 and 24 years have increased 56% between

2007 and 2017. This represents approximately 6.8 per 100,000 people. The suicide rate for children ages 10 to 14 years old nearly tripled during that same time frame. Stress and isolation during the COVID19 pandemic have compounded this issue. A significant percentage of pediatric transports are due to pediatric behavioral issues, of which suicidality is the most common.

Suicide emergencies are divided into two subtypes: attempts and ideations. Suicide attempts involve cases where the patient has acted upon their desire to hurt themselves, albeit unsuccessfully. This may or may not result in actual injury, however it should be noted that the patient acted with intent to harm themselves so severely that they would die from their actions.

Suicidal ideation is the thought, planning, and consideration of suicide. When taking the social history of a patient, if they disclose that they feel like the world would be a better place without them, and they have considered leaving their car running in the garage so they could go to sleep and end it all, that constitutes suicidal ideation. If they actually do sit in the garage with the car running and you arrive on scene and rescue them before they die from carbon monoxide poisoning, that constitutes an attempt.

Symptoms of suicidal ideation include discussions of guilt, speaking about hopelessness and no reason to live, wanting to die, or concern about being a burden to others. Excessive use of drugs and alcohol and withdrawal from family and friends along with these discussions is significantly concerning for suicidal ideation.

Risks for suicide include history of depression, chronic pain conditions, previous suicide attempt, family history of suicide, substance abuse, and history of violence. Having a firearm in the home significantly increases the risk of a child successfully completing a suicide attempt.

Treatment for patients who have attempted suicide or for those who have suicidal ideation includes medications and psychotherapy. Take measures to ensure your personal safety. Establish trust by reflective listening, and limit the number of caregivers who directly engage with the patient. Speak clearly and calmly when communicating. Contact law enforcement for assistance with transport. Make sure to transport the patient to a facility that has the resources necessary to provide inpatient treatment and stabilization of suicidal and homicidal patients. Not all hospitals have pediatric inpatient psychiatric services.

# Autism Spectrum Disorder

Autism spectrum disorder (ASD) is a lifelong, complex neurodevelopmental disability defined by a set of behaviors that affects individuals on a spectrum of severity. Some individuals may be very high functioning, with successful careers and families, while others may have such a large symptom burden that they require extensive care and support.

There is no single known cause for ASD; however, boys are 4.5 times more likely to be afflicted than girls. It is estimated that ASD occurs in 1 out of 59 individuals in varying degrees of severity. Most children with ASD have some form of sensory integration issue or sensitivity. The behavioral signs of autism are highly variable. They may include the initiation of social interactions different from the chronologic developmental age. Maintaining a typical back-and-forth conversation, along with appropriate eye contact is often difficult for individuals with ASD, as are facial expression recognition and social reciprocity. Abnormalities in body gestures, tics, body posture, vocal tone alteration, and difficulty with respect to personal space may be present in individuals with ASD. Individuals with ASD may be completely free of physical limitation or have severe physical disabilities.

Autism is often accompanied by other behavioral health conditions that can exacerbate or compound the underlying ASD. For example, ADHD is present in 28% of patients with ASD and anxiety is present in up to 20%. Depression, schizophrenia, bipolar disorder, and altered sleep–wake patterns are all more prevalent in individuals with autism spectrum disorder.

Prehospital management of ASD involves taking measures to maintain personal safety and the safety of the patient. Individuals with ASD are rarely violent unless they feel threatened. Children with severe developmental delay will often respond to redirection and distraction with toys such as fidget spinners and light spinners. Videos or games on a tablet can also help distract and deescalate patients with autism. The caregivers are an excellent resource for discussing what deescalation techniques work best for the patient. Avoid the use of flashing lights and siren, as the visual and auditory stimuli can be overwhelming to the patient. Limit the number of caregivers directly interacting with the patient. Carefully explain everything and keep in mind that patients with autism spectrum disorder have a very literal interpretation of the words and jargon you might use.

Be prepared to change your approach to accommodate the shifting mood of the patient. Some patients may adamantly refuse certain procedures due to fear or sensory issues. Blood pressure cuffs, for example, may cause severe discomfort due to sensory integration issues. In cases where the patient is clearly perfusing well, you may have to assess the risk versus benefit of forcing a blood pressure cuff onto a patient who may become acutely agitated because they feel threatened or are having difficulty integrating sensory input, leading to dysregulation. There are few interventions that *absolutely* must be done in EMS, and in most cases, when an intervention must take place, the patient is generally ill enough to comply.

Restraints for patients with ASD should be used only as a last resort and are rarely necessary when distraction and redirection techniques have been used appropriately. When physical restraints must be used,

papoose-style restraints may have a calming effect similar to that of a weighted blanket.

EMS practitioners should not assume a patient's complaints are completely attributable to an underlying behavioral health disorder. It is important to obtain a detailed history; appropriate vital signs, including cardiac and glucose monitoring; and to subsequently transport without delay.

# CASE STUDY

## Case 1

### Dispatch

You are dispatched to a local school for a 13-year-old male with difficulty breathing on a fall morning. The outside temperature is 56°F (13°C).

### Case Questions

- What are your initial concerns?
  - The primary concern for this patient is that he is having difficulty breathing.
- Based on the dispatch information, what is the possible differential diagnosis for this patient?
  - The causes of this respiratory distress could include asthma, respiratory infections such as pneumonia or viruses, chemical exposure, illicit drug use, seasonal allergies or anaphylaxis, or panic attack.

### Initial Observations

As you pull up to the school and unload your equipment you are met by the school nurse. She escorts you to the patient who is sitting outside in front of the school (**Figure 11-1**).

- Pediatric Assessment Triangle
  - Appearance
    - Alert
  - Work of breathing
    - **F**laring present
    - **R**etractions present
    - **A**udible airway sounds not present
    - **P**ositioning not present
  - Circulation
    - Skin warm and sweaty

The nurse tells you that she was advised by students that the patient was sitting on the bench in front of the school having trouble breathing prior to the morning bell ringing. She informs you that she has contacted the patient's mother who will meet you at the hospital.

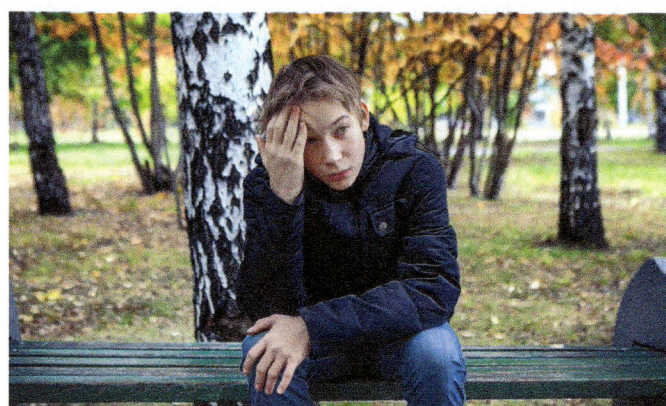

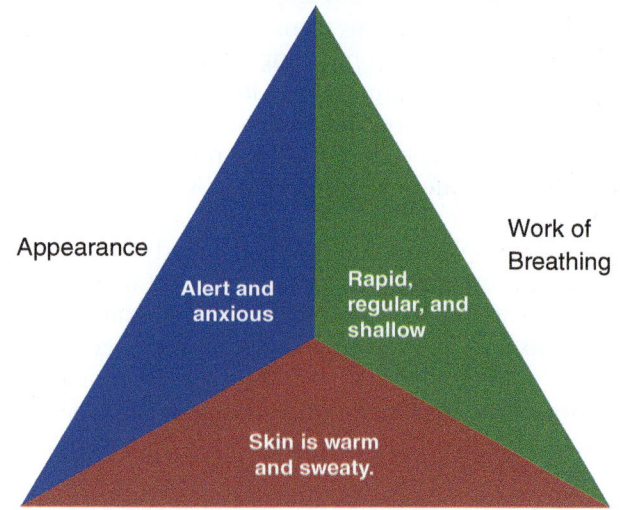

**Figure 11-1** The differential diagnosis for a 13-year-old with difficulty breathing can include both respiratory and behavioral health causes.

## Case Questions

- Based on your initial impression, is this patient "Quick" or "Not Quick"?

  - This patient is "Quick." He is in respiratory distress with rapid, shallow respirations. Although he appears to be stable currently, he is at risk for sudden respiratory decompensation.

## Primary Survey

The primary survey for this patient reveals the following:

**X**—No bleeding found

**A**—Patent

**B**—Regular, rapid, shallow breathing. The lung sounds are clear bilaterally.

**C**—Radial pulses are strong and rapid. The skin is warm, sweaty, and pink.

**D**—Glasgow Coma Scale (GCS) score is 15 (E4, V5, M6). The patient is alert and anxious.

**E**—Sitting on a school bench. Well-groomed with good hygiene.

## Case Questions

- Based on the findings noted in the primary survey, what would your initial interventions and treatment include?

  - The initial treatment for this patient should focus on supporting airway, breathing, and circulation. To that end, coached breathing techniques can be employed to optimize the patient's respiratory effort and work of breathing.

## Detailed Assessment

### History Taking

As your partner attaches the monitor and takes vital signs, you begin to take a detailed history from the patient.

**OPQRST:**

- **O**nset: Sudden
- **P**rovocation/palliation: Discussing the reason he is upset causes his symptoms to increase. When he is redirected, his symptoms decrease.
- **Q**uality: None
- **R**adiation: None
- **S**everity: None
- **T**iming: 20 minutes

**SAMPLER:**

- **S**igns/symptoms: Rapid, shallow breathing; anxiety; heart racing with palpitations
- **A**llergies: No known allergies to medications, foods, or the environment
- **M**edications: Zoloft
- **P**ast medical history: Depression
- **L**ast oral intake: Breakfast this morning before school
- **E**vents leading up to the emergency: Has had problems with being bullied this year and was made fun of this morning for not having a girlfriend
- **R**isk factors: History of depression and bullying

### Vital Signs

As you were discussing the history, the patient was attached to the monitor and the following vital signs were obtained (**Figure 11-2**):

**Heart rate:**

- 111 beats/min
- The patient is tachycardic. A 12-lead electrocardiogram (ECG) should be obtained to rule out any potential cardiac ectopy.

**SpO$_2$:**

- 100% on room air (RA)
- This speaks against a respiratory issue such as pulmonary embolism or asthma attack.

**ETCO$_2$:**

- 30 mm Hg
- This is appropriately decreased in the setting of hyperventilation.

**Respiratory rate:**

- 38 breaths/min
- This is very rapid for this patient, and the ETCO$_2$ reflects the hypocarbia that is developing. This can lead to numbness and tingling in the extremities and even syncope in severe cases.

**Blood pressure:**

- 126/72 mm Hg
- This is reassuring.

**Temperature:**

- 98.4°F (36.9°C)
- This speaks against infection as the etiology of the patient's respiratory distress.

**Blood glucose:**

- 88 mg/dL

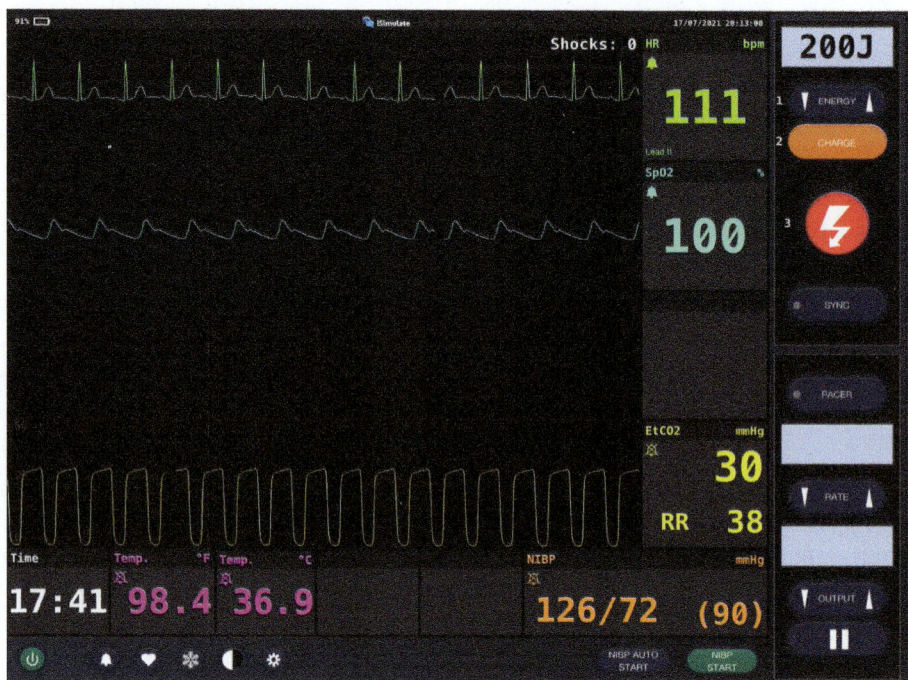

**Figure 11-2** The patient's vital signs indicate tachycardia.

Courtesy of iSimulate.

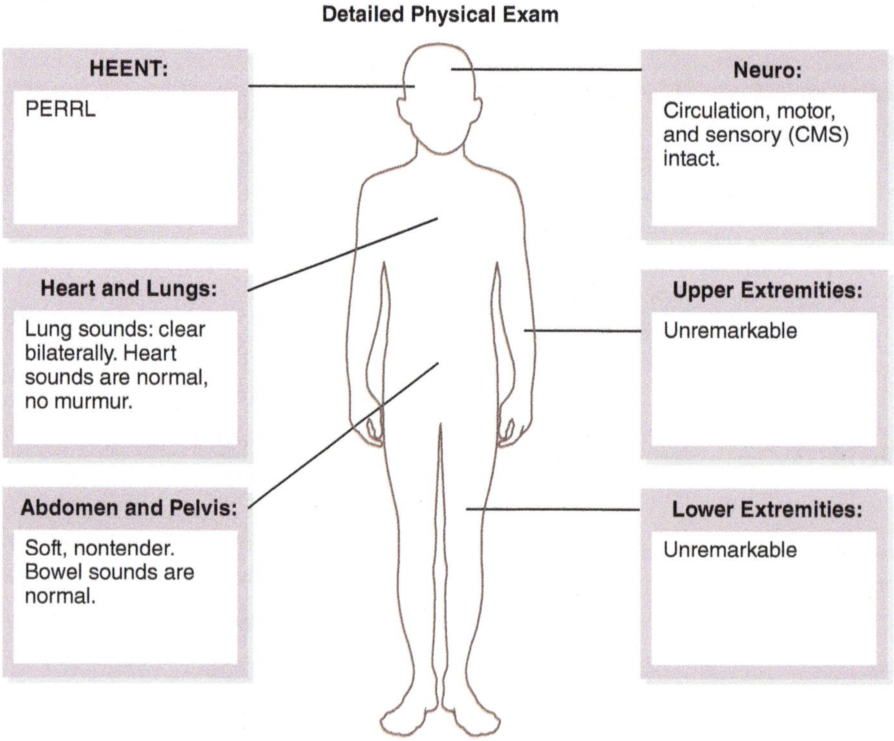

**Detailed Physical Exam**

**HEENT:**

PERRL

**Neuro:**

Circulation, motor,
and sensory (CMS)
intact.

**Heart and Lungs:**

Lung sounds: clear
bilaterally. Heart
sounds are normal,
no murmur.

**Upper Extremities:**

Unremarkable

**Abdomen and Pelvis:**

Soft, nontender.
Bowel sounds are
normal.

**Lower Extremities:**

Unremarkable

**Figure 11-3** Nothing remarkable is revealed in the patient's secondary survey.

© Jones & Bartlett Learning.

This is a 13-year-old male with sudden-onset tachypnea and tachycardia in the setting of emotional distress with no acute findings suggestive of cardiac or respiratory pathology (**Figure 11-3**). His hemodynamic and respiratory status is intact with the exception of hypocarbia.

When anxiety is suspected, the primary measures to slow the rate of respiration and reduce tachycardia include redirection and respiratory coaching. Having the patient slow their breathing along with you and redirecting them away from thoughts regarding the source of stress can be beneficial.

## Detailed Exam

**HEENT:**

- **H**ead: Unremarkable
- **E**yes: PERRL, unremarkable
- **E**ars: Unremarkable
- **N**ose: Unremarkable
- **T**hroat: Unremarkable

**Chest, heart, and lungs:**

- Pulses: Peripheral pulses readily palpable in all extremities
- Cardiac auscultation: Regular rate and rhythm with no rubs, gallops, or murmurs auscultated
- Lung auscultation: Clear bilaterally with good aeration. The patient is breathing with rapid shallow respirations, but there are no signs on pulmonary exam of air trapping or other pulmonary pathology.
- Chest exam: Symmetric rise and fall with good excursion

**Neurologic:**

- Neurovascular status intact

**Abdomen and pelvis:**

- Unremarkable

**Extremities:**

- Upper extremities: Unremarkable
- Lower extremities: Unremarkable

**Back:**

- Unremarkable

## Treatment

The initial treatment for this patient includes measures to increase comfort, redirect from stressful or anxiety-provoking thoughts, and respiratory coaching to reduce tachypnea. Oxygen may be applied as needed; however, the patient is saturating well on room air and it is likely not necessary. Therapeutic communication can be very helpful in cases of anxiety to reduce stress and ease tension.

The treatment provided by advanced life support (ALS) and critical care personnel is largely the same as basic life support (BLS) crews. Medications should be avoided in this patient if possible.

Additional diagnoses such as asthma and pulmonary infection were ruled out based on the absence of signs of lower airway obstruction and no clear evidence of infection such as fever. Chemical exposure is unlikely as a single individual is affected. Illicit drug use remains a possibility and can only be ruled out through comprehensive urinary drug screen, although that test may not capture all potential drugs ingested.

## Ongoing Management

The patient calms significantly with respiratory coaching and therapeutic communication. He remains stable throughout transport.

### Case Questions

- What is the most appropriate treatment destination and why?
  - You and your partner note that the local pediatric hospital has the appropriate resources available to manage behavioral health crises and you determine that this is the best transport destination. You contact the mother and update her regarding her son's status and let her know the transportation destination. She agrees to meet you there.
- Can you safely transport this child in your ambulance?
  - The patient was appropriately restrained to the stretcher.

## CASE WRAP-UP

Diagnosis: Panic attack

At the hospital the patient ultimately calmed down and the attack subsided. He discussed his issues with the social worker who provided outpatient behavioral health resources for follow-up. He was discharged within a few hours of arrival with no medications being administered and in his normal state of health.

## CASE TAKEAWAY POINTS

Anxiety affects 7.1% of children ages 3 to 17 years. There is a range of anxiety disorders in children and adolescents, including separation anxiety disorder, social phobia, panic disorder, agoraphobia, and generalized anxiety disorder. Some adolescents may choose to "self-medicate" feelings of anxiety by using substances such as alcohol or cannabis. However, some evidence indicates that cannabis consumption may lead to increased prevalence of anxiety disorders, depression, and suicidality.

## CASE STUDY

### Case 2

#### Dispatch

You are dispatched to a residence for a 16-year-old female with reported suicide attempt (**Figure 11-4**). A friend called 911 after she witnessed a social media post regarding the suicide attempt. The friend advised the patient posted an image of several pills with the caption "I'm going to die today; I hope you're happy." It is a spring Saturday afternoon with an outside temperature of 75°F (24°C).

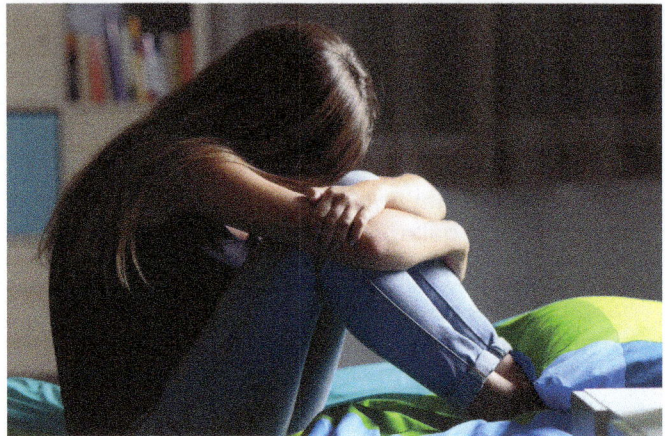

#### Case Questions

- What are your initial concerns?
  - The initial concerns for this patient are toxic ingestion. Scene safety will be a major concern, as it is anytime there is a potentially suicidal patient.
- Based on the dispatch information, what are the possible differential diagnoses for this patient?
  - The differential diagnosis for this patient includes suicidal ideation, suicide attempt, toxic ingestion, depression, anxiety, panic attack, and illicit drug use.

#### Initial Observations

As you approach the scene you see a police cruiser in front of the home. You are waved up by the officer who informs you that the scene is safe to enter.

- Pediatric Assessment Triangle
  - Appearance
    - Alert
  - Work of breathing
    - Nonlabored with adequate rate and depth
    - **F**laring not present
    - **R**etractions not present

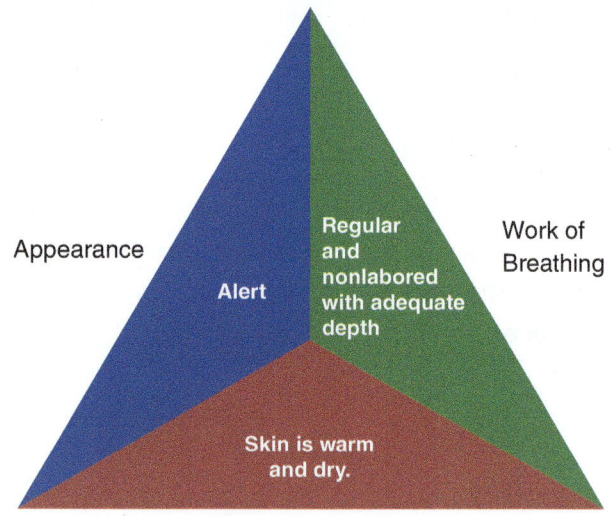

**Figure 11-4** Your patient is a 16-year-old female with reported suicide attempt.

- - - **A**udible airway sounds not present
    - **P**ositioning not present
  - Circulation
    - Skin warm and dry

The patient is crying and states she is tired of all the rumors at school that she and another girl are dating the same boyfriend. She states, "I just don't want to live anymore."

The patient's mother is on scene and explains that she was unaware of her daughter's problems at school. She advises you that the daughter has a history of self-harm in the form of cutting, but she thought "we were past that." She noticed that her daughter seemed more withdrawn today but did not think much of it. She hands you the daughter's prescription bottle of Zoloft (sertraline) that she found in the daughter's hand.

You examine the date on the bottle. It indicates that it was filled 4 days ago with a 30-day supply of 30 pills. You count 26 pills left, indicating that the patient has been taking the prescribed amount daily.

## Case Questions

- Based on your initial impression, is this patient "Quick" or "Not Quick"?
  - Currently the patient is stable from a cardiopulmonary perspective. Although she is exhibiting signs of suicidal ideation, a review of her medications indicates that she has not ingested any of the Zoloft. She is currently "Not Quick."
- Have you identified any red flags?
  - The patient is stating that she doesn't want to live.

## Primary Survey

The primary survey for this patient reveals the following:

  **X**—No bleeding found

  **A**—Open and patent

  **B**—Regular and nonlabored with adequate depth. Lung sounds are clear bilaterally.

  **C**—Radial pulses are strong and regular; the skin is warm and dry.

  **D**—GCS is 15 (E4, V5, M6).

  **E**—She is sitting on her bed. She is well groomed with good hygiene.

## Case Questions

- Based on the findings noted in the primary survey, what would your initial interventions and treatment include?
  - The initial treatment for this patient should focus on therapeutic interventions such as reflective listening, empathy, and redirection of harmful thoughts. Demonstrate understanding to the patient to build trust and rapport.

## Detailed Assessment

### History Taking

As your partner applies the cardiac monitor, you begin to obtain a history.

**OPQRST:**

- **O**nset: Sudden
- **P**rovocation/palliation: None
- **Q**uality: None
- **R**adiation: None
- **S**everity: None
- **T**iming: 30 minutes

**SAMPLER:**

- **S**igns/symptoms: Depressed mood, suicidal ideation
- **A**llergies: No known allergies to medications, foods, or the environment
- **M**edications: Zoloft
- **P**ast medical history: Depression, history of cutting
- **L**ast oral intake: Fruit chews, has not eaten much today
- **E**vents leading up to the emergency: Rumors and bullying at school leading to thoughts that she does not want to live anymore
- **R**isk factors: Depression, bullying and rumors at school

### Vital Signs

As you were discussing the history, the patient was attached to the monitor and the following vital signs were obtained (**Figure 11-5**):

**Heart rate:**

- 97 beats/min

**SpO$_2$:**

- 99% RA

**ETCO$_2$:**

- 38 mm Hg

**Respiratory rate:**

- 20 breaths/min

**Blood pressure:**

- 126/68 mm Hg

**Temperature:**

- 98.6°F (37°C)

**Blood glucose:**

- 100 mg/dL

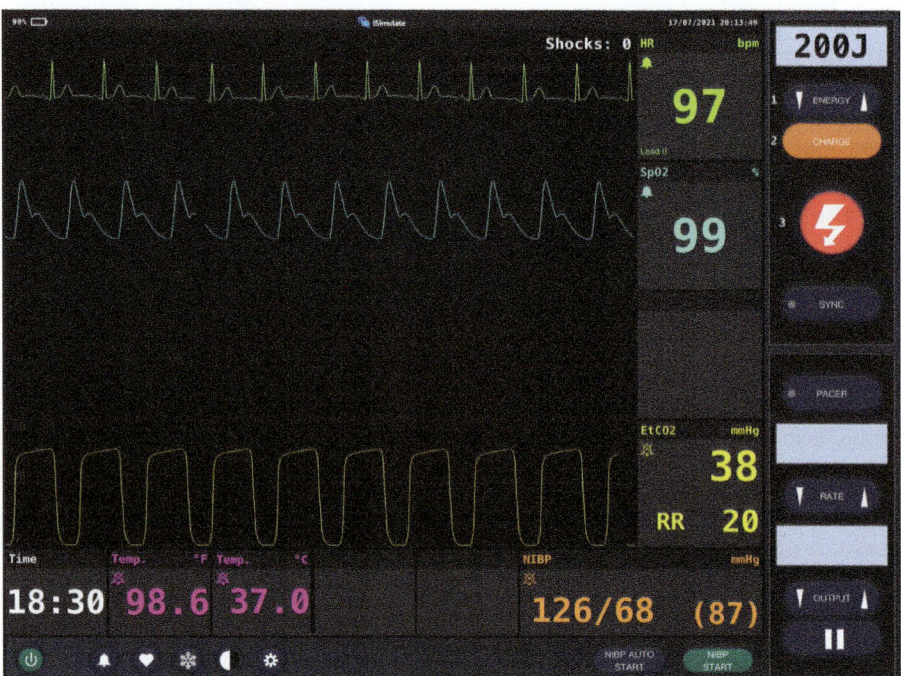

**Figure 11-5** This patient's vital signs are reassuring.
Courtesy of iSimulate.

This is a 16-year-old female with history of depression and cutting presenting with suicidal ideation and clinical signs and symptoms that do not support intentional ingestion of sertraline. She is currently stable but at risk for decompensation if her mood shifts and she becomes violent or angry.

This patient's vital signs, along with the accurate pill count, do not support the story that she ingested pills. She still has a medical emergency because she has suicidal ideation, but she is currently safe and does not require emergent treatment and stabilization of toxic ingestion (**Figure 11-6**).

## Detailed Exam

**HEENT:**

- **H**ead: Unremarkable
- **E**yes: PERRL, unremarkable
- **E**ars: Unremarkable
- **N**ose: Unremarkable
- **T**hroat: Unremarkable

**Chest, heart, and lungs:**

- Pulses: Peripheral pulses strong
- Cardiac auscultation: Regular rate and rhythm with no rubs, gallops, or murmurs
- Lung auscultation: Clear to auscultation in all fields
- Chest exam: Symmetric chest rise with good air entry

**Neurologic:**

- Neurovascular status intact

**Abdomen and pelvis:**

- Unremarkable

**Extremities:**

- Upper extremities: Old scars present consistent with history of cutting
- Lower extremities: Old scars present consistent with history of cutting

**Back:**

- Unremarkable

## Treatment

The initial treatment for this patient involves a low-stimulation environment and a caring, empathetic approach. Provide reassurance that she is in a safe place. Place her in a position of comfort for transport. Oxygen can be given as needed. Communicate with her therapeutically and redirect negative thoughts of self-harm. ALS and critical care will involve a similar approach. You likely do not need intravenous access for this patient.

## Ongoing Management

During transport you ask the patient about her plan of action and her suicidal thoughts. This is an important part of the history for patients presenting with suicide

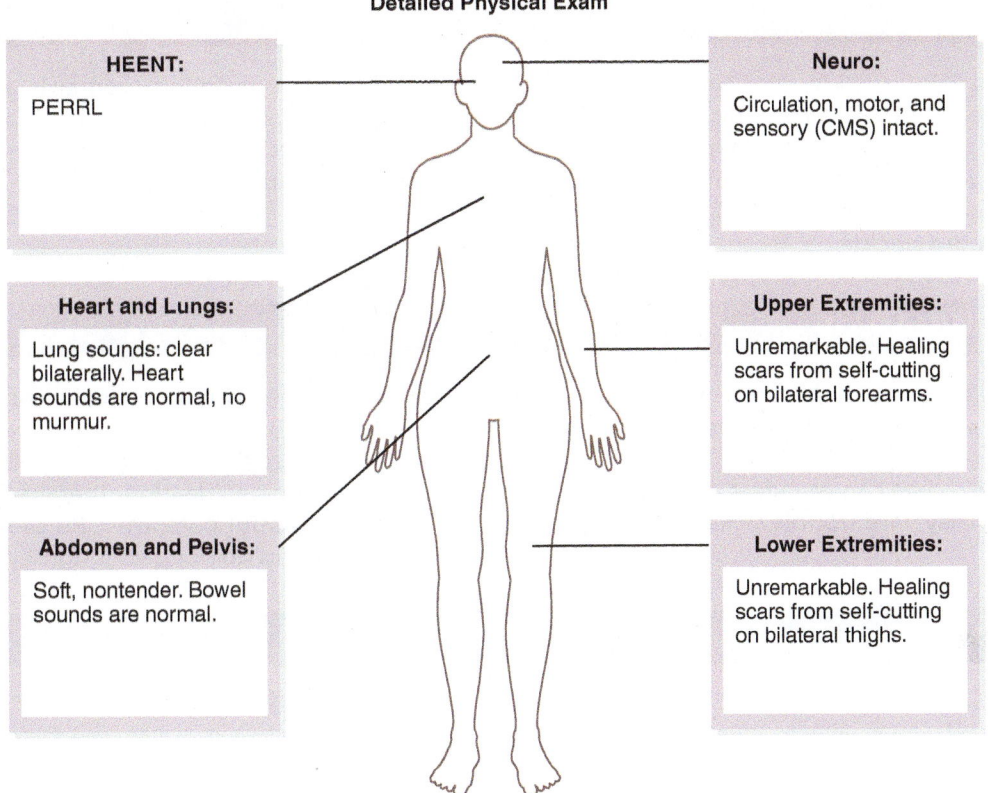

**Detailed Physical Exam**

**HEENT:**

PERRL

**Neuro:**

Circulation, motor, and sensory (CMS) intact.

**Heart and Lungs:**

Lung sounds: clear bilaterally. Heart sounds are normal, no murmur.

**Upper Extremities:**

Unremarkable. Healing scars from self-cutting on bilateral forearms.

**Abdomen and Pelvis:**

Soft, nontender. Bowel sounds are normal.

**Lower Extremities:**

Unremarkable. Healing scars from self-cutting on bilateral thighs.

**Figure 11-6** The patient's secondary survey reveals scars on the extremities that are consistent with a history of cutting.

© Jones & Bartlett Learning.

attempt or suicidal ideation. Important questions to ask include the following:

- Have you ever considered suicide?
- If so, for how long?
- Have you rehearsed or contemplated how you would carry out your suicide?
- Have you ever attempted suicide before?

The responses to these questions can help determine the risk level for suicide in a particular patient. Patients with a plan are at higher risk than those who have no plan. Patients with a prior suicide attempt are at higher risk than those who have never attempted before.

## Case Questions

- What is the most appropriate treatment destination and why?
  - You and your partner discuss with the patient's mother that the local children's hospital has adequate resources, including social work and inpatient therapy, to support the patient's recovery.
- Can you safely transport this child in your ambulance?
  - The patient is secured to the stretcher.

## CASE WRAP-UP

Diagnosis: Suicidal ideation

The patient remains stable throughout transport, and she is transferred to the pediatric hospital without incident. It is determined that she needs inpatient treatment, and she is placed in a short inpatient therapy program. She is discharged in approximately 7 days with intensive outpatient follow-up. She has transferred schools and is reportedly adjusting well.

## CASE TAKEAWAY POINTS

From 2009 to 2018, suicide rates for teens ages 14 to 18 years increased 61.7% in the United States. In 2019, 18.8% of high school students reported seriously considering suicide. Of those individuals, 24.1% identified as female. Nearly 1 in 10 high school students reported having attempted suicide.

Suicide prevention programs and practices, along with support and outreach to at-risk communities would reduce suicidal ideation and its associated consequences.

## LESSON WRAP-UP

Identifying differences in pediatric behavioral health disorders allows for proper treatment of each specific disorder.

Anxiety disorders can manifest in a variety of ways. A young child may have trouble sleeping, be irritable or angry, or even exhibit physical symptoms such as aches and pains.

Recognize and employ effective management strategies for suicidal ideation. Therapeutic management is key to successful outcomes. Be prepared to listen empathically, and do not pass judgment.

## REFERENCES

Autism Science Foundation. How common is autism? 2015. Accessed December 27, 2021. https://autismsciencefoundation.org/what-is-autism/how-common-is-autism/

Centers for Disease Control and Prevention. Anxiety and depression in children. Reviewed March 22, 2021. Accessed December 27, 2021. https://www.cdc.gov/childrensmentalhealth/depression.html

Centers for Disease Control and Prevention. Children and youth with special healthcare needs in emergencies. Reviewed January 6, 2021. Accessed December 27, 2021. https://www.cdc.gov/childrenindisasters/children-with-special-healthcare-needs.html

Centers for Disease Control and Prevention. Post-traumatic stress disorder in children. Reviewed March 22, 2021. Accessed December 27, 2021. https://www.cdc.gov/childrensmentalhealth/ptsd.html

Centers for Disease Control and Prevention. What is ADHD? Reviewed September 23, 2021. Accessed December 27, 2021. https://www.cdc.gov/ncbddd/adhd/facts.html

Erdmann J. Analysis pins down prevalence of mental health conditions in autism. Spectrum. October 2019. Accessed December 27, 2021. https://www.spectrumnews.org/news/analysis-pins-down-prevalence-of-mental-health-conditions-in-autism/

Gobbi G, Atkin T, Zytynski T, et al. Association of cannabis use in adolescence and risk of depression, anxiety, and suicidality in young adulthood: a systematic review and meta-analysis. *JAMA Psychiatry*. 2019 Apr 1;76(4):426-434. doi:10.1001/jamapsychiatry.2018.4500. Erratum in: *JAMA Psychiatry*. 2019 Apr 1;76(4):447.

Ivey-Stephenson AZ, Demissie Z, Crosby AE, et al. Suicidal ideation and behaviors among high school students—Youth Risk Behavior Survey, United States, 2019. *MMWR Suppl.* 2020;69 (Suppl 1):47-55. doi:10.15585/mmwr.su6901a6

Korioth T. Guns in child's home raise risk of suicide, unintentional death. *AAP News*. Published June 21, 2018. Accessed November 10, 2021. https://publications.aap.org/aapnews/news/10383

National Institute of Mental Health. Bipolar disorder in children and teens. Revised 2020. Accessed December 27, 2021. https://www.nimh.nih.gov/health/publications/bipolar-disorder-in-children-and-teens/index.shtml

National Institute of Mental Health. Post-traumatic stress disorder. Revised May 2019. Accessed December 27, 2021. https://www.nimh.nih.gov/health/topics/post-traumatic-stress-disorder-ptsd/index.shtml

National Institute of Mental Health. Schizophrenia. Revised May 2020. Accessed December 27, 2021. https://www.nimh.nih.gov/health/topics/schizophrenia/index.shtml

National Institute of Mental Health. Suicide. Accessed December 27, 2021. https://www.nimh.nih.gov/health/statistics/suicide.shtml

Rettew D. Is autism a mental illness? *Psychology Today*. Published October 8, 2015. Accessed December 27, 2021. https://www.psychologytoday.com/us/blog/abcs-child-psychiatry/201510/is-autism-mental-illness

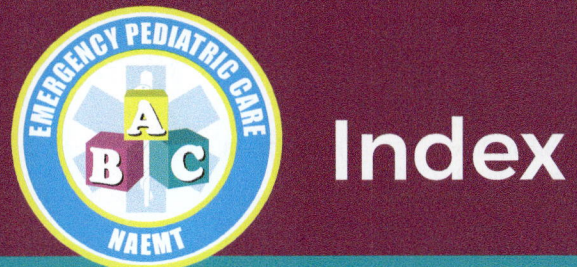

# Index

Note: Page numbers followed by *f* and *t* denote figures and tables, respectively.

## A

abnormal fetal presentation, 208–211, 208–210*f*
absorption, routes of exposure, 166
abuse, red flags for, 182–184
   caregiver behavior, 183–184, 184*t*
   child behavior, 184, 185*t*
   scene size-up, 183
abusive head trauma, 187–189, 188*t*, 189*f*
accessory muscle use, 7, 9
acidosis, 59–60
acyanotic heart defects, 229
adenosine triphosphate (ATP) molecules, 89
ADHD. *See* attention deficit/hyperactivity disorder
adolescents, 168
advanced life support (ALS), 262
aerobic metabolism, 89, 90*f*
airway injuries, 62–63
   management, 63
ALS. *See* advanced life support
altered mental status, 107–111, 108*t*
   AEIOU-TIPS, 108–111
   assessing mental status, 107–108
amiodarone/lidocaine, 144
anaerobic metabolism, 89
anaphylaxis, 29–30, 29*f*
   common triggers, 29*t*
   treatment, 30, 30*t*
antipyretics, for pneumonia, 36
anxiety, 256–257, 256*t*
apnea, 218
arterial bleeding, 61
ASD. *See* autism spectrum disorder
ASDs. *See* atrial septal defects
assistive technology, additional forms of, 241–242, 242*f*, 242*t*
asthma, 34
   case study, 44–54
asystole, 158, 158*f*
ATP molecules. *See* adenosine triphosphate molecules
atrial septal defects (ASDs), 229
atrial/ventriculoseptal defects, 229
atropine, 151
attention deficit/hyperactivity disorder (ADHD), 237, 255–256
audible breath sounds, 8–9, 9*t*
auscultation, 15, 16*f*
autism, 259
autism spectrum disorder (ASD), 237, 259–260

## B

behavioral health disorder, 255
benzodiazepines, 257, 258

bicycle collision injuries, 59
biphasic stridor, 8
bipolar disorder, 257
bleeding
   control, 62, 73
   external, 61–62
      arterial, 61
      capillary, 61
      hemostatic dressings, 62, 62*f*
      tourniquets, 61–62
      venous, 61
   internal, 62
*Bordetella pertussis*, 36. *See also* pertussis
bradycardia, 149–152, 150*t*, 151*f*, 176
breathing, difficulty, 243, 243*f*, 260, 260*f*
breech presentation, 210, 210*f*
bronchiolitis, 35
   case study, 37–44
bulging sac, 208–209, 208*f*
burn injury, 68–71
   assessment, 69–70
   full-thickness, 69, 69*f*
   partial-thickness, 69, 69*f*
   subdermal, 69, 70*f*
   superficial, 69, 69*f*
   treatment, 70–71
burns, 189–191, 190–191*f*
button battery ingestion, 168, 168*f*

## C

capillary bleeding, 61
cardiac arrest, 156–161
   non-shockable rhythms, 156–161
      cardiac arrest summary, 160–161, 160*f*
      pulseless electrical activity, 156–159, 157–158*f*
      shockable rhythms, 159–160, 159–160*f*
cardiogenic shock, 97–99
   management, 97–99, 98*f*
   symptoms and signs of, 98*t*
cardiopulmonary resuscitation (CPR), 28–29
caregivers, 238
CDC. *See* The Centers for Disease Control and Prevention
CDM. *See* congenital dermal melanocytosis
The Centers for Disease Control and Prevention (CDC), 258
central venous catheters, 239–240, 239*f*
cerebral palsy, 249–251
cerebrospinal fluid (CSF), 239, 239*f*
chemical burns, 189–190
chest decompression, 84–85, 85*f*

chest injuries, 63–66
  closed pneumothorax, 64–65, 64*t*
  hemopneumothorax, 65
  open pneumothorax, 65
child abuse, 182, 183*t*
child maltreatment, types of, 181–182, 181*t*, 182*f*
children, bruising in, 184–187, 185–187*f*
cigarette burns, 190, 190*f*
circulatory changes, 201
closed pneumothorax, 64–65, 64*t*
CoA. *See* coarctation of the aorta
coagulopathy, 60
coarctation of the aorta (CoA), 230
cognitive impairment, 237
cognitive symptoms, schizophrenia, 258
cognitive *vs.* physical disabilities, 237
coining (Cao Gio/Gua Sha/Kerikan), 192–193, 193*f*
cold *vs.* warm shock, 101*t*
common substances, 167, 167–168*t*
compassionate options for pediatrics (COPE), 163
compensated shock, 91–92, 91–92*f*
concussion, 66
congenital dermal melanocytosis (CDM), 192–193, 192*f*
congenital heart defects, 226, 226–227*t*
  sign and symptoms of, 230, 230*t*
COPE. *See* compassionate options for pediatrics
corticosteroids, for anaphylaxis, 30
COVID19 pandemic, suicide, 259
CPR. *See* cardiopulmonary resuscitation
crackles, 8
critical care personnel, 263
croup, 31–32, 31*f*
CSF. *See* cerebrospinal fluid
cuffed *vs.* uncuffed endotracheal tubes, 25
cupping, 193, 193*f*
Cushing reflex, 67
cyanosis, 10
cyanotic heart defects, 226–229
  Tetralogy of Fallot, 228–229, 228*f*
  transposition of the great arteries, 229
  tricuspid atresia, 229
  truncus arteriosus, 229
cystic fibrosis, 243

**D**

damage control resuscitation (DCR), 60
DCR. *See* damage control resuscitation
decompensated shock, 92, 92*f*
depression, 257
depressive episodes, 257
developmental milestones, 1, 2–3*t*, 4*f*
dexamethasone, for croup, 32
diabetic ketoacidosis (DKA), 115
digoxin toxicity, 176, 179, 179*f*
distributive shock, 94–96
  management, 96–97, 96*f*
DKA. *See* diabetic ketoacidosis
DWPSS (dry, warm, position, suction, stimulate)
  steps, 220

**E**

early shock. *See* compensated shock
eclampsia, 208
ECMO. *See* extracorporeal membrane oxygenation

electrical burns, 189
end-tidal carbon dioxide (ETCO$_2$), 47, 47*f*, 68, 257, 258
endocrine changes, 202, 202*t*
endotracheal tubes, cuffed *vs.* uncuffed, 25
epiglottitis, 33
epinephrine, 151, 157
  for anaphylaxis, 30
  for asthma, 34
  intramuscular, 30
  nebulized, 31–33
epistaxis, 15, 15*f*
expiratory breath sounds, 8
extracorporeal membrane oxygenation (ECMO), 128

**F**

FABO. *See* foreign body airway obstruction
family-centered care, 20
febrile seizures, 119–120
feeding tubes, 240–241, 240*f*, 241*t*
fever, 117–118
finger thoracostomy, 65
foreign body airway obstruction (FABO), 28–29
fractures, 68
FRAP, 7, 7*t*, 25. *See also* work of breathing
frenulum injuries, 187
full-thickness burn, 69, 69*f*
fundal height/viability, 202–203, 203*f*, 203*t*
  age of viability, 202

**G**

gastrointestinal changes, 201–202
GCS score. *See* Glasgow Coma Scale score
general anxiety, 256*t*
general assessment. *See also* TICLS
GFR. *See* glomerular filtration rate
Glasgow Coma Scale (GCS) score, 107
glomerular filtration rate (GFR), 201
G/P (gravida/para) nomenclature, 204
grunting, 8, 9*t*

**H**

hazardous material (HazMat) scene, 169
head injuries, 66–68
  concussion, 66
  Cushing reflex, 67
  herniation, 67
  intracranial hemorrhage, 66–67, 66*f*
  management, 67–68
Health Insurance Portability and Accountability
    Act (HIPAA), 169
heart rate, newborn, 221
HELLP syndrome, 208
hemopneumothorax, 65
hemorrhage, 61–62
  external, 61–62
    hemostatic dressings, 62, 62*f*
    tourniquets, 61–62
  internal, 62
hemostatic dressings, 62, 62*f*
herniation, 67
HFNC devices. *See* high-flow nasal cannula devices
HHS. *See* hyperglycemic hyperosmolar state
high-flow nasal cannula (HFNC) devices, 35

high-risk deliveries, 204–211, 205*t*
    abnormal fetal presentations, 208–211, 208–210*f*
    eclampsia, 208
    meconium, 205
    multiple gestation pregnancies, 204–205
    multiple previous births, 204
    placental abnormalities, 205–207, 206*f*
    preeclampsia, 207–208
    prematurity, 204
HIPAA. *See* Health Insurance Portability and
        Accountability Act
100-day cough. *See* whooping cough
hyperglycemia, 114–116
    diabetes mellitus, 114, 115*f*
    hyperglycemia management, 116
    hyperglycemic emergencies, 114–116, 116*t*
hyperglycemic hyperosmolar state (HHS), 115–116, 116*t*
hypoglycemia, 111–114
    hypoglycemia severity, 112
    mild to moderate hypoglycemia management, 112–113
    pathophysiology of, 112
    severe hypoglycemia management, 113–114
    signs of, 111–112, 111*t*
hypothermia, 59, 218
hypovolemic shock, 94, 94*f*
    management, 94, 95*f*
hypoxia, 110

**I**

illicit substance abuse, 168–169, 169*f*
ingestion, routes of exposure, 165–166
inhalation, 7
    routes of exposure, 166, 166*t*
injection, routes of exposure, 166
injury. *See also* trauma
    nonfatal, 57, 58*f*
    types of, 61–71
        airway, 62–63
        burns, 68–71
        chest, 63–66
        fractures, 68
        head, 66–68
        hemorrhage, 61–62
    unintentional, 57, 58*f*
intellectually disabled, 237
intracranial hemorrhage, 66–67, 66*f*
    epidural hematoma, 66
    intracerebral hemorrhage, 67
    subarachnoid hemorrhage, 67
    subdural hematoma, 66–67
intussusception, 135

**J**

"junctional" hemorrhage, 61

**K**

ketamine, 53, 258

**L**

labor, stages of, 214, 214*t*. *See also* stages of labor
Lactated Ringer's solution, for burns, 71
level of consciousness (LOC), 170, 171*f*

LOC. *See* level of consciousness
lower respiratory tract, 25, 26*f*
Lund-Browder chart, 71*f*

**M**

magnesium sulfate
    for asthma, 34
malignant hyperthermia, 110
manic episodes, 257
marijuana ingestion/intoxication, 174, 174*f*
meconium, 205, 218, 224, 224*f*
meningococcal septicemia, 128
mental retardation, 237
minute ventilation equation, 23–24
mother, post-delivery care for, 214–215
mottling, 10
multiple gestation pregnancy, 204–205
multiple previous births, 204
multiple subdural hematomas, 199

**N**

N95 respirators, 123
nasal flaring, 7
nasal suctioning, 39–40, 40*f*
needle decompression, for closed pneumothorax, 64–65
needle thoracostomy, recommended site for, 84, 85*f*
negative symptoms, schizophrenia, 258
neurogenic shock, 96
newborn care, initial steps for, 217–219, 217*f*
    Apgar scoring system, 218–219, 219*f*
    appearance, 219
    delayed cord clamping, 218
    work of breathing, 219
newborn pulse oximetry, 223–224, 224*t*
newborn resuscitation, 220–221
    chest compressions, 221
    medications, 221
    ventilations, 220–221
newborns, "quick" *vs.* "not quick" for, 220, 220*t*, 231
non-shockable rhythm treatment, 158–159, 158*f*
norepinephrine, 127
normal pediatric ECG, 137–144, 138*f*
    normal QRS and expected axis, 137–138
    Q waves, 138, 139*t*
    T waves, 138, 138*t*
nuchal cord, 209–210, 209*f*

**O**

obstetric/newborn care/congenital birth defects
    case study, 211–235
    circulatory changes, 201
    documentation of pregnancy history, 204, 204*t*
    endocrine changes, 202, 202*t*
    fundal height and viability, 202–203, 203*f*, 203*t*
        age of viability, 202
    gastrointestinal changes, 201–202
    high-risk deliveries, 204–211, 205*t*
        abnormal fetal presentations, 208–211, 208–210*f*
        eclampsia, 208
        meconium, 205
        multiple gestation pregnancies, 204–205
        multiple previous births, 204
        placental abnormalities, 205–207, 206*f*

obstetric/newborn care/congenital birth defects (*continued*)
    preeclampsia, 207–208
    prematurity, 204
  renal changes, 201
  respiratory changes, 201
obstetric emergencies, 204
obstructive heart defects, 230
open pneumothorax, 65
OPQRST, 17–18, 17t

**P**

pallor, 10
panic disorder, anxiety, 256t
Parkland burn formula, 71
partial-thickness burn, 69, 69f
PAT. *See* Pediatric Assessment Triangle
pattern marks, 187, 187f
peak end-expiratory pressure (PEEP) valve, 220
Pediatric Assessment Triangle (PAT), 5f, 5–10, 5t, 26f, 122, 122f,
     153, 153f, 161, 161f, 171, 171f, 195, 195f, 219, 221, 222f
  appearance, 6, 6f, 6t
  breathing, 6–10, 7t
    audible breath sounds, 8–9, 9t
    flaring, 7
    positioning, 9–10
    retractions, 7, 8f
  circulation, 10, 10f
pediatric behavioral health
  anxiety, 256–257, 256t
  attention deficit/hyperactivity disorder (ADD/ADHD),
     255–256
  autism spectrum disorder, 259–260
  bipolar disorder, 257
  case study, 260–268
  depression, 257
  posttraumatic stress disorder (PTSD), 258
  schizophrenia, 258
  suicide attempt/suicidal ideation, 258–259
pediatric cardiac events
  case study, 144–163
  normal pediatric ECG, 137–144, 138f
    normal QRS and expected axis, 137–138
    Q waves, 138, 139t
    T waves, 138, 138t
  pediatric cardiac rhythms, 138–144
    tachycardia, 139–144, 140t, 142f, 143t, 144f
pediatric development/assessment, 1–20
  developmental milestones, 1, 2–3t, 4f
  family-centered care, 20
  general impression, 4–5
    Pediatric Assessment Triangle, 5f, 5–10, 5t
    Pediatric Glasgow Coma Scale, 11, 11t
  primary survey, 14–17, 14t
    airway, 15, 15f
    breathing, 15, 16f
    circulation, 16
    disability, 16, 16f
    exposure and environment, 16–17
    exsanguination, 15, 15f
  scene size-up, 4
  secondary assessment, 17–18
  transport, 19–20, 19f
  treatment plan, 18
  vital signs, 1, 4, 4t

pediatric distributive shock, 127
Pediatric Glasgow Coma Scale (PGCS), 11, 11t
pediatric human trafficking, 191–192
pediatric intubation, for asthma, 53–54
pediatric maltreatment
  abusive head trauma, 187–189, 188t, 189f
  bruising in children, 184–187, 185–187f
  burns, 189–191
    abusive burns, 190–191, 190–191f
  case study, 194–199
  child maltreatment, types of, 181–182, 181t, 182f
  conditions mistaken for, 192–193
    coining (Cao Gio/Gua Sha/Kerikan), 192–193, 193f
    congenital dermal melanocytosis, 192–193, 192f
    cupping, 193, 193f
  epidemiology, demographics/risk factors, 182, 183t
  history taking, 193–194
    mandated reporting, 194
  pattern marks, 187, 187f
  pediatric human trafficking, 191–192
  red flags for abuse, 182–184
    caregiver behavior, 183–184, 184t
    child behavior, 184, 185t
    scene size-up, 183
Pediatric Management Diagram, 12–14, 12f
  "not quick" patient, 13, 13f
  "quick" patient, 13, 13f
  "quick" *vs.* "not quick" decision, 14, 14f
pediatric medical emergencies
  altered mental status, 107–111, 108t
    AEIOU-TIPS, 108–111
    assessing mental status, 107–108
  case study, 121–136
  fever, 117–118
  hyperglycemia, 114–116
    diabetes mellitus, 114, 115f
    hyperglycemia management, 116
    hyperglycemic emergencies, 114–116, 116t
  hypoglycemia, 111–114
    hypoglycemia severity, 112
    mild to moderate hypoglycemia management, 112–113
    pathophysiology of, 112
    severe hypoglycemia management, 113–114
    signs of, 111–112, 111t
  seizures, 118–121, 118f, 119t
    commonly encountered seizure emergencies, 119–120
    seizure management, 120–121, 120–121t
pediatric respiratory system, 23–25
  anatomy, 24–25, 24f
    lower airway, 25, 26f
    upper airway, 24–25, 24f, 25t
  physiology, 23–24
pediatric trauma. *See* trauma
PEEP valve. *See* peak end-expiratory pressure valve
pertussis, 36–37, 37t
PGCS. *See* Pediatric Glasgow Coma Scale
phobias, anxiety, 256t
physical disabilities, 237
placenta previa, 205–207, 206f
placental abnormality, 205–207, 206f
  hypertensive emergency, 212
pneumonia, 36, 36f
pneumothorax
  case study, 81–85
  closed, 64–65, 64t

hemopneumothorax, 65
open, 65
poison control, 170, 170*f*
posttraumatic stress disorder (PTSD), 258
prednisolone, for croup, 32
preeclampsia, 207–208
pregnancy history, documentation of, 204, 204*t*
prematurity, 204
primary survey, 14–17, 14*t*
    airway, 15, 15*f*
    breathing, 15, 16*f*
    circulation, 16
    disability, 16, 16*f*
    exposure and environment, 16–17
    exsanguination, 15, 15*f*
prolapsed cord, 209, 209*f*
psychotic symptoms, schizophrenia, 258
PTSD. *See* posttraumatic stress disorder
pulseless ventricular tachycardia, 159, 159–160*f*
PURPLE Crying, 188, 188*t*

**Q**

Q waves, 138, 139*t*

**R**

rapid sequence intubation (RSI), 96
reactive airway disease, 34
rectal diazepam, 120
rehydration therapy, 116
renal changes, 201
respiratory arrest, 27, 27*t*
respiratory changes, 201
respiratory distress, 25–26, 27*t*
respiratory emergencies, 23–54. *See also* pediatric respiratory system
    classification of, 27, 28*t*
    lower airway infection, 34–37
        bronchiolitis, 35
        pertussis, 36–37, 37*t*
        pneumonia, 36, 36*f*
    lower airway obstruction, 33–34
        asthma, 34
        reactive airway disease, 34
    severity assessment, 25–27, 26*f*
        respiratory arrest, 27, 27*t*
        respiratory distress, 25–26, 27*t*
        respiratory failure, 26–27, 27*t*
    upper airway infection, 31–33
        bacterial tracheitis, 33
        croup, 31–32, 31*f*
        epiglottitis, 33
        retropharyngeal abscess, 32
    upper airway obstruction, 28–30
        anaphylaxis, 29–30, 29*f*, 29–30*t*
        foreign body airway obstruction, 28–29
respiratory failure, 26–27, 27*t*
respiratory syncytial virus (RSV), 37–44
retractions, 7, 8*f*
retropharyngeal abscess, 32
return of spontaneous circulation (ROSC), 196
rhonchi, 8, 9*t*
ROSC. *See* return of spontaneous circulation
RSI. *See* rapid sequence intubation

RSV. *See* respiratory syncytial virus
rule of nines, 70, 70*f*

**S**

SAMPLER, for history taking, 17–18, 18*t*
SBS. *See* shaken baby syndrome
scald burns, 190–191, 191*f*
scene safety, 169, 169*t*
schizophrenia, 258
secondary assessment, 17–18
    OPQRST, 17–18, 17*t*
    SAMPLER, 17–18, 18*t*
seizures, 118–121, 118*f*, 119*t*
    commonly encountered seizure emergencies, 119–120
    seizure management, 120–121, 120–121*t*
separation anxiety, 256*t*
septic shock, 100–101
serum potassium, 116
shaken baby syndrome (SBS), 187. *See also* abusive head trauma
shock
    cardiogenic, 97–99, 98*f*, 98*t*
    case study, 99–105
    causes of, 89–90, 90*t*
    compensated, 91–92, 91–92*f*
    decompensated, 92, 92*f*
    defined, 89
    distributive, 94–96, 96*f*
    hypovolemic, 94, 94*f*
    progression of, 90, 90*t*
    types of, 92–93
    warm *vs.* cold, 101*t*
shockable rhythm treatment, 159–160
shoulder dystocia, 210–211, 210*f*
sinus tachycardia, 139–140, 140*t*
social anxiety, 256*t*
special healthcare needs, children with
    assessment, 238
    assistive technology, additional forms of, 241–242, 242*f*, 242*t*
    case study, 243–252
    central venous catheters, 239–240, 239*f*
    cerebrospinal fluid shunts, 239, 239*f*
    cognitive *vs.* physical disabilities, 237
    feeding tubes, 240–241, 240*f*, 241*t*
    tracheostomy tubes, 238–239, 238*f*
    vagal nerve stimulator, 241, 241*f*
stable supraventricular tachycardia, 140–142
stable ventricular tachycardia, 143
stages of labor, 214, 214*t*. *See also* labor, stages of
status epilepticus, 120
steeple sign, 31, 32*f*
stridor, 8, 9*t*
subdermal burn, 69, 70*f*
submersion burn injuries, 191
suicidal ideation, 258–259, 266, 267
suicide attempts, 258–259, 264, 264*f*
superficial burns, 69, 69*f*
supplemental oxygen, 235
supraventricular tachycardia (SVT), 140–142, 148
SVT. *See* supraventricular tachycardia

**T**

T waves, 138, 138*t*
tachycardia, 139–144, 140*t*, 142*f*, 143*t*, 144*f*

tachypnea/tachycardia, patient's vital signs, 245f, 262, 262f
TBI. *See* Traumatic brain injury
TEN–4 FACES P, 186, 187f
tension pneumothorax, 65
Tetralogy of Fallot (ToF), 228–229, 228f, 231, 232
TGA. *See* transposition of the great arteries
thermal burns, 189
TICLS, 6, 6t
ToF. *See* Tetralogy of Fallot
tourniquets, 61–62
   use of, 74–75, 74–75f
toxic exposures, assessment of, 166–167, 166f
toxicologic emergencies
   button battery ingestion, 168, 168f
   case study, 170–179
   common substances, 167, 167–168t
   illicit substance abuse, 168–169, 169f
   poison control, 170, 170f
   routes of exposure, 165–166
      absorption, 166
      ingestion, 165–166
      inhalation, 166, 166t
      injection, 166
   scene safety, 169, 169t
   toxic exposures, assessment of, 166–167, 166f
tracheostomy, suctioning, 244–245, 244t
tracheostomy tubes, 238–239, 238f
tranexamic acid (TXA), 60, 79
   in pediatric patients, 79t
transcutaneous pacing, 151
transport, 19–20, 19f
transposition of the great arteries (TGA), 229
trauma. *See also* injury
   case study, 72–80
   kinematics, 57–59
      bicycle collision injuries, 59
      falls, 58
      seat belts and motor vehicle crashes, 58
   trauma triad of death, 59–61, 59f
      acidosis, 59–60
      coagulopathy, 60
      hypothermia, 59
      management, 60–61
traumatic brain injury (TBI), 66
   concussion, 66
   Cushing reflex, 67
   herniation, 67
   intracranial hemorrhage, 66–67, 66f
   management, 67–68
TXA. *See* tranexamic acid
type 1 diabetes pathology, 114
type 2 diabetes pathology, 114, 115f

**U**

uncuffed *vs.* cuffed endotracheal tubes, 25
unstable supraventricular tachycardia, 142, 142f
unstable ventricular tachycardia, 144, 144f
upper airway infection, 31–33
   bacterial tracheitis, 33
   croup, 31–32, 31f
   epiglottitis, 33
   retropharyngeal abscess, 32
upper airway obstruction, 28–30
   anaphylaxis, 29–30, 29f, 29–30t
   foreign body airway obstruction, 28–29
upper respiratory tract, 24–25, 24f, 25t

**V**

vaccination
   for pertussis, 37
VADRS. *See* Vanderbilt ADHD Diagnostic Rating Scale
vagal nerve stimulators (VNS), 241, 241f
Vanderbilt ADHD Diagnostic Rating Scale (VADRS), 255
venous bleeding, 61
ventricular fibrillation, 159, 159–160f
ventricular septal defects (VSDs), 229
ventricular tachycardia (VT), 142–144, 143t
visual pain scales, 17, 18f
VNS. *See* vagal nerve stimulators
vocal cords
   pediatric *vs.* adult, 24, 24f
VSDs. *See* ventricular septal defects
VT. *See* ventricular tachycardia

**W**

warm *vs.* cold shock, 101t
waveform capnography, and asthma, 48–49
wheezing, 8, 9t
whooping cough, 36–37. *See also* pertussis
work of breathing